THE EMBRYONIC HUMAN BRAIN
Second Edition

THE EMBRYONIC HUMAN BRAIN

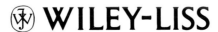

An Atlas of Developmental Stages
SECOND EDITION

RONAN O'RAHILLY, M.D., D.Sc., Dr.h.c.
FABIOLA MÜLLER, Dr.habil.rer.nat.

School of Medicine
University of California at Davis
Davis, California
and
Institut d'Embryologie Spéciale
Université de Fribourg, Fribourg, Switzerland

WILEY-LISS

A JOHN WILEY & SONS, INC., PUBLICATION
New York • Chichester • Weinheim • Brisbane • Singapore • Toronto

Published simultaneously in Canada.

For ordering and customer service, call 1-800-CALL-WILEY.

Library of Congress Cataloging-in-Publication Data:
O'Rahilly, Ronan.
    The embryonic human brain : an atlas of developmental stages /
Ronan O'Rahilly, Fabiola Müller. — 2nd ed.
          p.   cm.
    Includes bibliographical references and index.
    ISBN 0-471-25450-9 (cloth : alk. paper)
    1. Brain—Differentiation—Atlases. 2. Brain—Growth—Atlases.
I. Müller, Fabiola. II. Title.
    [DNLM: 1. Brain—embryology atlases. 2. Brain—growth &
development atlases.   WL 17063e 1999]
QM455.O73   1999
612.6'40181—dc21
DNLM/DLC   98-42193
for Library of Congress

Printed in the United States of America.

10 9 8 7 6 5 4 3 2 1

In memory of
Ernest Gardner, M.D.,
neuroscientist, colleague, and friend

. . . ce feroit vn grand bon-heur pour le genre humain, fi cette
partie, qui eft la plus delicate de toutes, & qui eft fujette á
des maladies tres-frequentes, & tres-dangereufes, eftoit auffi
bien connuë, que beaucoup de Philofophes & d'Anatomiftes
fe l'imaginent.

Niels Stensen, *Discovrs svr l'Anatomie du cerveau*, 1669.

C O N T E N T S

P R E F A C E

The main objective of this monograph is to provide drawings, photographs, and photomicrographs of the human embryonic brain, and to include summarizing statements of the morphological status of the brain at each stage. The staging used is the internationally accepted Carnegie system. The drawings include at least a lateral view and a median reconstruction of the brain at each stage, as well as a clear indication of the plane of section of further illustrations, either drawings or photomicrographs. The vast majority of the drawings are based on extremely precise graphic reconstructions. At the end of the description of the normal at most stages, a brief statement concerning relevant anomalous conditions is added.

The reasons for concentrating on the embryonic period proper (the first eight postfertilizational weeks) are:

1. The embryonic brain is extremely difficult to comprehend and to visualize;
2. Serial sections of first-class quality that show the human embryonic brain are rarely accessible;
3. The correct interpretation of the appropriate serial sections requires years of specialized work;
4. The time-consuming preparation of accurate three-dimensional reconstructions is essential for correct interpretation;
5. The embryonic period is of particular importance because most major congenital anomalies appear during that time;
6. Until the publication of the first edition of this book, in 1994, no accurate, detailed, well-illustrated account of the human embryonic brain was available in book form, or even in a chapter of a book.

A set of standardized abbreviations, mostly self-evident, is used throughout for the illustrations, and a list of them is placed immediately inside the front cover. A selection of references to the chief studies of the prenatal human brain is included, but is not intended to be complete. In the interest of brevity, as well as of immediate relevance, items from the profuse literature relating to other species have not been included.

This edition has been enlarged by the addition of 100 pages and the inclusion of more than 60 new illustrations, as well as a number of new tables. The ages assigned to the stages have been revised to conform to the latest ultrasonic findings. The definitions given in Chapter 6 have been expanded considerably and are an important prelude to the later chapters. Further details of neurulation and the neuropores are given. Neuromeres, which currently are of particular interest in relation to gene expression, are clarified for the first time in the human embryo, in line with recent investigations by the present authors. Several new figures showing the arteries, based on the well-known studies of Padget, are presented. More information concerning the cerebellum in both the embryonic and the fetal period is supplied, and the hippocampal formation is given special attention. The account of the fetal period has been expanded, thereby emphasizing the continuity of development, and a few postnatal images have been included. The Bibliography has been enlarged and brought up to date. A computer ranking of the sequence of appearance of features of the brain is provided in Appendix 1, and newly added appendices are concerned with median features, tracts, and the rhombencephalon.

Morphology has acquired ever increasing importance since the advent of imaging *in vivo,* and the emphasis in this book remains primarily morphological. By the same token, an atlas of the embryonic human heart along lines similar to those of the present work would be a very valuable contribution.

As stated in the first edition, the authors wish to acknowledge the great help given by the U.S. National Institutes of Health, which have supported their research (chiefly through Grant HD-16702, Institute of Child Health and Human Development). Except where otherwise indicated, the photomicrographs and photographs are reproduced by courtesy of the Carnegie Institution of Washington. It is a pleasure to thank all at Wiley-Liss for their cheerful assistance.

RONAN O'RAHILLY
FABIOLA MÜLLER
Rue du Coteau 57
CH-1752 Villars-sur-Glâne
Switzerland

CHAPTER 1

Historical Aspects

The Greek anatomist and physician, Erasistratus (ca. 300–250 BC), distinguished two convoluted parts of the brain, a greater and a lesser. Later, it became clear that "the cerebrum and cerebellum are different in function as in form," as Charles Bell wrote in 1811.

Although Malpighi in the 1670s observed the neural folds in the chick embryo, their significance escaped him, and he thought that the brain developed between them (Adelmann, 1966). Even von Baer was unaware that the neural folds are the primordium of the CNS, a role that was first appreciated by Rusconi and Reichert. Pander, however, understood that the neural folds form a tube. Nevertheless, the CNS was thought to be merely a fluid at first, and "the monotonous chronicle of vesicles and bubbles" (Adelmann) continued into the nineteenth century—if not, indeed, beyond it.

The *vesiculae cerebrales*, said to have been first noted by Coiter in 1573 (Tiedemann, 1816), were promoted by Meckel the younger, von Baer, and Bischoff, although the concept is largely a myth (Streeter, 1927). The current acceptance of three main divisions in the brain (prosencephalon, mesencephalon, and rhombencephalon) dates mainly from von Baer, who also identified the five subdivisions that appear a little later (telencephalon, diencephalon, mesencephalon, metencephalon, and myelencephalon). In 1893, Wilhelm His, senior, the founder of human embryology, added a sixth part, the isthmus rhombencephali, which becomes very evident during development.

Specific References to the Prenatal Human Brain

Some key studies are mentioned here for convenience, but the list is not intended to be complete.

One of the earliest specific accounts of the prenatal human brain is that by Friedrich Tiedemann (1816), which was translated into French (1823) and English within a decade. The monograph is arranged according to nine prenatal months, but early examples of the human embryonic brain were inevitably lacking.

In 1896, the detailed atlas of the gross morphology of the brain by Gustaf Retzius appeared. In addition to the adult organ, more than 35 plates included the fetal brain from "the third to the tenth month," the smallest being from two 35 mm fetuses. Retzius referred to the work of His on the embryonic brain, and he also cited Hochstetter.

In 1900 and 1901, Florence Sabin prepared solid (Born) reconstructions of the brain stem of a newborn, and the published illustrations were accompanied by a detailed description of some 90 pages.

In 1904, Wilhelm His, the real founder of human embryology, wrote an account of the human brain for embryos from 3.1 to 160 mm C-R. His had been very interested in photography, and a striking feature of his book is the high quality of the photomicrographs. It is to be regretted that neither this work nor his *Anatomie menschlicher Embryonen* has been translated into English.

In 1919, Ferdinand Hochstetter published a well-known monograph on the human brain from 23 somitic pairs (stage 12) to 125 mm C-R. It includes attractive illustrations of solid (Born) reconstructions and a series of photomicrographs of high quality. In 1923, the same author wrote an account of the development of the epiphysis cerebri. In 1929, he produced a further work, on the mesencephalon and rhombencephalon, based on a study of embryos from 6 mm GL to 250 mm C-R. The illustrations include solid (Born) reconstructions and many photomicrographs of first-class sections. Hochstetter wrote also on the choroid plexuses (1913) and on the development of the meninges (1939).

A classical study of the neuromeres in the human was completed by Bartelmez in 1923, and many further details were provided in a neglected study by Bartelmez and Evans in 1936. The neuromeres were investigated again in the 1950s and 1960s by Bergquist and Källén.

In 1938, a detailed investigation of the development of the human CNS was written by Barbé. This work, extending to 340 pages, covers the range from 14 mm C-H to 470 mm C-H (320 mm C-R). Many photographs and photomicrographs are included. Unfortunately neither His nor Hochstetter is mentioned.

In 1944, a richly illustrated work on the external features of the later fetal brain (from "4 months") was published by Fontes. A few years later (n.d.), some excellent external photographs (from "3 months") were included in a comparative study by Friant. The work of Fontes was unknown to Friant, as it still is to most authors.

In 1948, a very valuable series of reconstructions of the cranial arteries (in relation to the cranial nerves) was published by Padget, who subsequently (1957) produced a comparable work on the cranial venous system. The stages of the Carnegie embryos she studied are known. It needs to be appreciated

TABLE 1-1. Relationship Between Padget's Vascular Phases and Carnegie Stages

Arterial phases	Venous phases	Carnegie stages
—	1	13
1	—	13–14
2	2	14
—	3	15–16
3	—	16
4	—	17
—	4	17–18
5	—	18–19
—	5	19
6	6	20–21
7	7	40 mm GL
—	7a	60–80 mm GL

that her "age groups" (of Streeter) are now the Carnegie stages and that her "stages" are phases of vascular development (Table 1-1).

In 1962, the very important study by Bartelmez and Dekaban appeared and was based on the Carnegie Collection. This was the first detailed investigation of the internal structure of the human brain in staged embryos, from stage 10 to stage 22, with the omission of stages 9, 18, 21, and 23. The account is more complete than that of Streeter (revised by O'Rahilly and Müller, 1987a) and was not surpassed until the study of many embryos at each stage by Müller and O'Rahilly began to be published in 1981–1990.

In 1965, an excellent and well illustrated study of the globus pallidus and the corpus striatum was published by Richter. This important work was based on 13 embryos and 35 fetuses from 18.5 to 370 mm C-R.

In 1969, a very valuable and well-illustrated investigation of the development of the human cerebral hemispheres was published by Kahle. The work is arranged from the "second month" to the "eighth month" and includes examples from 3 mm GL to more than 275 mm C-R.

In 1970, Windle published a noteworthy study of the "development of neural elements in human embryos of four to seven (postovulatory) weeks." The examples range from about 3 to 16.5 mm GL. Although Streeter's "horizons" were stated to be "helpful," the embryos studied were unfortunately not staged. On the positive side, however, the use of Ranson's pyridine-silver method enabled early neurons and neurofibrillary differentiation to be investigated thoroughly.

In 1975, much useful information concerning the normal and abnormal development of the human nervous system was consolidated by Lemire, Loeser, Leech, and Alvord. Streeter's "horizons" and postovulatory ages were used.

Important studies that have appeared since 1980 will be cited in appropriate places in the various chapters of this text.

The present work is the first book devoted to the staged, embryonic human brain and serves as the necessary prolegomenon for accounts of the fetal period. It should be stressed, however, that very much further work on the fetal brain needs to be undertaken before a level of detail comparable with that now available for the embryonic brain can be attained.

C H A P T E R 2

Techniques

A number of matters related to human embryology in general, which also have particular relevance to human neuroembryology, will be summarized in the first few chapters.

The present work is based largely on personal investigations of the embryonic brain, stage by stage, carried out over some two decades and published in more than 30 research articles. The source material was mostly the Carnegie Embryological Collection and involved a careful study of 340 serially sectioned embryos (including 51 instances of silver impregnation), the preparation of graphic reconstructions from 89 brains, and the examination of 55 solid, three-dimensional reconstructions (modified method of Born).* No similarly detailed and adequately illustrated documentation of the developing human brain had been previously attempted, and a comparable study of the fetal brain has to await the future. Moreover, because most studies of the developing brain of other mammalian species are based on timing, but not on staging, comparative tabulation in neuroembryology is still in its infancy, and a standard for the human is an advisable preliminary.

When the first morphological indication of the nervous system is distinguishable, the greatest length of the embryo is only 1 mm. Hence histological study is essential. Throughout the embryonic period, serial sections of excellent quality are indispensable. The examination of isolated or haphazard sections, or of those of poor histological quality, is almost useless and is frequently misleading.

* Specimen numbers given in the legends (e.g., CEC 836) refer to the following sources: CEC, Carnegie Embryological Collection, D, Davis Collection, G, Peter Grünewald Collection.

At the end of the embryonic period proper, the diameter of the cerebral hemispheres is of the order of only 1 cm. This, coupled with the circumstance that many features are not at first sight identifiable (although most are present), as well as the rapidity with which changes occur, necessitates the preparation of enlarged reconstructions in order to investigate topographical relationships. Such reconstructions, which are made by projecting serial sections at a previously determined magnification, are of two kinds: solid and graphic.

Solid reconstructions are associated with the name of Gustav Born, who established the technique in 1876. It was adopted enthusiastically by Wilhelm His, the founder of human embryology (O'Rahilly, 1988). Such a reconstruction consists of stacked plates, each representing one or more enlarged serial sections. The laminae can be made of various substances. Originally wax was chosen, whereas those used here are made of plaster and were prepared by Mr. Osborn O. Heard. An example is shown in Figure 17-3. According to Carnegie usage, precise reconstructions are never referred to as "models."

Graphic reconstructions, which were also used extensively by His, are made by superimposing the outlines of structures—the contours being obtained by projecting serial sections. In this "point-plotting" method, hidden lines are omitted. An example is shown in Figure 10-4. All the median views in the embryonic period and many of the lateral views in the embryonic period in this book are carefully prepared graphic reconstructions based on detailed examination of serial sections. These drawings and reconstructions are the work of one of the authors (F.M.). A further technical advance, based on a modified pantograph, was introduced in the 1960s by Forster under the name *Perspektomat* and is patented. It was applied to human embryology by Müller and O'Rahilly (1980, Figs. 5-9) and is particularly useful for complicated structures, for correcting a markedly oblique plane of section, and for dissected views. Hidden lines can easily be omitted. Graphic reconstructions by computer are being used increasingly. Although most of those so far published are inadequate in precision and refinement, the standard may be expected to improve considerably.

It cannot be emphasized too strongly that first-class histological quality is essential for precise reconstructions, and that reconstructions are absolutely necessary for a valid three-dimensional interpretation. Moreover, examination of sections taken in the three major planes is needed in order to follow certain structures, especially tracts, which disappear completely from view when sectioned through a right-angled bend.

Additional techniques, such as histochemistry and electron microscopy, are being used to a limited extent in human neuroembryology. Immunocytochemistry is being applied to staged embryos and is being correlated with *in situ* hybridization for expression of genes. In addition, magnetic resonance imaging (MRI) and ultrasonic imaging, which are used extensively in clinical practice, confirm the results of embryological investigations and reconstructions.

Important

Imaging is valuable in prenatal diagnosis, but knowledge of the time of first appearance of various features, as well as the detailed morphology of the developing brain, depends on precise reconstruction from serial sections.

6

Prenatal Measurements

A considerable variety of measurements has been proposed and, as is also true of postnatal measurements, a range of values dependent on variability needs to be taken into account.

The most useful measurement in prenatal life is the greatest length (GL), taken as a caliper length without inclusion of the flexed lower limbs. The crown–rump (C-R) length, which is frequently similar, is a commonly cited but unsatisfactory measurement (O'Rahilly and Müller, 1984a). The term stage should not be applied to a mere measurement, nor to a supposed age. Thus, the "19 mm stage" should be replaced by "at 19 mm GL", and "the 7-week stage" by "at 7 (postfertilizational) weeks." The greatest length is replaced after birth by the sitting height.

The greatest length, as would be expected, shows variability in relation to age, and precision in estimating age can be increased by using several different measurements, as has been found in ultrasonographic studies. At $4\frac{1}{2}$ postfertilizational weeks the GL is about 5 mm, and at 8 weeks, the end of the embryonic period proper, it is approximately 30 mm.

The crown–heel (C-H) length includes the lower limbs and is replaced after birth by the standing height. Another useful measurement is the foot length (FL). At 8 postfertilizational weeks the C-H length is about 45 mm, and the FL is approximately 4.5 mm. Additional measurements used in imaging techniques include the biparietal diameter, the head circumference, the (calcified) femoral length, and the abdominal circumference.

Where the head is defective, e.g., in anencephaly, the fetal height can be estimated from the distance between the spinous process of thoracic vertebra

1 and the coccyx, and from measurements of the arm, thigh, and leg (Alexandre and Pineau, 1970).

Body weight, which is about 2 to 3 g at 8 postfertilizational weeks, is variable. Later, an estimate can be obtained *in vivo* by special formulae based on linear measurements (e.g., biparietal diameter and abdominal circumference).

Brain weight, which is also variable, has been studied in the fetal period by a number of authors (e.g., Tanimura et al., 1971; Gilles et al., 1983), and summarizing graphs are available (Lemire et al., 1975).

Important

The most useful single measurement in both embryonic and fetal development is the greatest length (GL) exclusive of the lower limbs.

C H A P T E R 4

Embryonic Staging

Prenatal life is conveniently divided into embryonic and fetal periods. The embryonic period is that during which new features appear with great rapidity, enabling subdivision to be made into morphological stages. It occupies the first 8 postfertilizational weeks. The vast majority of congenital anomalies appear during that time. The fetal period is characterized more by the elaboration of existing structures and, because of the less striking developmental changes, it has proved so far to be resistant to a morphologically based staging system.

In human embryology, staging, as distinct from mere seriation of embryos, was introduced by Mall in 1914. The system now used internationally, termed Carnegie stages by O'Rahilly, was prepared by Streeter in the 1940s and by O'Rahilly in the 1970s (O'Rahilly and Müller, 1987a). Other systems are now obsolete.

In the Carnegie system the embryonic period proper, i.e., the first 8 postfertilizational weeks of development, is subdivided into 23 stages based on external and internal morphological criteria. These stages are used throughout this book (Table 4-1).

The great advantage of morphological stages is that, in large measure, emancipation from the variables of age and measurement can be achieved for the embryonic period. As information concerning ages becomes more precise, no better example can be found of the value, indeed necessity, of the morphologically based staging system, which retains its validity throughout. Moreover, comparisons are made of a number of different features (e.g., somites, neuropores, eyes, limbs), so that individual differences are rendered

TABLE 4-1. Developmental Stages and Features of the Nervous System

Carnegie stage	Greatest length (mm)	Approximate age (days)	Key features of nervous system	First appearance of neuromeres	Pairs of somites
8	1	23	Neural folds and groove in stage 8b		
9	2	25	Mesencephalic flexure; neural groove evident; otic disc	P, M, Rh. A–D	1–3
10	3	28	Fusion of neural folds begins; optic primordium; otic pit	T, D1, D2	4–12
11	3.5	29	Rostral neuropore closes; optic vesicles and optic neural crest; nasal discs	Rh. 1–8	13–20
12	4	30	Caudal neuropore closes; secondary neurulation commences; adenohypophysial pouch	M1, M2	21–29
13	5	32	Closed neural tube; retinal and lens discs develop; hypothalamic cell cord; medial and lateral longitudinal fasciculi; primordium of cerebellum	Par., Syn., Isthmus	30–?
14	6	33	Future cerebral hemispheres; pontine flexure; torus hemisphericus & medial ventricular eminence; optic cup and lens vesicle	Rostral & caudal Par.; all 16 neuromeres present	
15	8	36	Nasal pit; di-telencephalic sulcus; lateral ventricular eminence; hippocampal thickening; medial forebrain bundle; longitudinal zoning in diencephalon (marginal ridge)		
16	10	38	Olfactory tubercle; dorsal thalamus; epiphysis cerebri; neurohypophysial evagination		
17	13	41	Vomeronasal organ and nerve; forebrain septum; 1 to 2 amygdaloid nuclei; subthalamic nucleus; posterior commissure; red nucleus; internal and external cerebellar swellings		
18	15	44	Paraphysis; future corpus striatum with intrastriatal sulcus; hippocampus C-shaped; inf. & superior cerebellar peduncles; primordium of nucleus dentatus		

10

TABLE 4-1. *(Continued)*

Carnegie stage	Greatest length (mm)	Approximate age (days)	Key features of nervous system	First appearance of neuromeres	Pairs of somites
19	17	46	Olfactory bulb; nucleus accumbens; globus pallidus; choroid plexus of fourth ventricle; substantia nigra; medial accessory olivary nucleus		
20	20	49	Choroid plexus of lateral ventricles; septal nuclei; interpeduncular nucleus; optic fibers in chiasmatic plate		
21	23	51	Cortical plate in area of future insula; optic tract & lateral geniculate body		
22	26	53	Olfactory tract; claustrum; internal capsule; adenohypophysial stalk incomplete		
23	29	56	Insula indented; external capsule; caudate nucleus & putamen discernible; anterior commissure begins; mesencephalic *Blindsäcke*; external germinal layer in cerebellum		

Note: The greatest lengths and the postfertilizational ages given are approximate only. The latter have been revised to conform to current ultrasonic information.

less significant and a certain latitude of morphological variation is taken into account.

Although external body form is of immediate access, and can even be recorded *in vivo* by ultrasonography, nevertheless it needs to be stressed that, particularly in certain stages (e.g., 20–22), internal morphology is an essential component of the Carnegie system.

Moreover, stages should not be assigned on the basis of mere length or age, both of which are too variable. An embryo of 20 mm, for example, could almost as easily belong to stage 19 as to stage 20, because the lengths usually given for the various stages are guidelines and do not show the complete range of values. Similarly, even were an embryo known to be precisely 49 postfertilizational days in age, it could as easily belong to stage 19 as to stage 20.

In addition, the admittedly subtle, arbitrary, but useful distinction between the embryonic and fetal periods is based on a histological criterion (the onset of marrow formation in the humerus), and neither length nor external form would be an adequate criterion.

In summary, staging is now an accepted procedure in human embryology, but it is essential to take both external and internal morphological criteria into consideration. Neither length nor age, nor a combination of them, defines a stage in the accepted embryological meaning of the term.

At present, staging is limited to the embryonic period proper. Despite attempts to do so, no satisfactory staging system has yet been devised for the fetal period. Prenatal life, however, can conveniently be considered in terms of trimesters: (1) including the embryonic period proper (up to about 30 mm GL), and extending to some 90 or 100 mm, (2) proceeding to about 250 mm, and (3) continuing until birth (very approximately 336 mm GL).

Staging systems are available for a number of species, two well known examples being Harrison's staging of *Ambystoma maculatus* and Hamburger and Hamilton's staging of *Gallus domesticus*. Such systems have arisen largely independently of each other and the numeration differs from one to another. Witschi, in the 1950s, was the major proponent of the attractive idea of a standard enumeration throughout vertebrate embryology, a suggestion that unfortunately was ignored. A more recent and valiant attempt at standardization is the atlas by Butler and Juurlink (1987). This is a praiseworthy effort to extend the Carnegie (i.e., human) staging system to a dozen mammalian species and even to the chick embryo. The Carnegie system had already been applied to a number of primate species, especially by Hendrickx and his coworkers, and this information was incorporated into the atlas. Unfortunately, however, most workers who study the developing mouse or rat continue to use ages instead of stages.

An ideal staging system, particularly from the viewpoint of experimental embryology, would be based entirely on external morphology. This is not always attainable, however. During some periods of development, external appearances may not change sufficiently rapidly to reflect adequately the accompanying internal changes. In the human, for example, difficulties may arise during the period from 7 to 8 postfertilizational weeks. Hence the internal structure is also important in staging. Details of internal development in staged embryos, however, seem to be incomplete or even lacking in most species other than the human. Furthermore, it should not be assumed that a given stage based on external appearances will reflect precisely similar internal features in different species. Even external features may vary among species. For example, the upper limb buds appear in the human at stage 12, whereas in the mouse they are said to begin at stage 11 and in the pig they are not distinct until stage 13; the pineal outgrowth appears in the human (and in other mammals) at stages 15–16, whereas in the chick it is said to be seen at what would correspond to stage 13.

It may be concluded that the study of "equivalent stages" should be pursued, but that present information is in many instances tentative. "Equivalent ages," on the other hand, are far less desirable insofar as a major objective of staging is to escape as far as is practicable from the variability of both ages and linear measurements.

Detailed studies of the embryonic brain of various species, comparable to the present work on the human, lie in the future. Such investigations are necessary in order to assess to what extent "equivalent stages" in the development of the brain parallel "equivalent stages" of the entire embryo, particularly those based on general external morphology. A relevant and valuable study of the brain of the rhesus monkey has been made already by Gribnau and Geijsberts. With reference to induced anencephaly, Müller and O'Rahilly (1984) offered preliminary tables of comparison of rat, mouse, and human embryos.

Important

The embryonic period is subdivided into 23 morphological (Carnegie) stages based on internal as well as external criteria. Morphological stages are not available for the fetal period.

C H A P T E R 5

Prenatal Age

Prenatal age should be given as postfertilizational weeks (or days). Ovulation is close to the time of fertilization (which, incidentally, is not a moment), so that postovulatory weeks or days (i.e., the time since the last ovulation) are an acceptable indication of age. The term "gestational age" should never be used, because three different starting points are possible: the last menstrual period (LMP), ovulation and/or fertilization, and implantation. In obstetrics, menstrual weeks are generally used and are assumed to be approximately a fortnight greater than the (postfertilizational) age. The designation menstrual "age," however, is obviously incorrect and should be abandoned. The use of the LMP measures the period of amenorrhea, when for the first two weeks no embryo existed (!), and hence menstrual weeks are not age.

In the embryonic period, once the stage of an embryo is known, its presumed postfertilizational age can be assessed from an appropriate table or graph (O'Rahilly and Müller, 1987a), such as Table 4-1. It is quite possible, however, that variation may be greater than previously thought, and some of the ages accepted for early embryos may perhaps be slightly too low. According to studies with transvaginal sonography (Dr. Josef Wisser, personal communication, 1992), embryos of stages 6 to 16 may commonly have ages 1 to 3 (more usually 3 to 5) days more than the previous embryological norms. When the embryonic length is within the range 3–30 mm, a very useful estimate of age in days can be obtained by adding 27 to the length.

It has already been pointed out that, in embryological usage, (1) external body form and (2) internal morphological status are the criteria for staging, and (3) embryonic length, although it is not a determining factor, is not entirely neglected. A further characteristic, (4) postfertilizational age, is rarely available and generally has to be estimated from the other three parameters.

Considerable progress in imaging (e.g., by the use of transvaginal sonography) has enabled an estimate, but frequently only an estimate, of the stage of a given embryo to be made *in vivo*. This is based on parameters 1 and 3 mentioned above, and No. 4 is sometimes also known. No. 2, internal morphological status, however, is not adequately identifiable, at least at the histological level, and hence precise staging remains an embryological rather than a clinical procedure. This distinction is particularly important in very early and in very late embryonic stages.

> Important
>
> Prenatal age is always postfertilizational by definition (or, as an acceptable alternative, postovulatory). Menstrual weeks are convenient in obstetrics but are not age. The term "menstrual age" is incorrect, and the ambiguous term "gestational age" should be abolished.

Terminology and Definitions

Terminology

The nomenclature used in this book is mostly that which is accepted internationally and is in current anatomical usage. Eponyms are by no means always justifiable historically: they convey no morphological information, they add unnecessary complications, and hence are to be avoided wherever possible. The island of Reil, for example, is much more simply rendered as merely the insula. Similarly, the fissures of Rolando and Sylvius, which are actually sulci (!), are much better given as the central and lateral sulci, respectively. A number of comparative terms that are inappropriate to the human (e.g., branchial) are also not used here.

In early development, such terms as anterior and posterior should be avoided. Appropriate terms for the embryo include rostral and caudal, dorsal and ventral. As in adult anatomy, the unofficial and unnecessary terms midsagittal, for median, and parasagittal, for merely sagittal, should not be used. Sagittal planes, including the median plane, are used as in adult anatomy. Transverse and coronal planes, however, generally refer to the trunk prenatally and are frequently unclear when applied to the flexed head, as found in the embryo.

Three main planes are used in anatomy: horizontal and two vertical planes, coronal and sagittal. One of the sagittal planes is median. One of the horizontal planes, the orbitomeatal, is used to ensure that the head is in the anatomical position. Strictly coronal planes are vertical planes that are at a right angle to both the orbitomeatal and the median plane. Prenatally, however, the situation is complicated by the curvature of the body and the flexion of the head. Consequently, a transverse section of the trunk (a horizontal section in the adult) is not parallel to the orbitomeatal plane (Fig. 24-13). Similarly, a coronal section of the prenatal trunk does not correspond to a coronal section of the adult head. These considerations, which are important in prenatal imaging, need to be kept in mind, even though a satisfactory resolution of the problem has yet to be achieved.

Definitions

A number of the terms used in this book may need a brief explanation, and such is provided in the following alphabetical list.

Archipallium: The cerebral cortex of the hippocampal formation. It is separated from the neopallium by the peri-archicortex (presubiculum), and it becomes distinguishable at stage 21 (Fig. 21-16).

Area dentata: The zone between the hippocampus *sensu stricto* and the area epithelialis. It develops into the dentate gyrus and, during the embryonic period, is characterized by having only a ventricular layer (Fig. 21-4).

Area epithelialis: The field between the area dentata and the lamina terminalis (Fig. 21-16). It consists of one to two, and later more, rows of cells, which, as development proceeds, contain dark inclusions. In the fetal period, a part of it becomes the lamina affixa.

Area hippocampi: This is characterized at first by an early appearing telencephalic marginal layer, and this is the only part of the telencephalon that possesses a marginal layer (q.v.). A little later, a ventricular thickening forms in the dorsomedial wall of the cerebral hemisphere (Fig. 15-6). It is C-shaped already at stage 18.

Area reuniens: A term used by His for the junctional region of the prosencephalon, the hypophysial primordium, the tip of the notochord, the roof of the foregut, and the oropharyngeal membrane.

Areae membranaceae: Two very thin areas of endothelioid cells in the roof of the fourth ventricle (Fig. 17-6). The epithelium is thinnest at 6 weeks, whereas at the end of the embryonic period, the thin cells become replaced by cuboidal cells. The area membranacea rostralis is adjacent to the cerebellar primordium. The area membranacea caudalis corresponds to the central bulge of Brocklehurst (1969) and to the saccular ventricular diverticulum of Wilson (1937), and is believed to be the site of the future median aperture of the fourth ventricle.

Bundles, forebrain: See Fasciculi, prosencephalic.

Canal, neurenteric: A more or less vertical passage (perpendicular to the embryonic disc) that appears during stage 8 as a result of increasing breakdown of the floor of the notochordal canal (q.v.). Both canals commence in common, dorsally in the primitive pit, and the neurenteric canal may be regarded as the remains of the notochordal canal at the level of the primitive node. The neurenteric canal connects the amniotic cavity (at the primitive pit) with that of the umbilical vesicle (or so-called yolk sac).

Canal, notochordal: An oblique passage that appears in the notochordal process during stage 8 (Fig. 8-2).

Cells, Cajal–Retzius: The embryonic Cajal–Retzius cells (Fig. 17-14) are tangentially arranged bipolar neurons within the primordial plexiform layer. These cells are said to possess a thick horizontal fiber (tangential fiber of Retzius) and an axon that descends vertically and gives off many horizontal collaterals in layer 1. Once the cortical plate develops, the Cajal–Retzius cells are external to ("above") it. The fetal Cajal–Retzius cells are transformed embryonic Cajal–Retzius cells. They have triangular, inverted pyramidal, or fusiform cell bodies from which two or more long horizontal dendrites emerge. The thick horizontal fiber extends throughout the surface of the cerebral cortex for a considerable distance and establishes contacts with the apical dendrites of all pyramidal neurons, regardless of their location (layers 6, 5, 4, 3, 2) or different functional role. The transfer of neuronal information from the Cajal–Retzius cells to all pyramidal neurons may be necessary for all of the latter to acquire and to maintain their funtional activity (Marín-Padilla, 1988a). Here, as in other regions, the use of immunological neuronal markers would enable such cells to become identifiable at earlier stages, as is being found already in other species.

Cerebellum: This part of the hindbrain is derived mostly from the entire alar laminae of rhombomere 1 and partly from the isthmus rhombencephali. The sources of cellular production are mainly the rhombic lip of rhombomere 1 and the ventricular layer of the alar laminae (Fig. 6-1). The cerebellar primordium, distinguishable at stage 13 (Fig. 13-3), becomes the cerebellar plate (q.v.) at about stage 18 (Fig. 18-2), by which time cerebellar swellings (q.v.) have appeared. The cerebellar hemispheres develop early in the fetal period, and the vermis is formed from the median portion of the hemispheres. See also Swellings, cerebellar.

Cerebrum: From Latin, meaning brain. In ancient usage the larger convoluted mass as distinct from the smaller (the cerebellum). At the time of His it included the mesencephalon (cf. cerebral peduncles), but became restricted to the prosencephalon, or to the telencephalon, or to the cerebral hemispheres. Hence the term has practically no scientific value, in contrast to the almost indispensable adjective (e.g., the middle cerebral artery).

Commissures of brain: In this book the term "commissure" is used as soon as fibers cross the median plane, although fibers growing medially are present long before they cross. Examples are the anterior and posterior commissures, and the corpus callosum. See also Decussation.

Cord, hypoglossal: A dense cellular prolongation formed by the dermatomyotomic material of at least the rostralmost three occipital somites caudal to the rostral cardinal vein. The dermatomic cells cannot be distinguished from the myotomic cells, nor can possible contributions from neural crest and epipharyngeal material of the vagus nerve be excluded. The relocation of the cells in the tongue is achieved before the arrival of the hypoglossal nerve. The hypoglossal cord forms (at least some of) the muscles of the tongue. Further details: O'Rahilly and Müller (1984b). A reconstruction of the hypoglossal cord (CEC 8943) at stage 12 (Müller and O'Rahilly, 1987, Fig. 6B) is in agreement with experimental findings in the rat, in which, at a similar stage, neural crest and dermatomyotomic cells of the occipital somites migrate within and dorsal to pharyngeal arches 3 and 4.

Cord, neural: The neural tissue in the caudal eminence (end-bud) of embryos with a closed caudal neuropore. It becomes canalized secondarily. The development of spinal cord (at stages 12 to about 17–20) from this solid material is termed secondary neurulation (Table 7-1).

17

Fig. 6-1. The sites of production and the migration of neurons in (**A**) the rhombencephalon, (**B**) the cerebellum, and (**C**) the mesencephalon.

(**A**) Block from the hindbrain showing migration from the floor plate to the raphe (1), from the ventricular layer for the motor and sensory (e.g., vestibular) nuclei (2), and from the rhombic lip, (e.g., for the cochlear nuclei (3)). The sensory areas are lateral to the sulcus limitans.

(**B**) Cerebellar migration from both the ventricular layer and the rhombic lip for the primordium of the dentate nucleus (stage 21). Cells from the ventricular layer give rise also to the piriform (Purkinje) cells, and those from the rhombic lip form the external germinal (or external granular) layer (stage 23).

(**C**) Migration in the mesencephalic tegmentum from the ventricular layer, producing first the interpeduncular nucleus and later the ventral tegmental area.

(**D**) The plane of the sections.

From Müller and O'Rahilly (1997a).

Fig. 6-1.

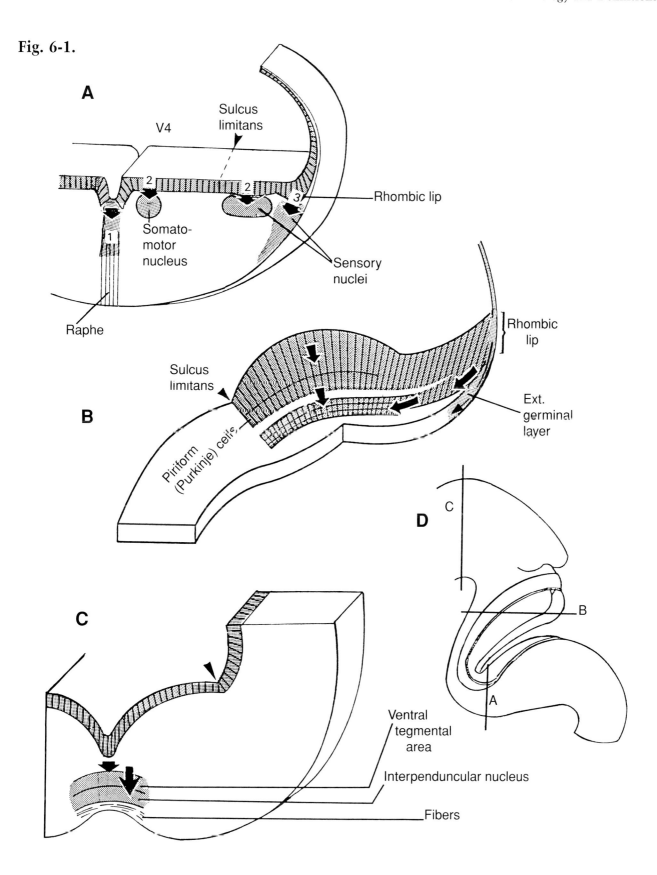

Cord, spinal: Embryologically, the part of the neural tube caudal to the last (the hypoglossal) rhombomere (Rh.D).

Corpus striatum (Fig. 6-2): The lentiform and caudate nuclei, which become connected by alternating striae of white and gray matter (hence the name). The putamen and the caudate nucleus are telencephalic and arise from the lateral ventricular eminence (experimental evidence exists in the rat), whereas the globus pallidus (externus and internus) is diencephalic and arises from the subthalamus.

Decussation: An intersection, the two lines of the letter X, as in the optic chiasma. Further examples are the pyramidal decussation, the decussation of the superior colliculi (e.g., of the tectobulbar fibers, Fig. 15-4), and that of the fibers of the trochlear nerves. See also Commissures.

Ectoderm, neural (or **neuroectoderm**): The pseudostratified epithelium derived from the embryonic ectoderm (which, in turn, comes from the epiblast) and that gives rise to the neural plate (Fig. 8-3) and to neural crest. The mitotic figures are found superficially, adjacent to the amniotic cavity initially and, as the neural tube develops, adjacent to the future ventricular cavity and central canal.

Eminences, ganglionic (or *Ganglienhügel*): Incorrect term for what are now termed the ventricular eminences (q.v.).

Eminences, ventricular (Fig. 15-3): The lateral ventricular eminence is a protuberance in the basolateral wall of the cerebral hemisphere. It represents the telencephalic part of the basal nuclei. The medial ventricular eminence is a thickening of diencephalic origin and it appears before the lateral swelling. The lateral eminence gives rise to the putamen and the caudate nucleus, the medial to most of the amygdaloid body. (Experimental evidence exists in the rat.) In the past the ventricular eminences were frequently but inaccurately termed ganglionic eminences.

Fasciculi, prosencephalic: Three chief bundles are described under this heading. The basal forebrain bundle (Fig. 19-16) contains descending fibers; it is "in part related to the olfactory system but also includes presumably non-olfactory channels of the vegetative nervous system present in macrosmatic, microsmatic, and anosmatic Mammals" and probably extends into the mesencephalic tegmentum (Kuhlenbeck, 1977). The lateral forebrain bundle contains ascending as well as descending fibers, and corresponds in large measure to the internal capsule (Fig. 19-16). The medial forebrain bundle (Fig. 19-16), which is predominantly descending, is described as the main pathway for longitudinal connections in the hypothalamus.

Fissures: (1) In the forebrain a term reserved for three grooves, the floors of which are not completed by cortical tissue, i.e., the longitudinal, transverse, and choroid fissures; (2) the numerous grooves on the surface of the cerebellum.

Floor plate: The ventromedial cells of the epinotochordal part (dorsal to the notochordal plate or notochord) of the neural plate or tube (Fig. 6-3). It is induced by the notochord. Whether the cells of the floor plate are exclusively glial is under discussion.

Formation, hippocampal: A convenient term used for the dentate gyrus, the hippocampus, the subiculum, and the parahippocampal gyrus. See also Hippocampus.

Ganglion, facio-vestibulocochlear: The common primordium (stage 10) that first appears for the ganglia of the facial and vestibulocochlear nerves

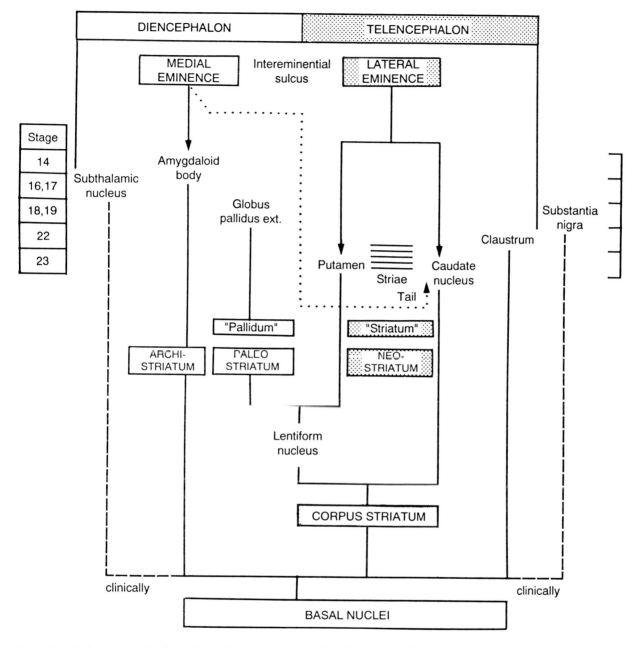

Fig. 6-2. Scheme of the basal nuclei showing the development of their diencephalic and telencephalic components. Stages of appearance are also included. Late in the embryonic period, the amygdaloid body as well as the globus pallidus externus moves into telencephalic territory. Whether the amygdaloid body and the claustrum should be included with the other basal nuclei is doubtful. The basal nuclei are best defined as the basal structures affected pathologically in so-called extrapyramidal motor diseases.

Precision

Basal nuclei is the correct term, not basal ganglia, because, by definition, ganglia are found only in the peripheral nervous system.

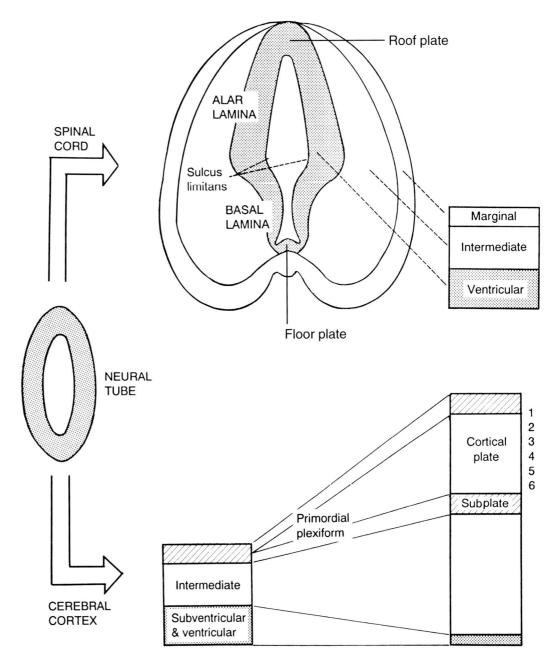

Fig. 6-3. Developmental comparison between the spinal cord and the brain wall as derivatives of the neural tube. The cortical plate develops within the primordial plexiform layer, so that it comes to lie between superficial and deep laminae, namely layer 1 and the subplate of the neocortex. The stages illustrated are 11 for the neural tube, and 17 for the spinal cord. The neocortical blocks are (left) up to stage 20, and (right) from stage 21.

(Fig. 11-2). It consists of neural crest to which the otic vesicle contributes. The facial and vestibulochochlear components become distinguishable from each other at stage 13. It is not clear whether, at that time, the non-facial part contains both vestibular and cochlear elements.

Glia or neuroglia (a singular noun): The non-neural interstitial tissue of the nervous system. Whether glial cells differentiate at the same time as, or following, neuronal differentiation has not been resolved. It is probable that in the spinal cord both neurons and glial cells arise from a common, pluripotent progenitor cell, whereas in the cerebral cortex it may be that neurons, astrocytes, and oligodendrocytes arise from different precursor cells. The first glial cells to arise are the radial glial cells, from which other types may develop (Marín-Padilla, 1995). Glia arises from two main sources: (1) the ventricular and subventricular layers in the prosencephalon (from the intermediate zone of the developing cerebral cortex in the ferret), and (2) the neural crest in the mesencephalon, rhombencephalon, and spinal cord. Glial growth factor, which is expressed by migrating cortical neurons, promotes their migration along radial glial fibers, and also aids in the maintenance and elongation of radial glial cells. The chief types of glial cells are astroglia, oligodendroglia, microglia, and ependymal, satellite, and neurilemmal cells. Glial cells are about 10 times more numerous than neurons.

Hippocampus (area hippocampi): The hippocampal primordium appears (at stage 14) as an early marginal layer (q.v.) (Fig. 16-17), followed by a ventricular thickening in the dorsomedial wall of the cerebral hemisphere. Its C-shaped form is soon evident (by stage 18, Fig. 18-3). It consists mainly of large pyramidal cells that are concentrated in a narrow band. The synapses per neuron are more than twice as numerous as elsewhere in the cortex. See also Formation, hippocampal.

Insula: The slight depression of the insula that becomes apparent in stage 23 is preceded by a flat area overlying the lateral ventricular eminence at stages 18–22 (Fig. 23-2).

Isthmus rhombencephali: A term introduced by His for an "independent part of the brain" (now acknowledged as a neuromere) during development and in the adult. At the beginning of its appearance (in stages 13 and 14) this is a short, narrow part of the neural tube between the midbrain and the hindbrain (Fig. 13-4). It contains nuclei and intramural and commissural fibers of the trochlear nerves. Then it expands and participates in the formation of the rostral medullary velum dorsally. Its basal portion contains cerebellar tracts. The isthmus is believed to be a source of morphogens.

Lamina reuniens (*Schlussplatte*): A term used by His (1904) for what is here called the embryonic lamina terminalis. Its ventral part becomes the *Endplatte* (lamina terminalis *sensu stricto*), which remains thin and forms the rostral wall of the telencephalon medium. Its dorsal part is the *Trapezplatte* or massa commissuralis (q.v.).

Lamina terminalis, embryonic: The median wall of the telencephalon (Fig. 11-3) rostral to the chiasmatic plate (future optic chiasma). The commissural plate appears as a thickening in the embryonic lamina terminalis, and the remainder of the lamina then constitutes the adult lamina terminalis (Fig. 6-4). Further details: Bossy (1966).

Laminae, alar and basal (Fig. 6-3): Terms used by His for the dorsal and ventral zones of the neural tube, separated by the sulcus limitans. In the spinal cord, the alar plate, which has a broader ventricular layer, is essentially

Fig. 6-4. A median view of the brain at stage 22 to show the termination of the alar and basal laminae, and that of the sulcus limitans. The asterisk indicates the junction of the brain and spinal cord. The chief interpretations of the ending of the sulcus limitans, as summarized by Richter (1965, Fig. 35), are: (1) the supramamillary recess (Kingsbury; Schulte and Tilney; Kuhlenbeck); (2) the prechiasmatic recess (His; Johnston; Streeter); (3) the interventricular foramen (Spatz; Kahle; Richter). The first interpretation is that supported by the present authors for the human embryo. The inset shows an enlargement of the commissural plate to show three subregions described in the rat: a, the future anterior commissure; b, the probable site of closure of the rostral neuropore; and c, the future hippocampal commissure and the corpus callosum. With further development of these commissures, the embryonic lamina terminalis becomes reduced to the adult type (Ad.), which extends from the caudal limit of the commissures to the optic chiasma.

Fig. 6-4.

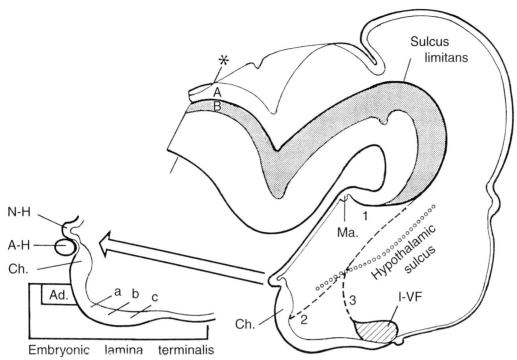

afferent, whereas the basal plate, which has a narrower ventricular layer but grows more rapidly, is fundamentally efferent (the "Bell–Magendie law"). An alar/basal distinction continues into the rhombencephalon and the mesencephalon, but not into the prosencephalon, where the sulcus limitans is absent. This point was long disputed in the past. The laminae express *Pax* genes (3 and 7 from the alar, 6 from the basal).

Layer, dural limiting (Fig. 22-14B):   A layer of condensed cells appearing in the peripheral mesenchyme and forming the external boundary of the leptomeningeal primordium. See also Meninx, primary. Further details: O'Rahilly and Müller (1986).

Layer, external germinal (or **external granular) of cerebellum** (Fig. 23-26D):   A lamina on the surface of the cerebellar primordium. It arises from the rhombic lip, mainly of the isthmic segment and of Rh.1. A special feature (at least in the rat) is that the migration of the cells in a lateromedial direction involves the use of axons as a substrate. It is frequently called the external granular layer because the granule cells arise from it. Sidman and Rakic (1982) have discussed the transformation and migration of the cells of the external germinal layer as they become granule cells. These cells are believed to be the origin of medulloblastoma.

Layer, primordial plexiform (Figs. 6-3 and 17-14):   The superficial stratum of the embryonic cerebral cortex. This layer contains horizontal (Cajal–Retzius) cells, unipolar as well as multipolar pluriform cells, tangentially arranged nerve fibers, horizontal branches of corticipetal fibers, and vertical cytoplasmic prolongations of the neuroepithelial cells. The long axes of the Cajal–Retzius cells run parallel to the cortical surface. Certain portions of the primordial plexiform layer are considered to be functionally active in the human embryo by stage 20 (Marín-Padilla and Marín-Padilla, 1982).

The earliest synapses seen in the human brain are in the primordial plexiform layer (Larroche, 1981; Choi, 1988) at about stages 17 to 19. They are formed by horizontal cells that correspond to those of Cajal–Retzius (Larroche and Houcine, 1982). After the subdivision of the primordial plexiform layer into subpial and subplate components, the synapses are present in those two layers, above and below the cortical plate but not within it (Molliver et al., 1973). Synapses have appeared within the cortical plate by 23 weeks (Molliver et al., 1973).

The primordial plexiform layer is thought to play a significant role in the structural organization of the neocortex by determining the unique morphology of its pyramidal cells. "However, the nature of layer I remains enigmatic" (Marín-Padilla, 1992).

A useful scheme of the development of the neocortical layers has been proposed by Rakic (1984, Fig. 3), although the primordial plexiform layer was not included.

Layer, subpial granular (of Brun):   A lamina that appears at about 15 weeks (Choi, 1988; Marín-Padilla, 1995), is fully developed at 25 weeks, begins to regress at 26 weeks, and has disappeared by about 35 weeks. It is formed from the subventricular layer of the olfactory bulb, does not show mitotic figures, and contains precursors of astrocytes that later migrate into the gray matter of the insular region.

Layer, subventricular (Fig. 6-3):   Present only after the establishment of the cortical plate (at stage 21), this layer consists of cells at the interface between the ventricular and intermediate layers. These cells divide without interkinetic nuclear migration, and the cellular production constitutes the secondary proliferative phase. The subventricular layer of the neopallium remains active in the adult (mouse). Many glial cells are produced in the subventricular and intermediate layers.

Layers, intermediate, marginal, and ventricular (Fig. 6-3): The *ventricular layer* of the neural tube, which is adjacent to the ventricular cavity, contains most of the mitotic figures that generate neurons and glial cells. Later it becomes the ependymal layer. Mitotic figures, however, are not restricted to the ventricular layer but can be found also more peripherally, in the *subventricular layer,* where cells apparently divide without movement of the nuclei during the mitotic cycle. It is believed that a temporal pattern of heterogeneity exists in the matrix. In early cerebral development, more neurons (Cajal–Retzius cells, subplate cells, secondary matrix cells of the subventricular layer) than glial cells are produced. The development continues with the production of neurons for layers 6 and 5, and finally of neurons for layers 4, 3, and 2. As development proceeds, the percentage of glial cells versus neurons increases. The *intermediate layer* consists of several rows of postmitotic cells that appear peripheral to the ventricular layer and it corresponds approximately to the term mantle layer. The intermediate layer is poorly defined in routine histological sections, but very distinct in Golgi preparations. It is composed mainly of corticipetal and corticofugal fibers and their collaterals (Fig. 23-19) and is crossed by migrating neurons. Because of its richness in fibers the layer was named embryonic white matter by Marín-Padilla (1988a). It is the precursor of the internal white matter of the adult cerebral cortex. The *marginal layer* is the cell-free peripheral zone of the neural tube. It is present in the spinal cord and in most parts of the brain. In the telencephalon it may be considered to be present in the hippocampal primordium, whereas in the neopallium a primordial plexiform layer (q.v.) is found.

Lip, rhombic: A proliferative area that persists in the most dorsolateral part of the rhombencephalic alar plate (Fig. 17-4). It becomes clearly defined in stage 17, when its mitotic figures become abundant and the remainder of the alar plate has differentiated into marginal and intermediate layers. The rhombic lip participates in the formation of the external germinal layer of the cerebellum (Fig. 23-26D). It produces three superficial streams: a pontine, a cochlear, and the so-called olivo-arcuate migration of Essick (1912). The last-mentioned layer (Fig. 20-16) is ill-named because it has been shown (in the monkey) that the olivary nuclei arise mainly from the ventricular layer. "Rhombic lip" should not be used as a synonym for cerebellum.

The term was introduced by His, who distinguished primary and secondary types (although the likelihood of artifact was pointed out by Hochstetter, 1929). Subsequent usage of the term is twofold: (1) morphologically the junction between the thin roof plate and the much thicker alar lamina, i.e., more or less equivalent to the taenia of the fourth ventricle; (2) functionally, as used in this book, the dorsolateral portion of the alar lamina, which (characterized by mitotic figures from stage 16 on) acts as a proliferative zone (Figs. 20-17, 22-13, and 23-26).

Massa commissuralis (of Zuckerkandl): A bed through which the fibers of two cerebral commissures pass: the commissura fornicis and the corpus callosum. It develops early in the fetal period from the commissural plate and also from proliferating cells of the mesenchyme between the medial hemispheric walls in the region of the hippocampal primordium.

Matrix, extracellular (ECM): Occupying 15–20% of the volume of the brain and associated with neurons and glia, the ECM preserves epithelial integrity and acts as a substrate for cellular migration and as a guide for axonal extension.

Meninx, primary: The loose mesenchyme (*meninx primitiva* of Salvi) adjacent to the brain (Fig. 14-6) and spinal cord. From stage 17 onwards the leptomeningeal meshwork contains fluid that is believed to be derived from the adjacent blood vessels. Its peripheral border is represented by the dural limiting layer (q.v.). Further details: O'Rahilly and Müller (1986).

Midline: An undesirable term for the median plane (O'Rahilly, 1996).

Migration: The cells for the cerebral cortex migrate both radially and tangentially.

In radial migration, cells within a given radial column, although they may arise from various progenitors, share the same birthplace, and migrate along a common pathway towards the pia mater. The number of radial columns determines the extent of the cortical surface, whereas the number of cells within the columns determines cortical thickness.

In tangential migration, which has been found in the intermediate and ventricular layers (in the ferret), clonally related cells are dispersed in a direction parallel to the pia mater. A special form of tangential migration occurs as cellular chains from the adult ventricular and subventricular layers of the olfactory bulb (in the mouse).

Neopallium: The cerebral cortex derived from the areas that possess a cortical plate, which latter begins to appear in stage 21 (Fig. 6-3).

Nerve, vomeronasal (Fig. 18-13): Nonmyelinated fibers from the vomeronasal organ (q.v.). The fibers enter the rostromedial wall of the olfactory bulb.

Nervus terminalis (Fig. 20-10): Fibers that enter the olfactory tubercle at stage 18 and that are probably autonomic. These fibers arise in the nasal mucosa and later will traverse the cribriform plate.

Neuroectoderm: See Ectoderm, neural.

Neuroglia: See Glia.

Neuromeres: Morphologically identifiable transverse subdivisions perpendicular to the longitudinal axis of the embryonic brain and extending onto both sides of the body (Müller and O'Rahilly, 1997b). The larger (primary) neuromeres appear early in the open neural folds (at stage 9), and the smaller (secondary) neuromeres are found both before and after closure of the neural tube. The full complement of 16 neuromeres is present at stage 14 (Table 14-1). Neuromeres are particularly clear in the hindbrain (Figs. 10-2 and 10-3), where they are termed rhombomeres (q.v.). In some instances the neuromeres are coextensive with domains of gene expression, whereas in others the domains cross interneuromeric boundaries.

Neuropores: Temporary rostral (stage 11, Fig. 11-6) and caudal (stages 11 and 12) openings that represent the remains of the neural groove before the fusion of the neural folds has been completed at each end. The neuropores close during stages 11 and 12, respectively. Further details of the rostral (or cephalic) neuropore: O'Rahilly and Müller (1989a).

Neurulation: The formation of the neural tube in the embryo (Fig. 9-5). Primary neurulation is the folding of the neural plate to form successively the neural groove and the neural tube. Secondary neurulation, which occurs without direct involvement of the ectoderm and without the intermediate phase of a neural plate, is the continuing formation of the spinal cord from the caudal eminence, which develops a neural cord (q.v.). Further details: Müller and O'Rahilly (1987, 1988a); O'Rahilly and Müller (1994).

Nuclei: The term is used here in the restricted meaning of areas of lower cellular density and slightly larger cellular size. As Dekaban (1954) pointed out, early and later neurons "group themselves into 'centers' or 'nuclei,' which will constitute functional systems or parts of the systems." Rakic (1974), on the other hand, in delimiting diencephalic nuclei, maintains that subdivisions into discrete nuclear groups "appears to be based initially on the establishment of boundaries by fascicles of nerve fibers."

Nuclei, amygdaloid: These are originally in a diencephalic position mostly in the medial ventricular eminence (Fig. 18-5B), but later become telencephalic.

Nuclei, basal (Fig. 6-2): An arbitrary group that generally includes the corpus striatum (q.v.), the amygdaloid body, and the claustrum. To these are added, from a clinical point of view, the subthalamic nucleus and the substantia nigra, to complete the basal structures affected pathologically in so-called extrapyramidal motor diseases. The region of the future basal nuclei, which becomes compartmentalized into three entities by stage 19, extends to the preoptic sulcus caudally and to the prosencephalic septal area rostrally. The three compartments are, in order of appearance: (1) the medial ventricular eminence, (2) the lateral ventricular eminence, and (3) the basal ventricular eminence (Fig. 19-5). From the lateral eminence arise the caudate nucleus and the putamen; from the medial the amygdaloid body; and from a basal thickening, the nucleus accumbens. The constituent cells of the basal nuclei are derived from the subventricular zone. These cells proliferate throughout the entire prenatal period (Kahle, 1969; Sidman and Rakic, 1982) by a special mode of division that has been investigated by Smart in the mouse. The basal nuclei are not ganglia, which, by definition, occur only in the peripheral nervous system.

Organ, vomeronasal: Epithelial pockets that appear bilaterally in the nasal septum in stage 18. They enlarge during the embryonic and fetal periods and are generally said to involute postnatally, although this has been queried (Smith et al., 1997). See also Nerve, vomeronasal.

Organs, circumventricular: Specialized ependymal regions in (chiefly) the third ventricle. They are practically all median in position and (with the exception of the subcommissural organ) are highly vascular and lack a blood–brain barrier. They vary in prominence and in structure with age, and some are difficult to find in the adult or may even disappear. Functions include secretion of substances (e.g., neuropeptides) into the cerebrospinal fluid, and transport of neurochemicals in both directions between neurons, glia, and blood cells and the CSF. The main structures that are generally included are (1) the median eminence of the tuber cinereum (around the base of the infundibulum); (2) the neurohypophysis; (3) the organum vasculosum of the lamina terminalis (OVLT; supraoptic crest; intercolumnar tubercle); (4) the subfornical organ (at the level of the interventricular foramina); (5) the paraphysis (a temporary ependymal thickening rostral to the velum transversum in trimester 1); (6) the epiphysis cerebri; (7) the subcommissural organ (modified ependyma in the roof of the aqueduct, beneath the posterior commissure); and (8) the area postrema (at the junction of the fourth ventricle and the central canal), which resembles the subfornical organ but differs from the strictly circumventricular organs in being related to the fourth rather than the third ventricle and in being bilateral.

Paleopallium: The cerebral cortex of the pyriform area, including the surface of the medial ventricular eminence with the amygdaloid body. The peripaleocortex is the transitional region between paleopallium and neopallium. It becomes apparent when the cortical plate appears in stage 21 (Fig. 21-8).

Paraphysis: A telencephalic formation appearing first as a knob (stage 18, Fig. 18-8) and later developing one or more evaginations, which are in communication with the ventricle of the telencephalon medium and are lined by a single layer of ciliated cells. Further details: Ariëns Kappers (1955); O'Rahilly and Müller (1990).

Parencephalon (Table 14-1): A part of the diencephalon (neuromere D2) which, together with the synencephalon (q.v.), becomes discernible at stage 13. Two portions can be distinguished at stage 14: the rostral parencephalon (including the infundibular region and the ventral thalamus) and the caudal parencephalon (containing the mamillary region and the dorsal thalamus).

Plane, median: This is considered to be a special region that is subject to a variety of anomalies, such as holoprosencephaly and agenesis of the corpus callosum. The median features of the developing brain are shown in Figures 17-6, 24-24, and 25-2.

Plate, callosal commissural: See Massa commissuralis.

Plate, cerebellar: A term used when the cerebellar primordium becomes coronally oriented and more or less at a right angle to the remainder of the rhombencephalon (Fig. 18-2). See also Cerebellum and Swellings, cerebellar.

Plate, chiasmatic (or **torus opticus**): A bridge between the optic primordia across the median plane (Fig. 10-2). Its rostral end corresponds to the tip of the former neural plate. The fibers of the preoptico-hypothalamic tract cross in its caudal part at stage 18 (Fig. 18-3) and the optic fibers in its rostral portion at stage 19 (Figs. 19-3 and 20-3).

Plate, commissural (Fig. 12-3): A thickening in the embryonic lamina terminalis (q.v.) at the situs neuroporicus (q.v.). It is considered by some to be the bed through which commissural fibers of the anterior commissure, corpus callosum, and commissura fornicis pass (Streeter, 1912; Hochstetter, 1929; Bartelmez and Dekaban, 1962). Others (e.g., His, 1904; Rakic and Yakovlev, 1968) have maintained that the commissuration is preceded by the development of a massa commissuralis (q.v.), which implies some fusion of the medial hemispheric walls at the level of the hippocampal primordium.

Plate, cortical (Fig. 6-3): A neopallial feature first found in the embryo at stage 21 (Fig. 21-7). It consists of three to five rows of cells that have migrated radially from the ventricular layer and are arranged vertically. It increases in thickness and persists for long into the fetal period. Although formerly it was thought that only layers 2 to 5 develop from the cortical plate, it is now generally believed that layer 6 is also derived from the plate (Mrzijak et al., 1988). The migrating neurons that accumulate within the primordial plexiform layer are arranged in an outside–inside order.

Synapses develop relatively late within the cortical plate, at about 23 weeks (Molliver et al., 1973), whereas they are already present in the primordial plexiform layer at stages 17–19.

Plate, neural (Fig. 9-5): The neural primordium that appears during stage 8 and is present in caudal areas up to stage 10. At the time of its first appearance it is slightly vaulted on each side of the neural groove. The prenotochordal part of the neural plate is the diencephalic region (neuromere

D1 and the future rostral parencephalon). The epinotochordal portion of the neural plate (that overlying the notochord) develops a floor plate (q.v.).

Plate, optic: The median region that unites the optic primordia of the two sides (Fig. 10-2). It represents the rostral end of the neural plate, and it participates in the formation of neuromere D1.

Plate, prechordal: A multilayered accumulation of endodermal cells in close contact with the median part of the future prosencephalon in the human embryo (Figs. 8-3 and 8-5). The plate differs appreciably in the mouse and in the chick embryo.

Plates, alar and basal: See Laminae, alar and basal.

Plexuses, choroid: Intraventricular invaginations at stages 18–20 of choroidal (as distinct from ventricular) ependyma derived from the ventricular layer of the neural tube and characterized by tight junctions and tela choroidea (vascular pia mater). The plexuses are relatively very large in the embryo (Fig. 23-16). They produce cerebrospinal fluid (in contrast to the ependymal fluid of earlier stages) and probably a variety of growth factors.

Preplate: A term that is sometimes used for the primordial plexiform layer.

Recess, postoptic: The site where the optic sulci meet in the median plane (Fig. 10-2). This is the caudal limit of the chiasmatic plate.

Recess, preoptic: In later stages this depression indicates the rostral limit of the chiasmatic plate (Fig. 14-3).

Rhombomeres: The transverse swellings in the neural tube, known as neuromeres, are termed rhombomeres in the developing rhombencephalon, where they are clearly visible up to stage 17. They are originally four in number (Fig. 9-2C) and are termed A, B, C, and D. They increase in number by subdivision during stage 10 and are numbered 1, 2, 3 (from A), 4 (corresponding to B), 5, 6, 7 (from C), and 8 (corresponding to D and related to somites 1–4). Eight rhombomeres are generally identifiable from stage 11 to stage 17; in addition, the isthmus rhombencephali (q.v.) becomes apparent from stage 13 onwards. They are believed to result from transverse bands of high mitotic activity and they are maintained by cytoskeletal components, although their significance is still disputed. Cranial nerves 5 to 10 have a clear relationship to specific rhombomeres; the otic vesicle, however, changes its position with regard to the rhombomeres, shifting from Rh.4 (in stage 10) to Rh.6 (in stages 14–17).

Roof plate: The plate consists of the dorsomedial cells of the neural tube (Fig. 6-3). It is believed to be induced by a morphogenic protein of ectodermal origin, and it may be important in causing differentiation of the dorsal part of the spinal cord.

Septum, prosencephalic: The septum verum (Andy and Stephan, 1968) is the basal part of the medial wall of the cerebral hemispheres. Hence it is formed at the time when the hemispheres expand beyond the lamina terminalis, beginning at stage 17. It is the area between the olfactory bulb and the commissural plate (Fig. 18-3). The nuclei arising in it during the embryonic period are the medial septal nucleus, the caudal nucleus of the diagonal band, and the nucleus accumbens.

Situs neuroporicus (Fig. 12-6): The site of final closure of the rostral neuropore. It corresponds later to an area within the commissural plate. Further details: Müller and O'Rahilly (1984).

Stalk, hemispheric: The original connection (*Streifenhügelstiel, Hemisphärenstiel:* His, 1904) between the diencephalon and the telencephalon,

31

which becomes a stalk from about stage 17. It becomes greatly enlarged by fibers and tracts, especially by the continuation of the internal capsule (Figs. 21-6, 22-10, and 22-11), namely the lateral prosencephalic fasciculus (q.v.). Further details: Sharp (1959), Richter (1965).

Stammbündel: The term used by His for the fibers (lateral prosencephalic fasciculus, q.v.) connecting the dorsal thalamus and telencephalon and continuing also to the epithalamus and to the mesencephalon.

Subplate (Figs. 6-3 and 23-20):   A derivative of the primordial plexiform layer (q.v.), which may participate in the specification of the cortical plate (q.v.). It has been termed by Rakic a waiting compartment for incoming afferent axons.

A clear anatomical separation does not exist between the subplate and the intermediate layer; both are characterized by an abundance of fibers (Figs. 23-19 and 23-20). The subplate gradually disappears during early infancy (Kostović and Rakic, 1990). However, the original components of the primordial plexiform layer are believed neither to decrease nor to disappear, but rather to undergo a significant and progressive dilution (Marín-Padilla, 1988a). The early subplate cells undergo regressive changes and they are progressively replaced by new projection neurons (Marín-Padilla, 1988a).

Sulcus, hypothalamic (Table 20-1):   An internal groove between the thalamus *sensu lato* (comprising the dorsal and ventral thalami) and the hypothalamus *sensu lato* (comprising the subthalamus and hypothalamus *sensu stricto*). It begins and ends in the diencephalon.

Sulcus, intereminential: A term used by the present authors for the slight groove that appears at stage 18 between the lateral and medial ventricular eminences (Fig. 22-6A).

Sulcus limitans (Fig. 6-3 and 6-4):   An internal groove found bilaterally in the developing mesencephalon, rhombencephalon, and spinal cord. It is present at stage 12 and is the boundary between the alar and basal laminae (q.v.). In the human embryo the sulcus limitans ends rostrally near the rostral end of the mesencephalon (Fig. 17-5). This point was long disputed in the past (Fig. 6-4). See also Laminae, alar and basal.

Swellings, cerebellar: Bulges that are parts of the cerebellar plate, i.e., the alar lamina of the isthmic segment together with that of rhombomere 1. The earlier appearing internal cerebellar swelling (*innerer Kleinhirnwulst* of Hochstetter, 1929) is inside the fourth ventricle (Fig. 17-5). The external cerebellar swelling (*äusserer Kleinhirnwulst*) forms as an expansion at the site of the rhombic lip (Fig. 17-4). It is delimited by a groove that corresponds to the later posterolateral fissure of the cerebellum. The internal and external cerebellar swellings are sometimes referred to, respectively, as the intraventricular and extraventricular portions of the developing cerebellum.

Synencephalon (Fig. 13-4):   The caudalmost part of the diencephalon, the portion that gives rise to the prerubrum and the pretectum. It is delineated rostrally by the habenulo-interpeduncular tract (fasciculus retroflexus) and caudally by the di-mesencephalic borderline passing between the two constituents of the posterior commissure.

Telencephalon medium or impar: The first part of the telencephalon to appear (at stage 10, Fig. 10-2) is lateral in position. Only later (stage 14) do the lateral walls become domed and form the future cerebral hemispheres. The median part of the telencephalon persists throughout life, so that a portion of the third ventricle remains telencephalic. Further details: Müller and O'Rahilly (1985).

Torus hemisphericus: A ridge at the ventricular surface between the telencephalon and the diencephalon, and along which the cerebral hemispheres are evaginated (Fig. 14-3). An external di-telencephalic sulcus develops and accompanies it.

Torus opticus: See Plate, chiasmatic.

Velum transversum: A transverse ridge in the roof of the forebrain marking the limit between telencephalon and diencephalon (Fig. 14-3).

Ventricle, olfactory (Fig. 22-12): A prolongation of the lateral ventricle into the growing olfactory bulb at approximately stages 19 to 23, and also in the fetal period.

Ventricle, optic: At first (stage 13), the cavity of the optic vesicle, which is a prolongation of that of the diencephalon. Later it becomes the intraretinal slit between the external and internal strata of the optic cup, and ultimately the potential space (along which so-called detachment of the retina occurs) between layer 1 and layers 2–10 of the retina (Fig. 23-13).

Zona limitans intrathalamica: A zone that parallels the marginal ridge and sulcus medius between the dorsal and ventral thalami and is at first recognizable as a thicker marginal layer at this site. Fibers of the zona limitans intrathalamica are visible at stage 19 (Fig. 19-15). The zona is believed to form later the lamina medullaris externa. The marginal ridge, sulcus medius, and zona limitans intrathalamica are seen in Figure 21-12.

Important

To use this atlas most effectively it is advisable to refer frequently to the definitions given in this chapter.

C H A P T E R 7

Early Stages

Because the first morphological indication of the nervous system appears at stage 8 (approximately 3 postfertilizational weeks), the following brief statement concerning stages 1 to 7 is provided. Full details of these early stages have been published in a monograph by O'Rahilly and Müller (1987a).

Stage 1 is the unicellular embryo that is formed at fertilization, normally in the lateral end (ampulla) of the uterine tube. A new, genetically distinct human organism is thereby formed, although the embryonic genome does not become activated until the next stage.

Stage 2 (2–3 days) is the cleaving embryo that proceeds along the uterine tube.

Stage 3 (4–5 days) is characterized by the appearance of a cavity within the cellular mass, at which time the embryo is termed a blastocyst and lies in the uterine cavity. The embryonic disc now presents dorsal and ventral surfaces.

Stage 4 (6 days) is the attachment of the blastocyst to the uterine lining (endometrium), an event that heralds the beginning of implantation within the uterine mucosa.

Stage 5 (7–12 days), the continuation of implantation, is complicated and is subdivided into three substages, according to whether (5a) the trophoblast is solid, (5b) the trophoblast contains lacunae, or (5c) the lacunae form a vascular circle. The amniotic cavity and umbilical vesicle (so-called yolk sac) appear during stage 5.

Stage 6 (about 17 days) is marked by the appearance of chorionic villi. During this stage, at approximately $2\frac{1}{2}$ postfertilizational weeks, axial features (particularly a cellular proliferation termed the primitive streak) develop, and hence the embryo acquires right and left sides, as well as rostral and caudal ends. The embryonic disc is now about 0.2 mm in length. Twins (other than certain conjoined examples) arise before the appearance of axial features, i.e., during approximately the first fortnight. Retinoic acid is believed to be implicated in the patterning of the rostrocaudal axis and the induction of the expression of *Hox* genes.

Stage 7 (about 19 days). An axial structure known as the notochordal process is characteristic of this stage, when the embryonic disc measures approximately 0.4 mm. Although no morphological sign of the nervous system is yet present, the site of the future neural plate around the notochordal process can be assessed (O'Rahilly and Müller, 1987b, Fig. 1), based on autoradiographic studies of the chick embryo.

Stage 8 (about 23 days) is the subject of the following chapter. Canalization of the notochordal process occurs (i.e., the notochordal canal develops) in embryos approximately 1 mm in length. When, during stage 8, the notochordal process attains a length of 0.4 mm, the neural groove, which is the first morphological indication of the nervous system, becomes recognizable.

The cells and tissues that give rise to the nervous system are given in Table 7-1.

The most frequently encountered errors in descriptions of the initial development of the human brain have recently been listed (O'Rahilly and Müller, 1999).

Important

The embryo acquires dorsal and ventral surfaces at about $1\frac{1}{2}$ postfertilizational weeks, and right and left sides, as well as rostral and caudal ends, at about $2\frac{1}{2}$ weeks.

TABLE 7-1.   The Origin of the Central Nervous System (CNS) and Peripheral Nervous System (PNS)

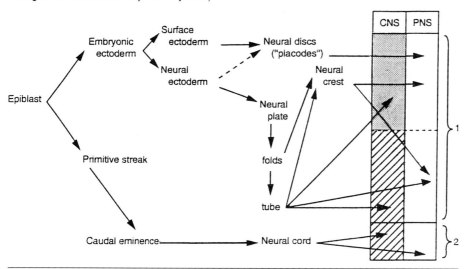

The stippling indicates the brain, the diagonal hatching represents the spinal cord, and the interrupted horizontal line is the cerebrospinal junction. Primary and secondary neurulation are marked 1 and 2 respectively. The neural discs, which appear in the surface ectoderm, were regarded by Streeter as islands of neural ectoderm.
Modified from O'Rahilly and Müller, 1996.

Comments on Neuroteratology (Stage 6)

Spina bifida aperta. It has been shown experimentally in the mouse that excessive cell death in the primitive streak plays a major role in spina bifida aperta caused by non-closure of the neural folds.

Stage 8: The First Appearance of the Nervous System

Approximately 1–1.5 mm in Greatest Length
Approximately 23 Postfertilizational Days

The embryo is an ovoid (frequently pear-shaped) disc with a longitudinal axis and distinct cephalic and caudal ends. In one-quarter of examples, referred to as stage 8b, the neural groove can be detected in the neural plate as a very shallow sulcus bounded by faint neural folds. This is the first visible sign of the future nervous system, and most of the folds represents the brain. The neural plate is closely related to two median features: the prechordal plate and the notochordal process. Further details: O'Rahilly and Müller (1981).

Stage 8 has been generally listed as 18 days, but is probably more usually about 23 days.

Although few morphological features are visible at the time of initial development of the brain, stage 8 and its organization are of crucial importance for an understanding of the developing nervous system. It is of interest that the primordium of the brain appears before the heart or any other organs become visible.

Although little is known concerning neural induction in mammalian embryos, studies of early neurogenesis suggest that differences among vertebrate classes are present from the beginning of neurulation, and that mammalian neurulation is extremely complex.

Fig. 8-1. Dorsal view of an embryo (CEC 5960) of stage 8. The rostral end is at the top of the page; the caudal end is below and is anchored by the connecting stalk, at the end of which two chorionic villi have been sectioned. The amnion has been cut and removed in order to expose the dorsal surface of the embryo. X and Y are the levels of the sections shown in Figures 8-3 and 8-4.

The embryo at stage 8 is a slightly vaulted, pear-shaped disc that displays a longitudinal axis. The axis is indicated (1) by the primitive groove, which begins at the primitive node and proceeds caudally, and (2) by the neural groove, which is situated in the median plane at level Y. This is the region of the neural plate, which, although sharp boundaries are not evident, comprises (a) a peripheral rim, the alar plate, and (b) a more central part capping the notochordal process and primitive node, namely the basal plate or lamina (Fig. 9-5). The neural groove, which is shown in Figure 8-4, is the first visible sign of the future nervous system and, for the most part, it indicates the site of the brain.

This beautiful drawing of the Heuser embryo is by James F. Didusch, whose "work is unexcelled in the anatomical literature" (Crosby and Cody, 1991). In 1917 Max Brödel referred to Didusch as "my first pupil."

Important
The first indication of the neural groove and folds is found during this stage.

Fig. 8-1.

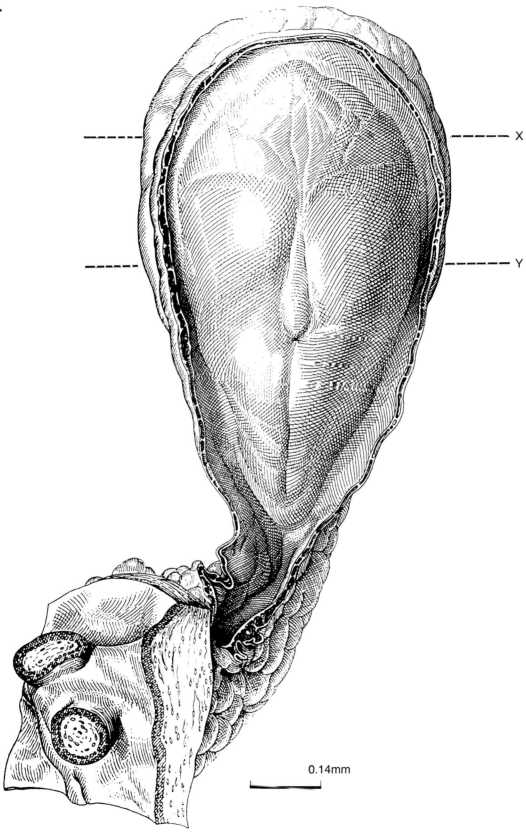

X

Y

0.14mm

Fig. 8-2. Graphic reconstruction prepared from transverse sections of an embryo (CEC 5960) of stage 8. The rostral end is to the right. From rostral to caudal, the following are indicated: prechordal plate, epiblast (dorsally), and endoderm.

The neural plate, situated dorsally in the general region of line Y, is in close contact rostrally with the prechordal plate, and ventrocaudally with the notochordal process. The rostralmost portion of the neural plate corresponds to the optic area of the diencephalon, neuromere D1.

Fig. 8-3. Transverse section at the level of the prechordal plate (CEC 7545), corresponding to line X in Figures 8-1 and 8-2. This figure and Figure 8-4 were selected from a histologically superior embryo. The prechordal plate is a multilayered accumulation of cells in close contact with the floor of the neural groove. It is involved in neural induction, which is probably maximal at stage 8. The plate also furnishes mesenchyme for the orbital muscles and probably for the tentorium cerebelli. The location of the prechordal plate in the human would seem to correspond to the axial mesoderm between the first pair of "somitomeres" in the mouse, in which species seven such segmental units have been detected rostral to the first somite. Bar = 0.05 mm.

The prechordal plate is an important source of prenotochordal tissue. It is maintained that the prechordal plate is ventral to a single retinal field at the rostral end of the neural plate and that normally it suppresses the median part of that field, thereby causing bilateral retinal primordia to develop.

Fig. 8-4. Transverse section at the level of the notochordal plate (CEC 7545), corresponding to line Y in Figures 8-1 and 8-2. The shallow neural groove, present in one-quarter of embryos of stage 8, is bounded on each side by a slightly elevated neural fold. Numerous mitotic figures are present in the neural plate and are adjacent to the amniotic cavity, i.e., near the future ventricular surface of the later-appearing neural tube.

The notochordal plate is the roof of the notochordal process at levels where the floor has already disappeared during the process of intercalation of the plate in the endoderm. The notochordal process is a cellular rod that contains the notochordal canal and is in close contact with the neural ectoderm dorsally and the mesenchyme laterally. Its canal begins as a pit in the primitive node and then proceeds more or less vertically, as the neurenteric canal, before continuing rostrally. The primitive streak is situated caudal to the primitive node, and it gives rise to numerous mesenchymal cells. The multilayered mesoderm interposed between ectoderm and endoderm is separated by the basement membranes of the two epithelia. The median part of the neural epithelium is the future floor plate. It is firmly attached to the notochordal plate and is as thick as the lateral portion of the neural plate. Bar = 0.05 mm.

Fig. 8-2.

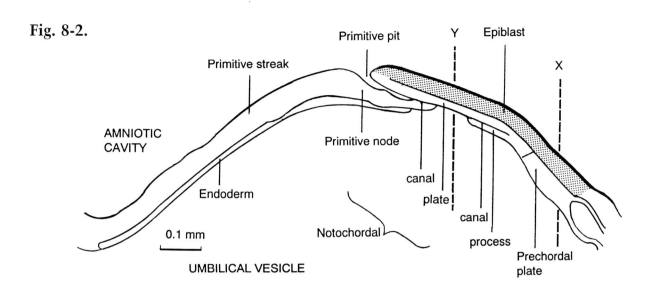

Fig. 8-3.

Fig. 8-4.

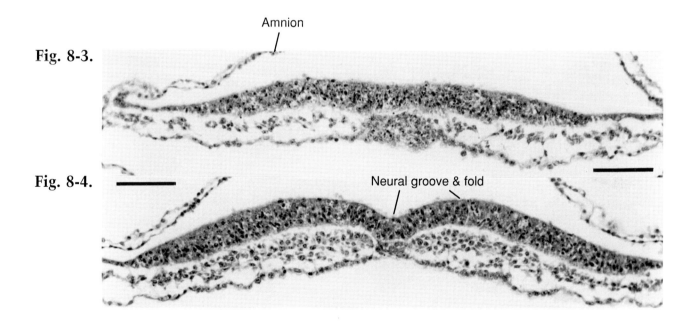

43

Fig. 8-5. Serial sections through an excellent example (CEC 7666) of stage 8. The level of the sections is indicated on the reconstructed median section and dorsal view.

(**A**) The prechordal plate in transverse section shows as many as eight rows of cells that differ from the endodermal cells in being larger and more nearly spherical, and in containing numerous granules. The neural ectoderm at this level shows a very faint indentation, the beginning of the neural groove. The prechordal and neural plates are separated by a basement membrane.

(**B**) The neural groove (arrow) in an area rostral to the notochordal process.

(**C**) The primitive pit and its continuation with the notochordal canal of the notochordal process.

(**D**) The primitive node.

(**E**) The primitive groove and streak. At this caudal level the mesenchyme between the surface ectoderm and the endoderm is far greater in quantity than at rostral levels. Blood vessels are not yet present. Bar = 0.03 mm.

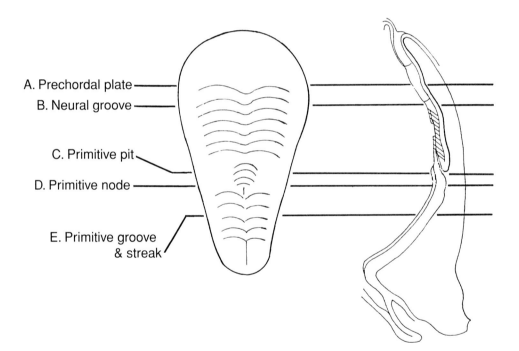

A. Prechordal plate

B. Neural groove

C. Primitive pit

D. Primitive node

E. Primitive groove & streak

Fig. 8-5.

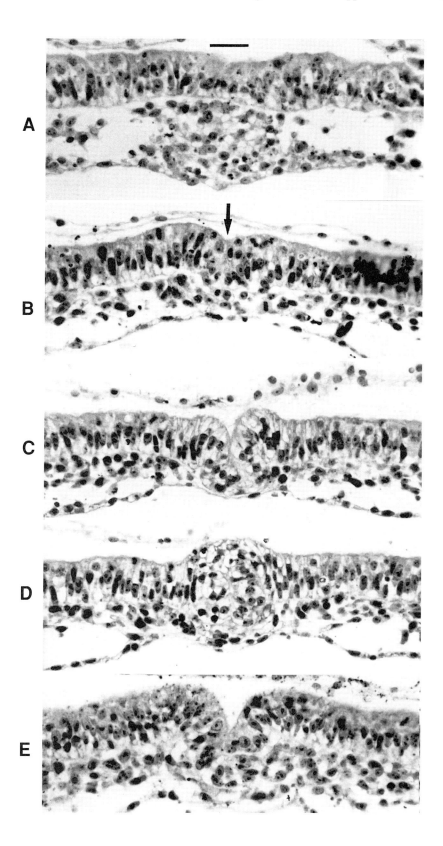

Comments on Neuroteratology (Stage 8)

Holoprosencephaly is a term used for a graded series of cerebral and facial anomalies that range from cyclopia to the almost normal. The "entire prosencephalon remains holospheric rather than becoming hemispheric" (DeMyer, 1987); i.e., the prosencephalon remains as a whole, a single, more or less undifferentiated sphere, incompletely cleft into complex halves. The basal parts of the brain are absent in holoprosencephaly. In the telencephalon the future septal area and the commissural plate (future anterior commissure and corpus callosum) are missing, and the telencephalic portion of the corpus striatum is not formed (Müller and O'Rahilly, 1989c). At the diencephalic level, disturbances are less evident, except at the level of the optic primordia. The adenohypophysis may be absent or may merely become detached. Its absence may perhaps be related to a disturbance of the prechordal plate. Holoprosencephaly may be autosomal dominant, autosomal recessive, or X-linked recessive, and about half of affected newborns have chromosomal disorders (chiefly chromosome 13, 18, or 21, deletions in chromosome 7 may be implicated). Association with trisomy 13 and triploidy may also occur. Absence of the rostral part of the notochord (with consequent cranial defects) could also result from faulty interaction with the prechordal plate. At stage 8 a mesenchymal disturbance could already be active. Faulty development of the paraxial mesenchyme from the primitive streak or node could interfere with the elevation of the neural folds. Defective prechordal mesenchyme may fail to produce the normal facial structures and to induce adequate morphogenesis of optic primordia and of the brain. The prosencephalon fails to "diverticulate" into cerebral hemispheres. Such conditions, although variable in their manifestation, would arise during the first 4 or 5 weeks (Fig. 16-19E, F). Holoprosencephaly is more than 60 times more frequent prenatally than in live births.

Cyclopia (the term is based on a mythical race of Sicilian giants) is characterized by a single median eye and orbit. The *sine qua non* is the presence of a single median (bony) orbit. The condition is accompanied by holoprosencephaly, and the nose is usually represented by a proboscis placed above the median eye. The impression of a fusion of formerly paired optic primordia is no longer considered to reflect the origin of the condition. In cyclopia *sensu stricto* the ocular structures are single rather than paired. The prosencephalon fails to "diverticulate" into the right and left optic evaginations. Such a disturbance could arise as early as stages 6 to 8 if the single eyefield, which is normally converted to paired optic primordia, is not so transformed because of a lack of inhibition of the median part by the prechordal plate. The teratogenetic termination-point is probably 3 weeks for cyclopia *sensu stricto* (a median eye in a single orbit) and 4 weeks for cyclopia *sensu lato* (paired ocular structures in a single orbit, Fig. 16-19). A parallel situation in the development of the limbs (the origin of symmelia) has been noted (O'Rahilly and Müller, 1989b).

Stage 9: The Major Divisions of the Brain

Approximately 1.5–2.5 mm in Greatest Length
Approximately 26 Postfertilizational Days

The embryonic disc is now an elongated body characterized by a long and deep neural groove. The first somites have appeared and are occipital. The three major divisions of the brain are distinguishable in the folds of the completely open neural groove: prosencephalon (mostly diencephalon), mesencephalon (at the mesencephalic flexure), and rhombencephalon (comprising four subdivisions, A to D). Rhombomere D is related to the (occipital) somites and was not recognized by previous authors. No neural tube has yet formed, and "brain vesicles" are not present. Neural crest is beginning to develop. The otic discs, which are the first indication of the (internal) ears, are first visible at this stage. Further details: Müller and O'Rahilly (1983).

The main subdivisions of the brain listed by His are given in Table 9-1.

TABLE 9–1. The Main Developmental Subdivisions of the Brain as Given by His in Preparation for the *Basel Nomina anatomica* of 1895 (based on von Baer, with the addition of the isthmus rhombencephali)

E n c e p h a l o n

Prosencephalon	6. Telencephalon
	5. Diencephalon
Mesencephalon	4. Mesencephalon
	3. Isthmus rhombencephali
	2. Metencephalon
Rhombencephalon	Cerebellum
	Pons
	1. Myelencephalon
	Medulla oblongata

Fig. 9-1. Left lateral and dorsal views of an embryo (CEC 1878) of stage 9. Striking changes have occurred since the prceding stage. The embryonic disc is now clearly an elongated embryonic body, set off from the surface of the umbilical vesicle (the so-called yolk sac).

In the lateral view, the "waist" of the embryo can be seen to be the site of considerable lordosis. The cephalic and caudal portions of the body are elevated from the surface.

In the dorsal view, the region of the head, which is broadest at the level of the mesencephalon, is clearly joined to the caudal eminence by a "waist," in which the first (occipital) somites are appearing. Caudally the greatest width is at the level of the primitive node, the site of which is shown in Figure 9-2. (In the present figure the artist has placed it too far caudally.) Cephalic to the node, the embryo has elongated greatly. Beyond the embryo, the umbilical vessels and the allantoic diverticulum have been sectioned. The neural folds bound a long and deep neural groove. Preotic and postotic sulci are very faint (compared with those in rodents).

This is another example of an elegant drawing by James F. Didusch, artist to the Carnegie Collection.

Fig. 9-1.

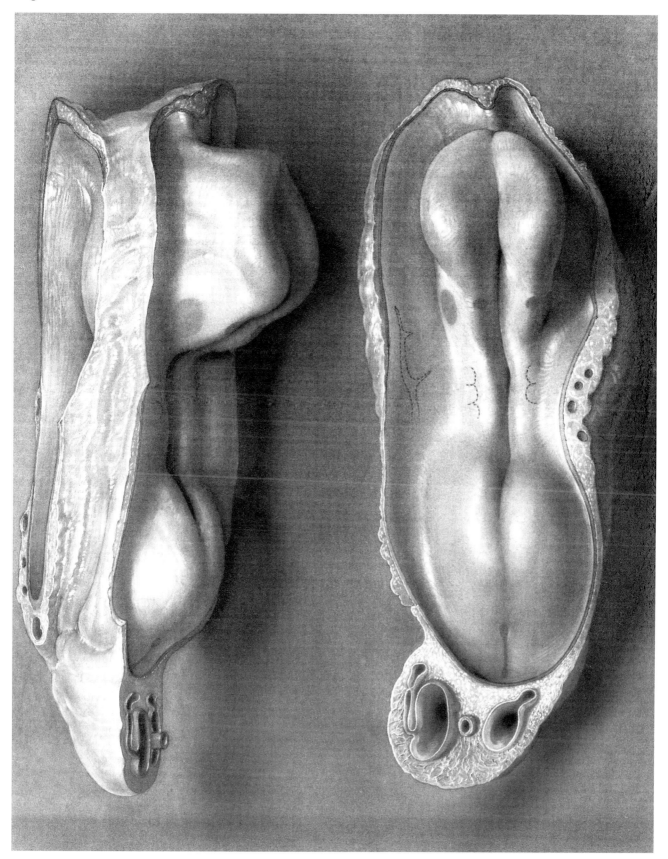

Fig. 9-2. (**A**) dorsal, (**B**) right lateral, and (**C**) median views of an embryo (CEC 1878) of stage 9. The cephalic end is to the right. The first (occipital) somites are stippled. The otic discs are indicated by interrupted lines; C is a graphic reconstruction prepared from transverse sections.

Although no part of the neural tube has yet formed and no so-called brain vesicles are present, the three major divisions of the brain recognized by von Baer are distinguishable. The prosencephalon is almost exclusively diencephalic. The mesencephalon is at the site of a marked bend, the mesencephalic flexure. In C, the rhombencephalon, which extends from the otic to the somitic region, can be seen to comprise four subdivisions: rhombomeres A, B, C, and D, the last (first recognized by Müller and O'Rahilly, 1983) representing the hypoglossal region. These rhombomeres are real entities (as shown by immunological methods in the chick). The asterisk indicates the future cerebrospinal junction. A vertical line shows the junction between primitive streak and primitive node. A faint groove is visible between the mesencephalon and Rh.A. It is clearest in a dorsal view (Fig. 9-2A), where it separates the wider midbrain from the narrower hindbrain. It corresponds to the preotic sulcus in rodents.

The first sign of the production of neural crest can be found in a few embryos of stage 9. It occurs at the level of the mesencephalon and the rhombencephalon. In addition, the production of general mesenchyme continues. The prechordal plate participates in the formation of the head and probably provides cardiac mesenchyme. The primitive streak, however, seems to have ceased as a site of proliferation, and its functional role has been replaced by that of the caudal eminence. The primitive node is shown in its correct position (more rostrally than in Fig. 9-1).

Fig. 9-3. Transverse section of an embryo (known as Ludwig's Da 1) of stage 9 through the rhombencephalic region. The neural groove is widely open to the amniotic cavity. The neural folds show a median hinge-point at the floor plate, which is in contact with the notochordal plate and has the same thickness as the lateral walls of the future neural tube. The thick ectoderm lateral to the summit of each neural fold is the otic plate. Mesenchyme is visible bilaterally. Until the neuropores close, the neural plate and early neural tube are nourished not by blood vessels, which have yet to appear, but through the amniotic fluid. Bar = 0.2 mm.

Fig. 9-2.

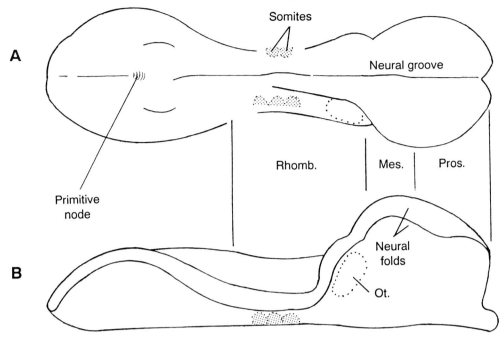

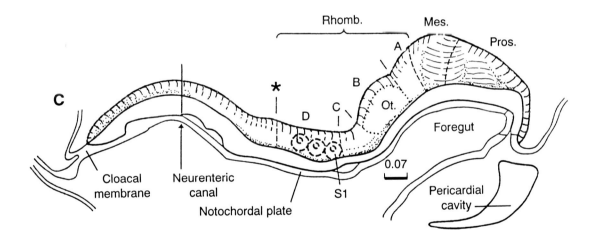

Fig. 9-3.

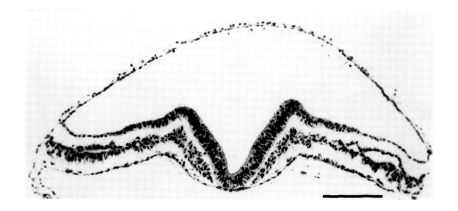

Fig. 9-4. Sections through an embryo (Ludwig's Da 1) of stage 9, a stage that is rarely seen.

Key drawings, a median section and a dorsal view, are the authors' reconstructions. The levels of the sections reproduced are indicated from A to H. The degree of lordosis of human embryos of this stage seems to be less pronounced than in the embryos of some other primates and of rodents.

(**A**) The head fold, including the most rostral part of the neural plate, a little caudal to the prechordal plate and rostral to the cardiac primordium. The foregut is a closed tube at this level. The amniotic cavity is well shown in this and in the subsequent section.

(**B**) The deep neural groove here is at the level of the mesencephalon. The floor plate lies on the broad notochordal plate, which is intercalated into the endoderm. The paired pericardial cavities are clearly visible.

(**C**) Rhombomere B is shown in Figure 9-3 (q.v.) and is not repeated here.

(**D**) Rhombomere D at the level of the caudal part of somite 1. This embryo possessed two somitic pairs.

(**E**) The primitive pit and the umbilical vesicle communicate with each other through the neurenteric canal.

(**F**) The primitive node and the beginning of the primitive groove. Venous channels on each side are the umbilical veins and that on the left side of the embryo (right side of the photograph) is wider, an asymmetry also seen in other embryos of this stage (e.g., CEC 7650).

(**G**) The primitive grove is deeper here. Mesenchyme invaginating from the primitive streak is visible.

(**H**) The caudal eminence (or end-bud) and its proliferating mesenchyme. The caudal portion of the neural tube does not arise by fusion of neural folds but from the cellular mass known as the caudal eminence. The allantoic diverticulum can be seen below in cross section.

Important

The three major divisions of the brain can be distinguished in the completely open neural folds, when no so-called vesicles are present.

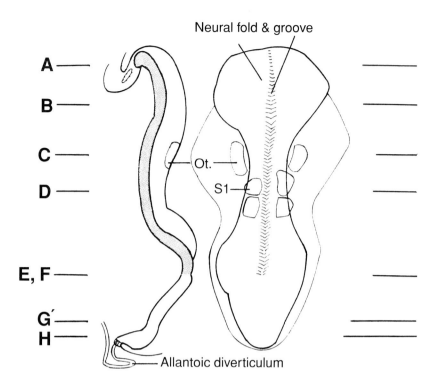

Neural fold & groove

A —

B —

C —

Ot. —

D —

S1—

E, F —

G´—

H —

Allantoic diverticulum

Fig. 9-4.

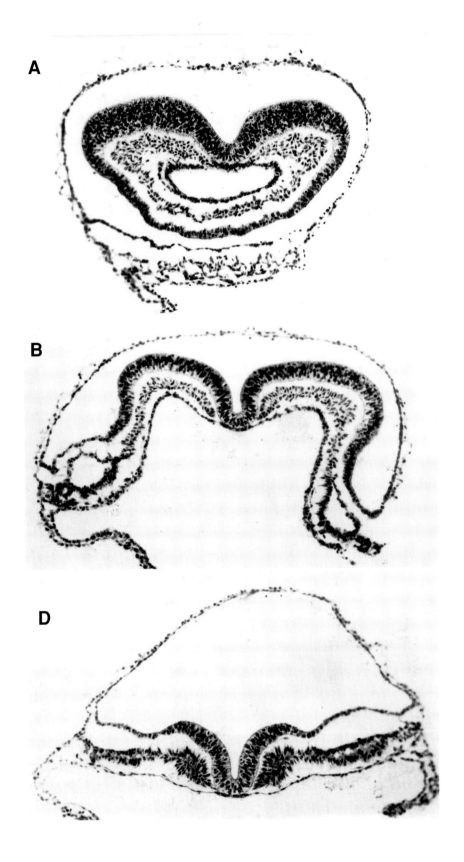

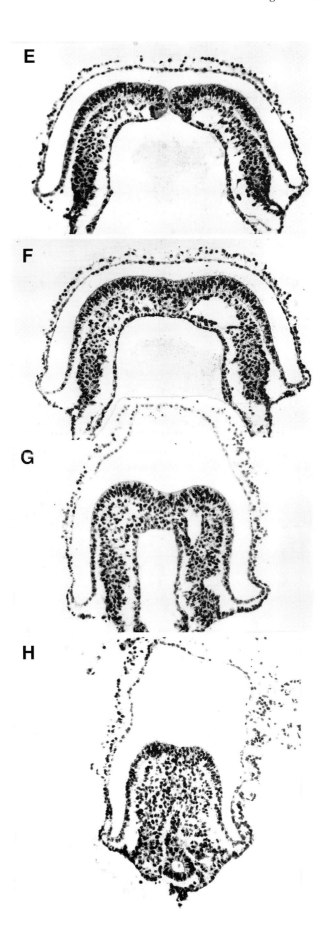

Fig. 9-5. Transverse sections at stages 8 to 11 to show the formation of the neural tube and the notochord. The neural primordium is closely related ventrally to the precursor of the notochord (stages 8–10). Later, when the notochord becomes surrounded by the developing centra of the vertebrae, the latter become and remain an important ventral relation of the spinal cord. A, the future alar plate (dorsal lamina); B, the future basal plate (ventral lamina) of the neural tube. The floor, basal, alar, and roof plates all express different genes. Further details: O'Rahilly and Müller (1993).

Inductional processes between the future notochord and the neural tube would likely be greatest during stages 8 and 9, when the future notochord is present as a plate and hence presents a relatively wide surface. The contact is particularly close at stages 8–10 because, as has been shown in the macaque, a basement membrane is lacking between the two tissues at that time.

56

Fig. 9-5.

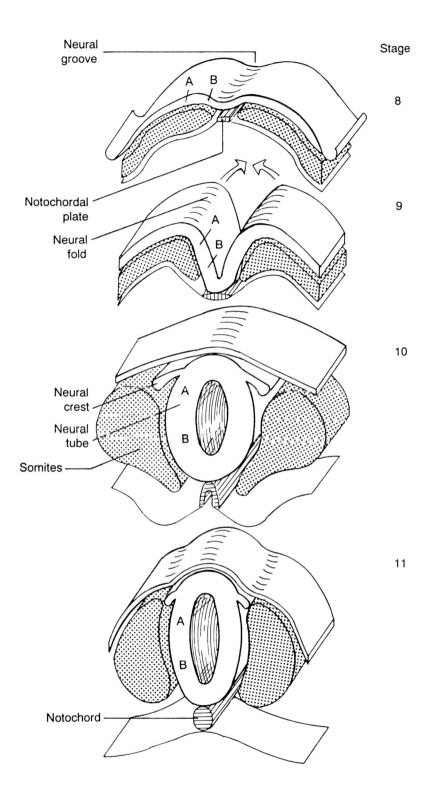

Neural groove

Notochordal plate

Neural fold

Neural crest

Neural tube

Somites

Notochord

Stage

8

9

10

11

Comments on Neuroteratology (Stage 9)

Synophthalmia is a variety of cyclopia *sensu lato* in which some or all of the ocular structures are paired within a single globe. Although the prosencephalon "diverticulates" into two optic primordia, these fail to lateralize. Such a disturbance could arise as early as stage 9, when the future optic area is probably changing from a median to bilateral regions (see Fig. 10-9).

Cerebral Dysraphia. Anencephaly develops in three phases. The first, cerebral dysraphia (encephaloschisis), is believed to arise as a failure of closure of the neural groove rostrally, an idea supported by many authors. Rupture of the already closed neural tube cannot be entirely excluded in some instances. Cerebral dysraphia arises early, probably as a mesenchymal defect, even as early as stages 8 or 9, i.e., before fusion of the neural folds begins, because elevation of the folds depends on the production of sufficient mesenchyme.

Stage 10: The Neural Tube and the Optic Primordium

Approximately 2–3.5 mm in Greatest Length
Approximately 29 Postfertilizational Days

When approximately five somitic pairs are present, the neural folds begin to fuse in the adjacent rhombencephalic and spinal regions, frequently in several places simultaneously. A portion of the neural tube is thereby formed, and mitotic figures are found near its cavity. The caudal part of the future neural tube, however, develops from the caudal eminence and not from the neural plate. The diencephalon consists of the future thalamic region (D2) and an optic portion (D1) in which the optic sulcus appears. The right and left optic primordia, which are visible for the first time at this stage, are connected by the chiasmatic plate (primordium chiasmatis; torus opticus). The lateral parts of the forebrain beyond the chiasmatic plate belong to the telencephalon, which is visible for the first time at this stage. Several regional components of the neural crest can now be distinguished, and the formation of the crest in the head is probably at its greatest. Further details: Müller and O'Rahilly (1985).

Stage 10 is usually listed as 22 days, but may be as much as a week older.

Fig. 10-1. Dorsal and right lateral views of an embryo (CEC 5074) of stage 10. The number of somitic pairs at this stage ranges from 4 to 12; the Corner embryo, shown here, has 10 pairs. An extensive portion of neural tube has already formed, leaving parts of the neural groove exposed.

(**A**) The dorsal view shows the neural folds fused in the adjacent rhombencephalic and spinal regions. Fusion begins in one or both of these regions, usually when approximately 5 somitic pairs are present. The fusion may occur in several different places independently and simultaneously. The neurenteric canal is still present in the least advanced embryos. The caudal eminence (a continuation of the primitive streak) constitutes about one-fifth of the embryonic length. It continues the production of mesenchyme and forms the caudal part of the future neural plate during stage 10.

(**B**) The right lateral view shows the developing pharyngeal arches and the cardiac region, represented here by the pericardial cavity. The surface ectoderm is contributing to the otic plate (dotted outline) and the epipharyngeal area of the future vagal ganglia.

(**C**) Schematic view of the more caudally situated somites and the corresponding vertebrae. The caudal neuropore will close at the level of somitic pair 31 (stippled), which corresponds to sacral vertebra 2.

Fig. 10-2. Graphic reconstruction prepared from transverse sections (CEC 5074) to show a median view. An end-on view is shown on the right. The major divisions of the brain are distinguishable in the largely still-open neural groove. The mesencephalic flexure has decreased (from approximately 150° to 104°) since the previous stage, contributing to a ventral bending of the prosencephalon and the shaping of the future head. The diencephalon comprises two portions: D2, the future thalamic region, and D1, in which the (left) optic sulcus can be seen for the first time. D1 possesses a thick floor that forms the median bridge between the two, laterally placed, optic primordia. This is the chiasmatic plate (primordium chiasmatis) or torus opticus. The optic sulci may extend to the median plane and end in a pit, the "postoptic recess" (Johnston, 1909), which is the caudal boundary of the chiasmatic plate. The lateral parts of the forebrain extend further rostrally than the chiasmatic plate. This is the telencephalon, evident for the first time at this stage in embryos of 7–12 somitic pairs. At this stage the notochordal plate extends rostrally to the oropharyngeal membrane (Müller and O'Rahilly, 1985), so that induction of the floor plate is possible as far rostrally as neuromere D2. This is the future epinotochordal part of the brain. Neuromere D1, which is induced by the prechordal plate (Fig. 10-6), is prenotochordal in position. *Pax 3* is expressed in the neural groove and in the closed part of the neural tube at stage 10 (and at stage 15 in the brain stem and spinal cord) in the human embryo (Gérard et al., 1995). *Pax 6* is important for the development of the eye.

Fig. 10-1.

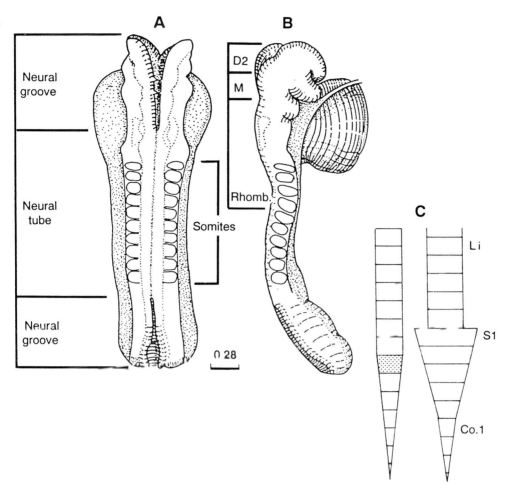

Fig. 10-2.

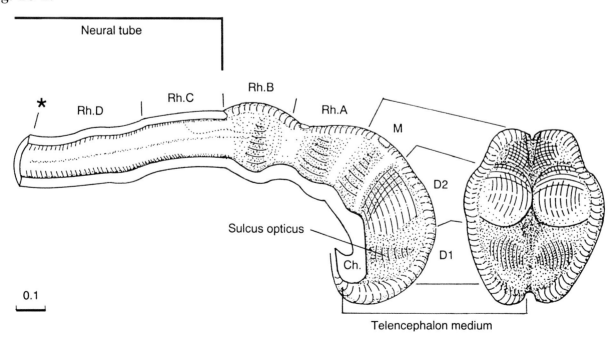

Fig. 10-3. The neuromeres of the human embryo. Neuromeres are morphologically identifiable transverse subdivisions perpendicular to the longitudinal axis of the embryonic brain and extending onto both sides of the body.

(**A**) Primary neuromeres are six larger divisions that appear early (stage 9) in the open neural folds: prosencephalon (P), mesencephalon (M), and rhombomeres A, B, C, and D.

(**B**) Secondary neuromeres are smaller subdivisions that are found both before (stages 10 and 11) and after (stages 12–14) closure of the neural tube.

(**C**) In all, 16 secondary neuromeres develop: telencephalon medium (T), diencephalon 1 (D1), rostral parencephalon, caudal parencephalon, synencephalon, mesencephalon 1 (M1), mesencephalon 2 (M2), isthmus rhombencephali, and rhombomeres 1 to 8. These are detectable at stages 14 to 17. A longitudinal organization begins to be superimposed on the neuromeres at stage 15, and five longitudinal zones can be discerned in the diencephalon (Table 18-1). Although in some instances territories of gene expression follow the morphological neuromeres, in others they may cross interneuromeric boundaries. Further details: Müller and O'Rahilly (1997b).

Important

The telencephalon medium can be distinguished from the diencephalon at this stage, i.e., much earlier than commonly stated.

Fig. 10-3.

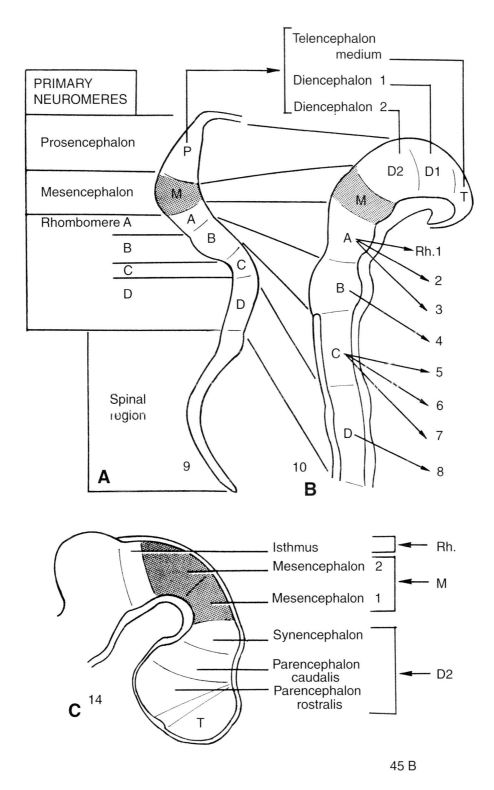

PRIMARY
NEUROMERES

Prosencephalon

Mesencephalon

Rhombomere A
    B
    C
    D

Spinal
region

Telencephalon
medium

Diencephalon 1

Diencephalon 2

Isthmus
Mesencephalon 2
Mesencephalon 1
Synencephalon
Parencephalon
caudalis
Parencephalon
rostralis

Rh.
M
D2

45 B

Fig. 10-4. The early development of neural crest in relation to the formation of the neural tube in an excellent embryo (CEC 5074) of stage 10. The left-hand column shows the levels (shaded by horizontal lines) of the neural tube. In the right lateral view the neural crest is indicated by stippling, and further detail is provided in the transverse sections at the right. At rostral levels (**A**), crest material is formed before closure of the neural groove occurs, whereas at levels **B** to **E**, closure of the neural folds takes place before migration of crest material. The thick interrupted line indicates the junction of cerebral and spinal parts of the CNS. Formation of the neural crest in the head is now probably at its peak. In addition to contributing to ganglia of cranial nerves, the cells migrate into the general mesenchyme, thereby contributing ectomesenchyme to the skull and the face. The crest cells leave the neural plate at areas where the basement membrane is interrupted. After closure of the neural groove (**B, C**), neural crest still seems to be derived from the neural ectoderm. The probable succession of appearance of the components of the neural crest is: facial, mesencephalic, trigeminal, vagal, occipital, glossopharyngeal, and spinal. In C, D, and E, bilateral dorsolateral hinge-points have given the lumen a diamond shape. Pharyngeal arch 1 contains a mixture of neural crest cells from the midbrain and from rhombomere 2. From Müller and O'Rahilly (1985).

Figures 10-5 to 10-8 are transverse sections (CEC 5074), the planes of which are shown in the key above Figure 10-7. The bars represent 0.15 mm.

Fig. 10-4.

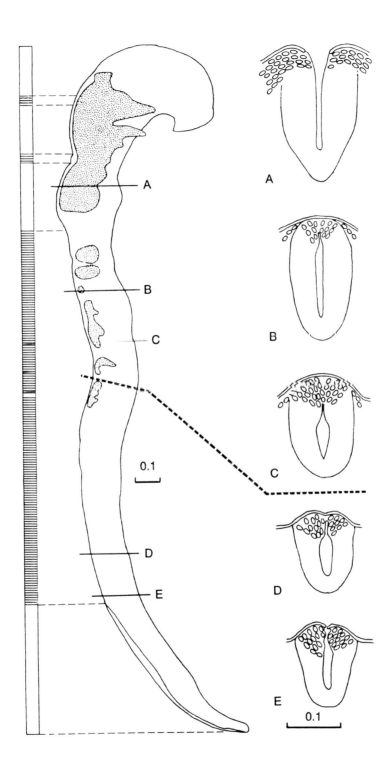

Fig. 10-5. In the upper part of the photomicrograph, the mesencephalic neural crest can be seen migrating on each side from the neural ectoderm. The sites of neural crest emigration show discontinuity of the basement membrane. The optic sulcus is indicated by an arrow.

Fig. 10-6. Neural crest is visible above as it emerges from rhombomere 1. The median plane is occupied by the floor of the neural groove. The prechordal plate shows as a small dark projection on each side of the lower portion of the photomicrograph above the chiasmatic plate. The very large bilateral blood vessels on each side of the neural plate are the first aortic arches, which arise from the paired dorsal aortae, visible in Figures 10-7 and 10-8.

Fig. 10-5.

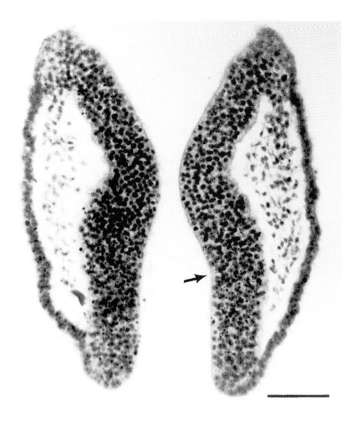

Fig. 10-6.

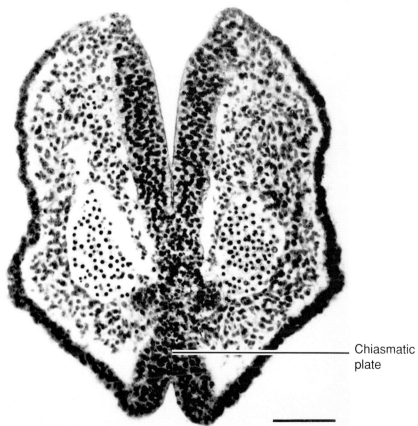

Chiasmatic plate

Fig. 10-7. The neural groove of rhombomere 2. Ventral to it, the notochordal plate is visible and, on each side, a dorsal aorta. Transverse anastomoses between the right and left dorsal aortae have been recorded at stage 11, and fusion has definitely begun at stages 13 and 14.

Fig. 10-8. The neural tube of rhombomere 5. Mitotic figures are visible near the cavity of the tube. The otic plates appear on each side as ectodermal thickenings. Extramural blood vessels are forming ventrally and laterally, adjacent to the wall of the brain, but they do not yet give off intramural branches. A histological distinction between the perineural arteries and veins becomes apparent by stage 20 and for the intramural vessels during trimester 2.

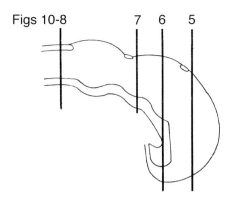

Fig. 10-7.

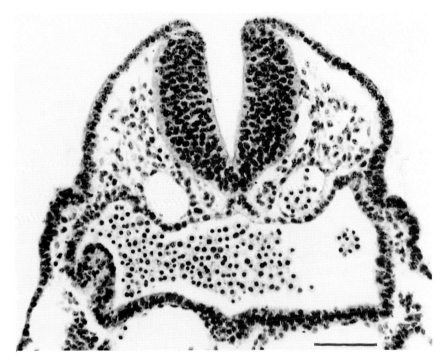

Fig. 10-8.

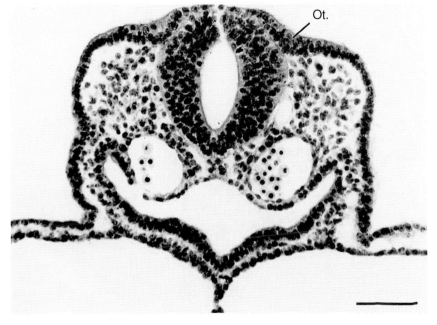

Fig. 10-9. Early development of the optic primordia and the floor plate.

(**A**) Dorsal view of the embryonic disc at stage 8 and a projection of the prechordal plate, which occupies about 15–20% of the width and 12% of the length of the embryonic disc. It is maintained that a single optic primordium (retinal field) exists at the rostral end of the neural plate (the future neuromere D1).

(**B**) Subsequently (although probably still in stage 8), the prechordal plate is believed to be responsible for suppressing the median part, so that bilateral optic primordia are formed. Lack of inhibition of the median component would lead to cyclopia.

(**C**) Dorsal view of an embryo of stage 10 (such as CEC 5074) in which the optic primordia occupy neuromere D1.

(**D**) Median view at stage 10 showing neuromere D2, distinguishable from its relationship to the neurophyophysial (N-H) and adenohypophysial (A-H) primordia. The notochordal plate extends as far rostrally as the caudal boundary of N-H and it induces the floor plate in the overlying neural ectoderm. The prenotochordal part of the brain comprises neuromeres T, D1, and the rostral portion of D2.

Bars: 0.2 mm.

Fig. 10-9.

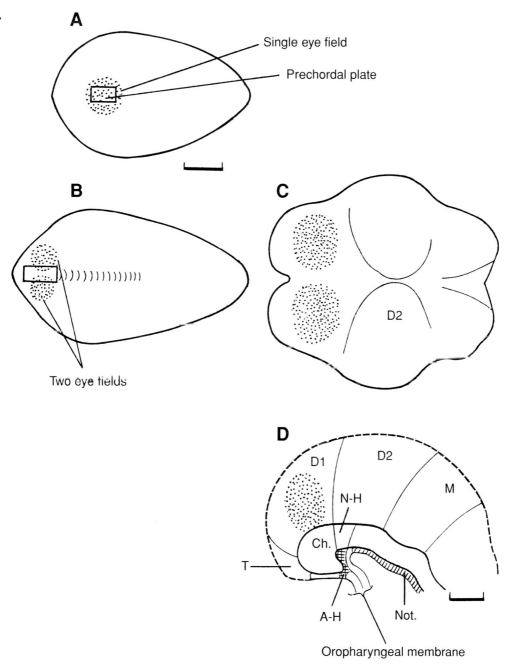

A

Single eye field

Prechordal plate

B

Two eye fields

C

D2

D

D1

D2

M

N-H

Ch.

T

A-H

Not.

Oropharyngeal membrane

Comments on Neuroteratology (Stage 10)

Cerebral dysraphia, the preliminary phase of anencephaly, may arise (at stages 8 and 9) even before fusion of the neural folds begins. The fusion commences during stage 10, and that stage is also relevant, because production of neural crest is then only starting. The ganglia of the cranial nerves, derived largely from neural crest, are only minimally affected in anencephaly. A reduction in the size of the ganglia, however, as well as an incomplete chondrocranium, would point to defective distribution of the cephalic mesenchyme, caused probably by a derangement of the mesencephalic neural crest in stages 10 and 11. Moreover, stage 10 is characterized by the first appearance of the optic primordium, and, rarely, anencephaly may be combined with anophthalmia. Usually, however, the eyes are very well developed in anencephaly, indicating that development of the diencephalon at first proceeds normally, although later it degenerates.

Holoprosencephaly may arise as early as stage 8. Stage 10 is also of interest, however, because production of the neural crest is then beginning. The ganglia of the cranial nerves derived from rhombencephalic neural crest are smaller in holoprosencephaly.

Holoprosencephaly is commonly graded into **alobar** (a holotelencephalon that lacks division into hemispheres; it can be detected ultrasonically by the demonstration of a single ventricle), **semilobar** (incomplete cerebral hemispheres), and **lobar** (well-formed cerebral hemispheres and longitudinal fissure). Further details: Siebert et al. (1990).

Encephalo(meningo)cele may arise, at least in some instances, from a failure in separation of the brain from the surface ectoderm in later stages. This failure in separation would be caused by a disturbance of the mesencephalic neural crest, which is at the height of its formation at stage 10. This mesenchyme is believed to be the main source for the development of the face, and insufficient production of it may lead to a narrow facies, as seen in the fetal alcohol syndrome.

Stage 11: Closure of the Rostral Neuropore

Approximately 2.5–4.5 mm in Greatest Length
Approximately 30 Postfertilizational Days

The rostral, or cephalic, neuropore closes during stage 11. The closure, in which the neural ectoderm also participates, is basically bidirectional; i.e., it proceeds from the region of D2 (its "dorsal lip") and simultaneously from the telencephalon (its "terminal lip"). Also during this stage, the floor of the telencephalon medium becomes distinct as the future lamina terminalis and commissural plate. The optic vesicle is being formed from the optic sulcus in D1, and is providing optic neural crest. Both adenohypophysial and neurohypophysial primordia can be distinguished, and they are in contact from the beginning of their development; the hypophysis develops as a single organ. Notochordal and neural axial structures are still closely related. Further details: Müller and O'Rahilly (1986a).

Fig. 11-1. Right lateral view of an embryo (CEC 6784) of stage 11 with the brain superimposed (interrupted line), and showing the rostral and caudal neuropores. The number of somitic pairs was 17; the range in number at this stage is 13–20. The umbilical vesicle and the body stalk have been sectioned at the right.

Fig. 11-2. Right lateral view of the brain (CEC 2053). The features shown are the optic vesicle, the trigeminal and facio-vestibulocochlear ganglia, the otic vesicle, the glossopharyngeal and vagal ganglia, and the hypoglossal crest, which will form the connective tissue of the tongue. Cells given off from the wall of the developing otic vesicle appear to be neural crest cells that form a ventral sheath; these latter will contribute perhaps more to the otic capsule than to the facio-vestibulocochlear ganglia. Trigeminal and otic arteries are present and later (stages 13–15) form parts of the caroticobasilar anastomosis (Fig. 19-17).

Fig. 11-3. Graphic reconstruction prepared from transverse sections showing a median view of the brain (CEC 7702). The asterisk indicates the junction with the spinal cord. The rostral, or cephalic, neuropore is indicated by a thick line between two arrowheads. Each of the two neuropores, rostral and caudal, measures about 0.5 mm in length (mean of 24 embryos). The rostral neuropore closes within a few hours during stage 11, when about 20 somitic pairs are present. (The embryo illustrated here has 17.) The thin surface ectoderm overlying the dorsal aspect of the neural tube has not been included in the drawing.

D1 still consists mostly of optic primordium. The chiasmatic plate is first at the rostral end of the neural plate (CEC 318; 13 pairs of somites), as in stage 10. When 14 or more somitic pairs have appeared, however, fusion at the "terminal" lip (Fig. 11-6A) of the neuropore results in the formation of a floor for the telencephalon medium. This represents the future lamina terminalis and commissural plate.

In D2, the neural floor adjacent to the adenohypophysial primordium is the neurohypophysial region. Both components of the hypophysis cerebri develop in contact with each other, so that no migration or growth of one to meet the other occurs. The level of the adenohypophysial primordium is caudal to that of the chiasmatic plate, and its site is clearly defined by the oropharyngeal membrane, which has not yet ruptured (in 11 out of 16 embryos).

The percentage of length occupied by the mesencephalon in relation to that of the whole brain remains almost constant from stage 9 up to and including stage 11. The rhombencephalon takes up approximately three-quarters of the brain in length. The relative increase in prosencephalic length is slightly less than in stage 10. Cranial ganglia and neural crest are projected onto the median view. Eight rhombomeres (1–7 and D) are distinguishable.

The notochord or the notochordal plate is still closely related to the neural tube or the plate, so that it is possible that induction could continue along almost the whole length of the neural axis.

Fig. 11-1.

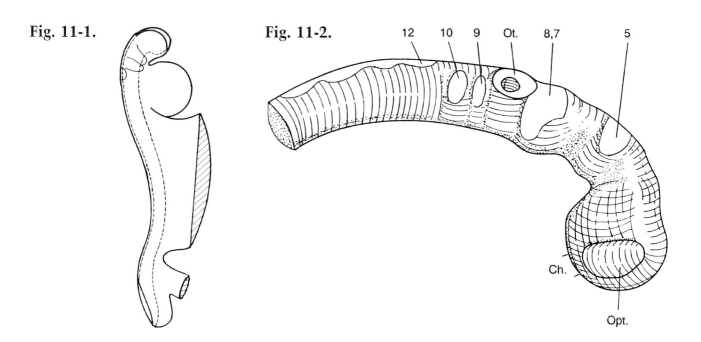

Fig. 11-2.

12   10   9   Ot.   8,7   5

Ch.

Opt.

Fig. 11-3.

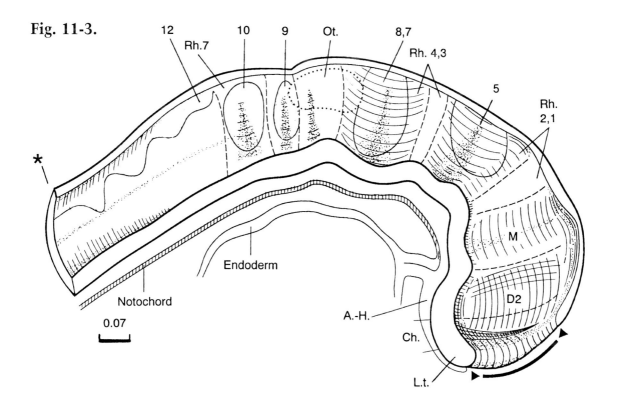

12   10   9   Ot.   8,7
Rh.7   Rh. 4,3
                                              5
                                                  Rh.
                                                  2,1

*

M

D2

Endoderm

A.-H.

Notochord   Ch.

0.07

L.t.

75

Fig. 11-4. Drawings of the rostral end of the neural tube in seven embryos of stage 11, to show the progressive closure of the rostral neuropore. Under each is shown a horizontal section taken at the level indicated by the horizontal lines. The embryos shown had 13, 14, 16, 17, 17, 17, and 20 somitic pairs, respectively. Modified from Streeter, as reproduced by O'Rahilly and Müller (1987a). The rostral neuropore, which is still open when 19 pairs of somites are present, is closed when 20 pairs have formed (O'Rahilly and Gardner, 1979, Table 2). See also Figure 12-11.

The rostral neuropore is not considered to be the "front" end (*das wahre ursprüngliche Ende*) of the neural tube, which is frequently taken to be the infundibulum or the infundibular recess (Dart, 1924, in agreement with von Baer). There is much to be said, however, for Johnston's (1909) view that "in all vertebrates the anterior end of the head is the point at which the brain plate meets the general ectoderm at the same time that it comes into contact with the anterior end of the entoderm. This point is marked in the adult by the optic chiasma."

Abbreviations: A-V, atrioventricular canal; C-T, conotruncus; LV, left ventricle; RA, right atrium; RV, right ventricle; SV, sinus venosus.

Precision
The neuropores are rostral (or cranial) and caudal, not anterior and posterior, which have specialized meanings in human anatomy. There is at present no embryological evidence in the human that a specific pattern of multiple sites of closure of the neural tube exists, such as has been described in the mouse.

Fig. 11-4.

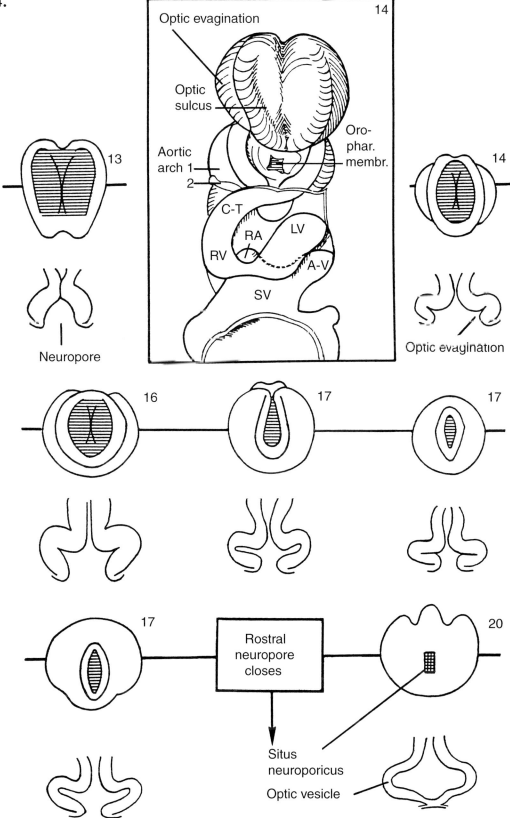

Fig. 11-5. Drawings and photomicrographs to illustrate the closure of the rostral neuropore in an embryo of stage 11 (CEC 6784). Basically, the neuropore closes bidirectionally, i.e., from its "dorsal lip" (near D2) and simultaneously from its "terminal lip" (in the telencephalon, adjacent to the chiasmatic plate). The surface ectoderm (unshaded) participates in the closure at the terminal lip, and the area of fusion of the neural folds lies between the two nasal discs. The right and left components of the neural ectoderm and those of the surface ectoderm seem to fuse simultaneously across the median plane. The bar represents 0.02 mm. A key drawing showing the lips and the plane of sections A and H is provided in Figure 11-6A. From O'Rahilly and Müller (1989a).

The phenomenon of closure at the "terminal lip" is ignored in most publications on embryology. In the chick embryo, near the time of fusion of the neural folds, occlusion of the lumen of the neural tube occurs and has been considered to be necessary for the growth of the brain. In the human embryo, however, occlusion is infrequent during stage 11 and has been found only when the rostral neuropore is still open (Müller and O'Rahilly, 1986a, thereby precluding any hydrodynamic function. Moreover, growth of the brain is practically at a standstill during stages 11 and 12 (Müller and O'Rahilly, 1987, Table 3).

Fig. 11-5.

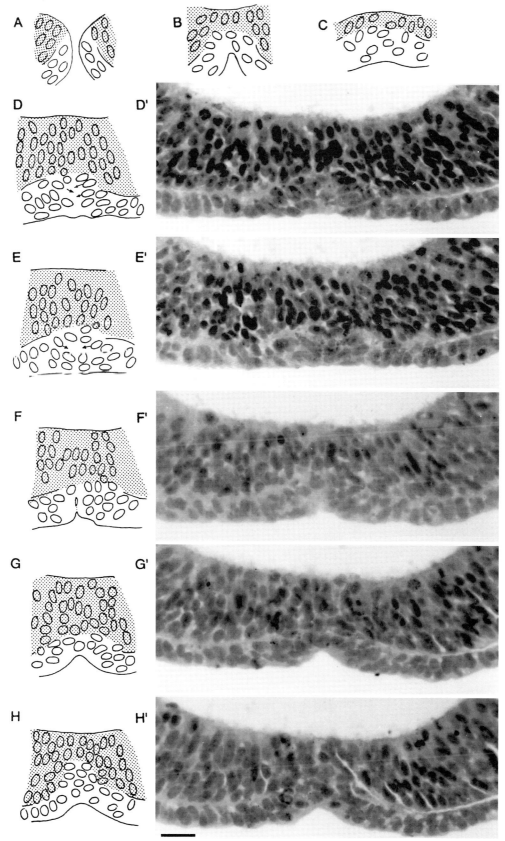

Fig. 11-6. Views of the rostral neuropore and the beginning optic vesicles at stage 11.

(**A**) End-on and median views as a key to Figure 11-5. Tel. indicates the surface ectoderm overlying the telencephalon. In the median view, the thin surface ectoderm overlying the dorsal lip has not been included in the drawing. The two horizontal lines show the plane of sections A and H.

(**B**) End-on and right lateral views as a key to the plane of section of the photomicrograph, C.

(**C**) A section through the optic vesicles (CEC 7611). The optic vesicle is being formed by further deepening of the optic sulcus in D1. Optic neural crest is developing from the external layer of the optic vesicle and is met by migrating mesencephalic neural crest. The two form the sheath of the optic vesicle, i.e., of the future optic cup. The basement membrane is interrupted where the cells of the optic crest leave the neural ectoderm. Optic neural crest is formed by mitotic division in the superficial cells of the optic vesicle, an exception to the general rule that mitosis in the neural tube occurs adjacent to the ventricle. The rostral neuropore is visible at the bottom of the photomicrograph. Bar: 0.15 mm.

Fig. 11-6.

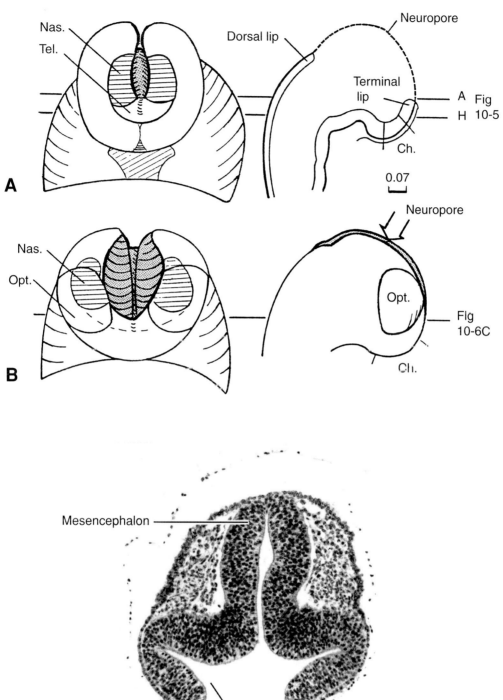

Fig. 11-7. Development of the notochord and the floor plate.

(**A**) After the notochord has developed from the dorsal part of the notochordal process of stages 7 and 8, its cross-sectional shape changes. It appears as the notochordal plate in stage 9 (Figs. 9-5B and 11-7A,b) and has the form of an inverted U in stage 10 (Figs. 10-7 and 11-7A,c,d, and 11-7B). Next it appears as a rod in stage 12 (Fig. 11-7A,e). A correlation seems to be present between large contact zones and newly formed neural tissue, probably facilitating the occurrence and efficiency of induction of the floor plate.

(**B**) The notochord in this embryo (CEC 7611) of stage 11 with 16 pairs of somites still has the form of an inverted U at the level of rhombomere 5. Bar: 0.05 mm.

Fig. 11-7.

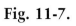

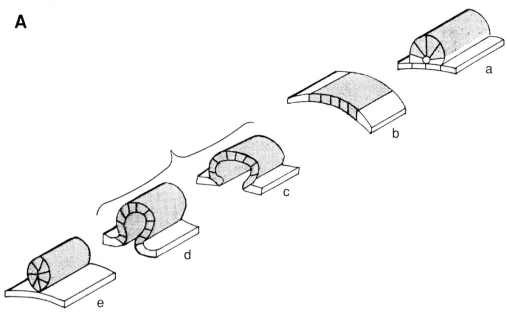

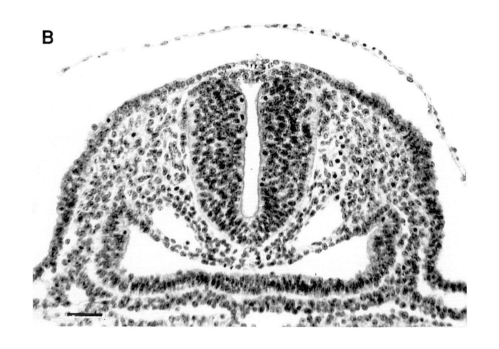

Fig. 11-7, continued   (C) The caudal part of the notochord, caudal to the site of the former neurenteric canal, which is formed from the caudal eminence, in an embryo (CEC 8116) with 17 pairs of somites. Here the neural groove is still open. Bar: 0.04 mm.

Fig. 11-7C.

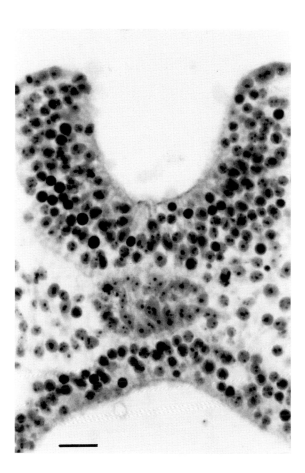

Comments on Neuroteratology (Stage 11)

Cerebral dysraphia, the first phase of anencephaly, probably arises early (stages 8–10). It would be extremely difficult to detect a pure cerebral dysraphia at stage 11, however, because it is only during that stage that the rostral neuropore normally closes. Nevertheless, an example of complete cerebrospinal dysraphia at stage 11, presumably the forerunner of craniorhachischisis totalis, has been described in detail (Dekaban, 1963; Dekaban and Bartelmez, 1964).

Arhinencephaly. This term *sensu stricto* refers to absence of the olfactory bulbs and tracts, irrespective of associations with other developmental malformations, such as holoprosencephaly, which is commonly combined with arhinencephaly. Isolated arhinencephaly would be expected to arise at the time when the nasal discs should begin to form: thickenings normally appear at stage 11, and a nasal field is outlined at stage 12 (Bossy, 1980). This timing, however, depends on the unproven assumption that the olfactory bulb is induced by the olfactory nerve. Holoprosencephaly and arhinencephaly may develop independently of synophthalmia, probably at about stage 11, or perhaps even 10. Although they are commonly linked, holoprosencephaly and arhinencephaly can also arise independently of each other. Siebert et al. (1990) studied 103 cases of this condition and found that arhinencephaly is extremely heterogeneous both clinically and pathologically.

Encephalocele. It has been speculated (by Hoving, 1993) that insufficient cell death (apoptosis) at the terminal lip of the rostral neuropore (e.g., from retinoic acid deficiency) might result (immediately after fusion of the neural folds) in persistent attachment of the surface ectoderm to the neural ectoderm, producing a subsequent cranial defect and a fronto-ethmoidal encephalocele. An interesting example of a telencephalic diverticulum in a 35 mm fetus has been recorded (Bossy, 1966). It was situated in the region of the former situs neuroporicus and was considered to represent cerebral dysraphia with secondary encephalocele. Usually, however, encephaloceles are, in the Western Hemisphere, much more frequently in the occipital region.

Nasal Glioma. Insufficient cell death in the region of the rostral neuropore causes a persistent "surplus of unintended surviving cells" that "might be represented by heterotopias like nasal gliomas" (Hoving, 1993).

Myelomeningocele. This serious defect of the neural tube appears probably at stage 10 or stage 11 when the cervical or thoracic region is involved. Lumbosacral myeloschisis, believed by many to be a precursor of myelomeningocele, begins also during primary neurulation (stages 8–12), although it is not a simple failure of neural closure.

CHAPTER 12

Stage 12: Closure of the Caudal Neuropore and the Beginning of Secondary Neurulation

---

Approximately 3–5 mm in Greatest Length
Approximately 31 Postfertilizational Days

The rostral neuropore is closed, although the situs neuroporicus can frequently be detected and is probably at the future commissural plate in the middle of the embryonic lamina terminalis. The closure (during stage 11) allows the formation of the telencephalon medium to occur. The mesencephalon consists of two neuromeres (M1 and M2), and the mesencephalic flexure is a right angle. The rhombomeres have important relationships to the cranial ganglia: Rh.5 is associated with the otic vesicle, and Rh.D is level with the four occipital somites. The first nerve fibers are differentiating, particularly those of the future lateral and ventral longitudinal fasciculi. The hypoglossal nucleus has appeared and four to five intramural hypoglossal roots are present. The caudal neuropore closes during stage 12, and its final site is at the level of somitic pair 31 (future vertebral level S2). Further details: Müller and O'Rahilly (1987).

Fig. 12-1. Right lateral view of an embryo (CEC 5923) of stage 12 with the brain superimposed. The number of somitic pairs was 28; the range in number at this stage is 21–29.

Fig. 12-2. Right lateral view of the brain (CEC 6097). The features shown are the optic vesicle, the trigeminal and facio-vestibulocochlear ganglia, the otic vesicle, and the glossopharyngeal and vagal–accessory ganglia. The brain now occupies about 40% of the length of the neural tube.

Mesenchyme and ectomesenchyme have various sources. Mesenchyme is penetrating laterally and dorsally between the surface and the brain; medially, however, areas of the forebrain are still in direct contact with the surface ectoderm (Figs. 12-4 and 12-6). Expansion of the brain stretches the surface ectoderm (O'Rahilly and Müller, 1985) so that entrance of mesenchymal cells may be hindered. The prechordal mesenchyme is caudal to the optic vesicles, where the orbital muscles will develop. The optic neural crest (Fig. 12-4) is now at the height of its development. The neural crest contributes to the facio-vestibulocochlear ganglia. Crest cells from the region of ganglia 9–11 migrate, by way of pharyngeal arch 3, towards the aortic sac. Moreover, the surface (epipharyngeal) ectoderm gives rise to cells that may contribute to the inferior glossopharyngeal and vagal ganglia. The hypoglossal cord is forming from the occipital somites and, in the more advanced embryos of this stage, it begins to enter pharyngeal arch 4.

Fig. 12-3. Reconstruction of the brain (CEC 7852). The asterisk indicates the junction with the spinal cord. The rostral neuropore has closed. The site of final closure (the situs neuroporicus) is probably at the future commissural plate in the middle of the embryonic lamina terminalis.

The initial formation of the telencephalon medium normally depends on the closure of the rostral neuropore during stage 11. The prosencephalon now consists of three parts: the telencephalon, D1, and D2. The telencephalon medium, which is rostral to the well-defined neuromere D1, is recognizable externally by its situation between the nasal discs (Fig. 12-6). D1 is still characterized mainly by the optic vesicles. The semilunar opening of the optic ventricle into the third ventricle is indicated by shading. D2 is related to the adenohypophysial primordium and now shows the first sign of the mamillary recess.

The mesencephalon consists of two neuromeres: M1 and M2. The mesencephalic flexure is a right angle between the forebrain and the hindbrain. The sulcus limitans is seen to traverse the midbrain.

The various rhombomeres have distinctive features. For example, the floor is expanded at the level of Rh.2, 4, and 6. Rh.5 is related to the otic vesicle, and the ganglia of the future cranial nerves (which are projected onto the median view) are important relationships of Rh.2, 4, 6, and 7. Rh.D is at the level of somites 1–4. The first nerve fibers are now differentiating. Apart from short fibers in ganglia 5 and 7/8, the fibers are mostly related to cells that will form the nucleus of the lateral longitudinal fasciculus. Moreover, fibers of the future ventral longitudinal fasciculus are discernible in Rh.7. Four intramural hypoglossal roots are present; i.e., the hypoglossal nucleus has developed and some hypoglossal neural crest is still present dorsally. In addition, fine cellular strands of crest pro-

Fig. 12-1.

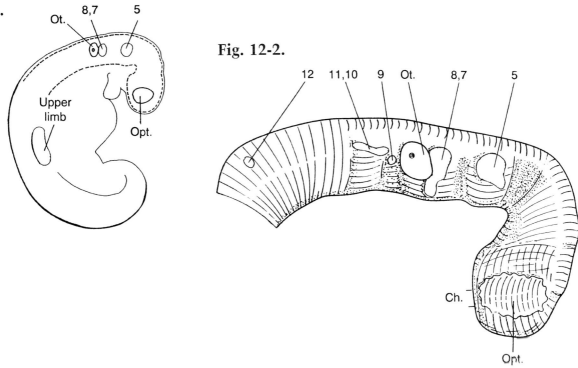

Fig. 12-2.

Fig. 12-3.

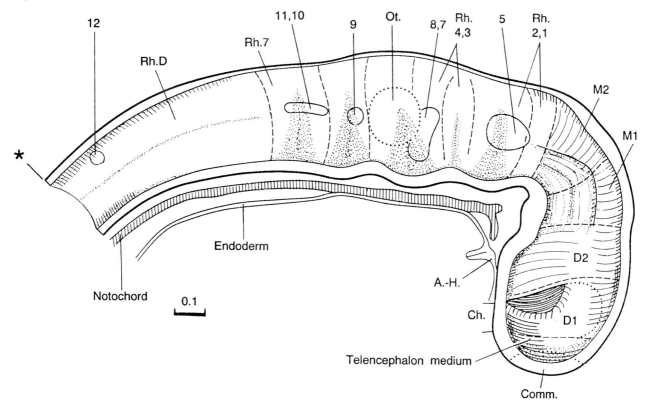

ceed towards the somites. The relative length of the rhombencephalon has been decreasing since stage 9.

Mesenchyme develops basally between the brain and the notochord. Sclerotomic material from the occipital somites is wedged between the rhombencephalon and the myotomes, and these sclerotomic cells will later participate in the formation of the basioccipital and exoccipital parts of the skull.

Precision

A double m is not used in mamillary because the term is derived from the Latin *mamilla,* which in turn is a diminutive of *mamma,* which does have a double m.

Figures 12-4 to 12-7. In contrast with the previous stages, it has now been found that the figures become more comprehensible if the orientation is changed so that the rostral end of the sections appears above in the reproductions. The levels of the sections are shown in a key drawing adjacent to Figure 12-7. The bars represent 0.1 mm.

Fig. 12-4. Optic vesicles and D1 in a horizontal section (CEC 6097). A mesenchymal sheath separates the optic vesicles from the surface ectoderm. Optic neural crest is evident and gives the optic vesicle the appearance of a "frightened hedgehog" (Bartelmez) externally (Fig. 12-2). Little or no mesenchyme is present between the dorsal part of D1 and the surface ectoderm. From Müller and O'Rahilly (1987).

Fig. 12-5. Rhombencephalon (CEC 6097). Several cranial ganglia and the otic pits are visible. The surface ectoderm covering the ventral part of pharyngeal arch 1 (arches 2 and 3 are also visible here) is thicker and gives off cells that join the trigeminal ganglion. The ectoderm is a part of the ectodermal ring (O'Rahilly and Müller, 1985).

Fig. 12-4.

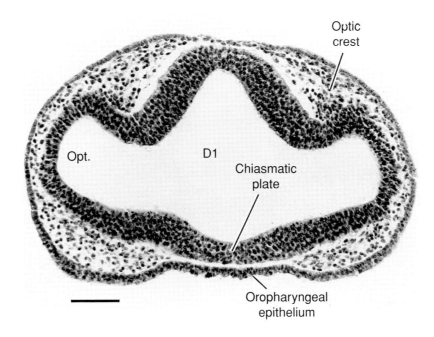

Optic crest

Opt.

D1

Chiasmatic plate

Oropharyngeal epithelium

Fig. 12-5.

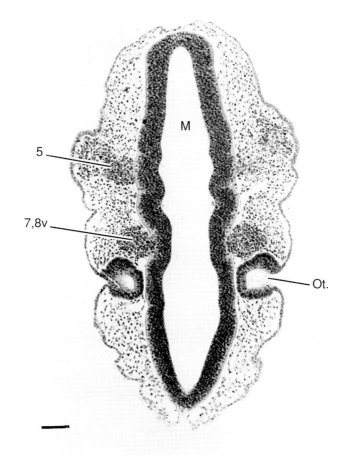

M

5

7,8v

Ot.

Fig. 12-6. Optic vesicles and D1 in a horizontal section of another embryo (CEC 8943). Optic neural crest is evident. At this time the diencephalon consists of two neuromeres: D1, related to the optic vesicle, and D2, related to the adenohypophysis. The site of the closed rostral neuropore is conspicuous. From Müller and O'Rahilly (1987).

Sternberg (1927), who placed the rostral neuropore in the region of, and probably dorsal to, the commissural plate, ventured to identify the situs neuroporicus even up to the end of the embryonic period, at which time he showed it between the eyes and at the root of the nose.

Fig. 12-7. Rhombencephalon of still another embryo (CEC 7852). Several cranial ganglia and the otic vesicles are visible. The uppermost part of the photomicrograph depicts the mesencephalon and is followed by rhombomeres, which are clearly delimited by evaginations. The trigeminal ganglion is related to Rh.2, the facial to Rh.4, the glossopharyngeal to Rh.6, and the vagal and accessory to Rh.7. The part of the brain that is related to the four occipital somites is Rh.D. Bars: 0.1 mm.

The key drawing shows the plane of section of Figures 12-4 to 12-7.

Fig. 12-6.

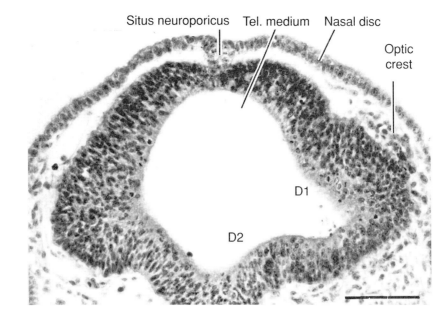

Situs neuroporicus   Tel. medium   Nasal disc   Optic crest

D1

D2

Fig. 12-7.

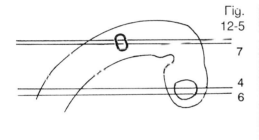

Fig. 12-5

7

4
6

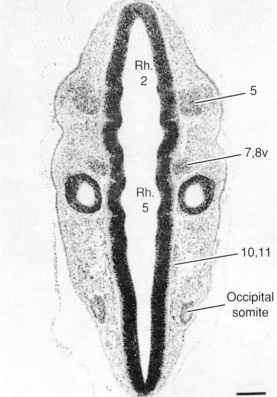

Rh. 2

5

7,8v

Rh. 5

10,11

Occipital somite

Fig. 12-8. The optic vesicles and the optic neural crest.

(**A**) In an embryo (CEC 7611) of stage 11, when the rostral neuropore is still open (arrow), as shown also in Figure 11-6C. The neuropore is covered by amnion, and the ependymal fluid within the future ventricular system is continuous with the amniotic fluid. Mesenchyme is not yet visible between the optic vesicle and the surface ectoderm. Some cells of the optic crest are emerging caudally, but are seen better in B. The vesicle is limited by the caudal limiting sulcus (O'Rahilly, 1966), beyond which blood vessels can be seen. ×214.

(**B**) In an embryo (CEC 8943) of stage 12, when the rostral neuropore has already closed. The striking feature of the optic vesicle here is the emergence from its wall of cells of the optic neural crest. ×450.

Fig. 12-8.

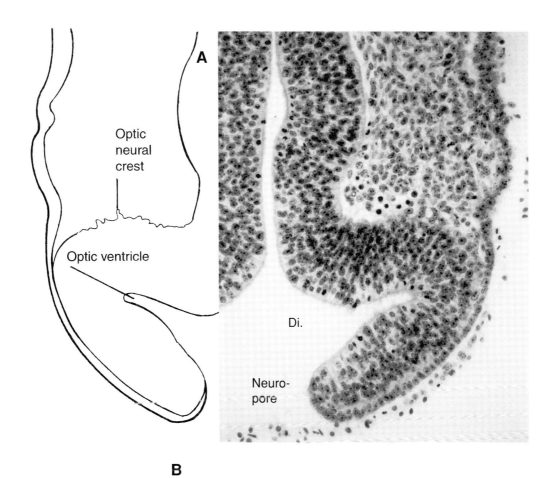

Optic
neural
crest

Optic ventricle

A

Di.

Neuro-
pore

B

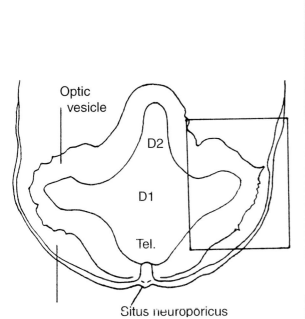

Optic
vesicle

D2

D1

Tel.

Situs neuroporicus

Mesenchymal sheath

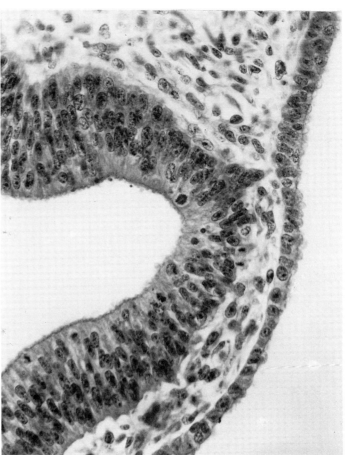

95

Fig. 12-9. Development of the ganglia of cranial nerves. Neural crest gives rise to the main, proximal portions of the ganglia of nerves 5, 7, 9, and 10, whereas epipharyngeal discs (incorporated in the ectodermal ring) contribute to the distal portions. Shown here are examples from an embryo (CEC 8943) of 22/23 pairs of somites.

(**A**) Transverse section through rhombomere 7 and the pharynx, showing the superior vagal ganglion (10s), which arises from neural crest, and the inferior ganglion (10i), which is arising from the epipharyngeal disc (asterisk) of pharyngeal arch 3. Bar: 0.15 mm.

(**B**) A more rostral section, through a part of the otic vesicle (Ot.), showing the geniculate (or facial) ganglion, which arises from both neural crest and the epipharyngeal disc (asterisk) of pharyngeal arch 2. Bar: 0.2 mm.

Abbreviations: Ao., dorsal aorta 5, 7/8, 9/10, cranial ganglia; 10s, superior vagal ganglion.

Fig. 12-9.

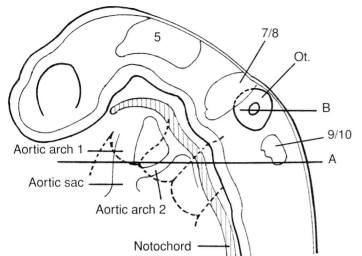

5

7/8

Ot.

B

9/10

A

Aortic arch 1

Aortic sac

Aortic arch 2

Notochord

A

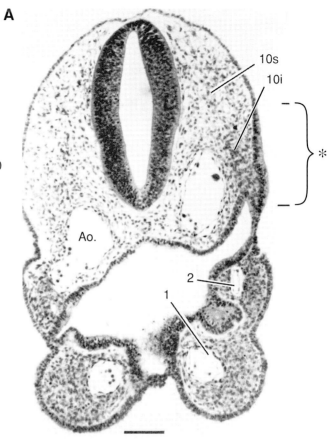

10s

10i

∗

Ao.

2

1

B

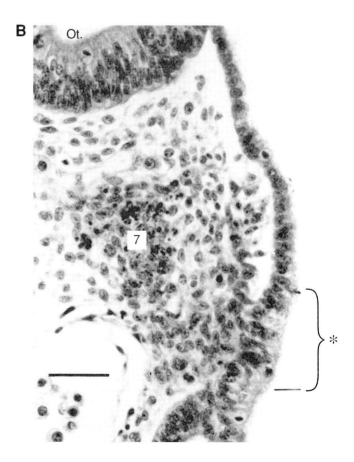

Ot.

7

∗

Fig. 12-10. The early blood vessels of the head.

(**A**) The vascular system (simplified) at stage 11 in an embryo with 14 paired somites (CEC 4529). The movement of the blood here would be merely ebb and flow. The still open brain would not yet be dependent on a blood supply. The capital venous plexuses are forming. Bar: 0.15 mm. Based on Streeter in O'Rahilly and Müller (1987a) and on Padget (1957).

(**B**) The vascular system (simplified) at stage 12 in an embryo with 28 paired somites (CEC 5923). The surface of the brain and the cranial ganglia have a good blood supply. Three aortic arches (the second is marked 2) are present. The capital plexuses (a, b, c) and the capital vein are now well developed, and the cardinal venous system is established: precardinal, postcardinal, and common cardinal. Bar: 0.15 mm. Based on Streeter in O'Rahilly and Müller (1987a) and on Padget (1957).

Abbreviations: a, b, c, rostral, middle, and caudal capital venous plexuses; Ao., dorsal aorta; C-T, conotruncus; LA, left atrium; LV, left ventricle; Ot., otic vesicle; RA, right atrium; RV, right ventricle; SV, sinus venosus.

Fig. 12-10.   **A**

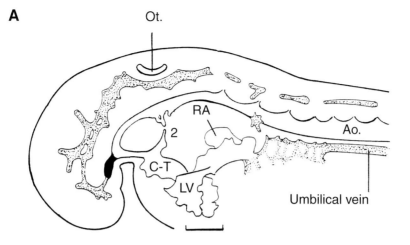

B

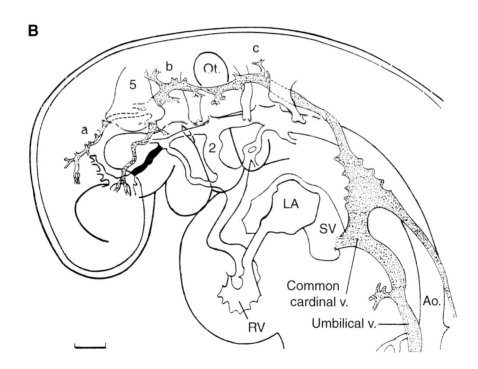

99

Fig. 12-11. The closure of the neuropores in the human, based on data from 19 embryos. The future neuropores are recognizable as soon as fusion of the neural folds begins, when approximately five to seven pairs of somites are visible (Heuser and Corner, 1957).

In the rostral region the dorsal lip formed by the roof progresses rapidly and has a much longer track than the terminal lip, formed by the floor. This can be seen from the steep rise of the line representing the roof. The line of the floor, by contrast, remains horizontal during stage 10 and then rises during stage 11, indicating the bidirectional closure of the rostral neuropore. Although closure seemingly may occur in several places independently, at least in some instances, no regular pattern of multiple sites, such as has been described in the mouse, has yet been shown in the human embryo.

Two instances of dysraphia (open circles) are included for comparison. In the first example an embryo of 14 somitic pairs showed complete failure of fusion of the neural folds (Dekaban, 1963), although the terminal lip had progressed normally. In the second case, believed to be future anencephaly (Müller and O'Rahilly, 1984), an embryo of stage 13 showed a well-developed terminal lip but a marked deficiency in the progression of the dorsal lip. Both these examples show that development of one lip can proceed more or less independently of the other. The triangles represent the situs neuroporicus; the asterisk, the cerebrospinal junction. The caudal region differs considerably from the rostral. Both the floor and the roof become increasingly elongated as further pairs of somites (the stepwise line) become visible. They remain approximately parallel, however. The neuropore, which remains small throughout, becomes displaced more and more caudally until it disappears at a level corresponding approximately to future sacral vertebra 2. This is taken to be the level of the junction between primary and secondary neurulation. Although both lips may contribute at the last moment to the final neuroporal closure, nothing has been found comparable to the bidirectional closure of the rostral neuropore, which extends throughout all of stage 11.

Once the caudal neuropore is closed, the whole caudal area of the embryo is covered by surface ectoderm. The continuing formation of the spinal part of the neural tube takes place without involvement of ectoderm and is termed secondary neurulation. The caudal part of the tube is present first as a concentration of tissue in the caudal eminence. **Secondary neurulation** is the continuing formation of the sacrocaudal part of the spinal cord without direct involvement of the surface ectoderm, i.e., without the intermediate phase of a neural plate. It begins once the caudal neuropore has closed during stage 12. The caudal eminence (or end-bud) is a mass of pluripotent mesenchymal tissue covered by ectoderm. It is recognizable already at stages 9 and 10, and gradually replaces the primitive streak. It provides structures that are comparable to those formed more rostrally by the three germ layers. The derivatives include the caudal portion of the digestive tube and coelom, blood vessels, notochord, somites, and spinal cord. At stage 12 the caudal eminence gives rise to a compact cellular mass known as the neural cord, which forms the nervous system in the sacrocaudal part of the body. The cavity (central canal) of the spinal cord, present already more rostrally, extends into the neural cord. The caudal eminence gives rise to at least somitic pair 32 (corresponding to future sacral centra 3 and 4) and those following. The mesenchyme for somitic pairs 30–34 is the material for sacral vertebrae 1–5. Secondary neurulation is important in regard to timing and localization of spina bifida aperta.

Fig. 12-11.

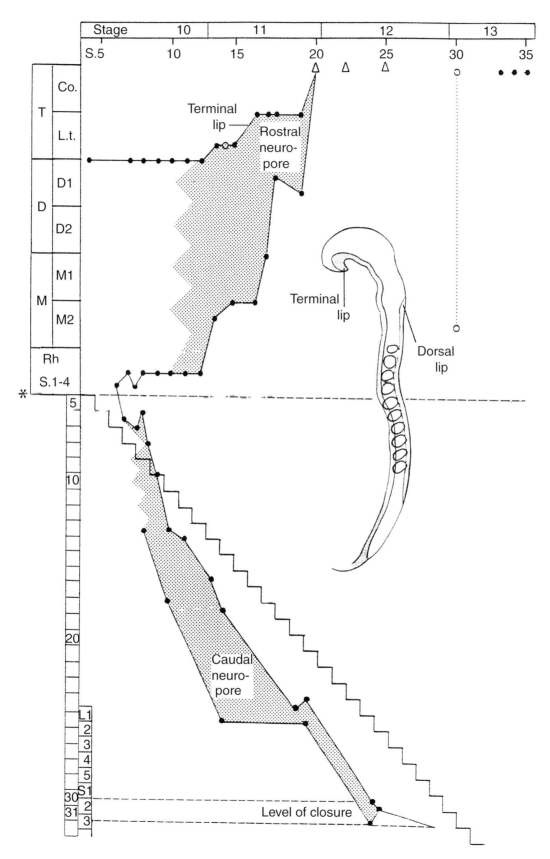

Fig. 12-12. Secondary neurulation.

(**A**) A reconstruction of the caudal end of an embryo (CEC 1062) of stage 12 with 29 pairs of somites. The site of the now closed caudal neuropore is indicated by an arrow. Somite 25 is shown as a dotted oval outline, and the position of the more caudal somites, including future No. 30, is shown. The closure of the neuropore is opposite future somite 31. The cross sections, from an embryo (CEC 8505a) with 24 pairs of somites, show some of the structures derived from the caudal eminence, e.g., the neural cord, spinal cord, and notochord of the caudal region.

(**B**) An embryo (CEC 9297) of stage 13 with 33 pairs of somites. The somites have not been included. The cross section, from an embryo (CEC 8967) also with 33 pairs of somites, shows the somitic plates that unite ventral to the hindgut.

Bars for A and B: 0.08 mm; for A', A", and B': 0.05 mm.

Fig. 12-12.

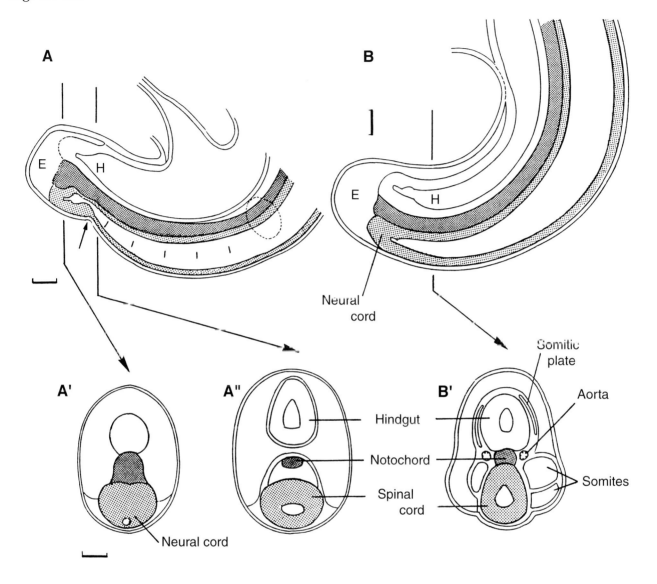

Comments on Neuroteratology (Stage 12)

Encephalo(meningo)cele in a fronto-ethmoidal position may be at or near the situs neuroporicus (as proposed by Hoving from studies of the rat). Occipital encephaloceles may perhaps be caused by a lack of the basal mesenchyme that forms at stage 12, originally between the neural tube and the notochord; its quantity is accumulating rapidly even at this stage.

Agenesis of the hypoglossal nerve would be expected from an isolated absence of the hypoglossal nucleus at stage 12. Although the lingual musculature would not be affected primarily, lack of innervation would lead to atrophy and fasciculation. The hypoglossal cord, which becomes recognizable at stage 12, gives rise to the muscles of the tongue and possibly to some of those of the larynx, although their connective tissue is believed to come from the neural crest.

Albinism is related to a defect in the production of neural crest, including probably the optic neural crest, which latter is noticeable at stage 12.

Myelomeningocele involves the neural tube and hence appears early, e.g., at stage 10 or 11 in the cervical and thoracic regions. At the lumbosacral level, where it is believed by many to be converted from a **myeloschisis**, myelomeningocele arises also during the period of primary neurulation (stages 8–12), although it is not a simple failure of neural closure. Lumbosacral lesions covered by intact skin are believed to appear during secondary neurulation (Lemire et al., 1975), but it should be stressed that lesions in the transitional zone between primary and secondary neurulation are not well understood. It is of interest that neural tube defects at stage 12 are more than 40 times more frequent than the number found at birth, so that most of the affected conceptuses are lost before birth, probably mainly within the embryonic period (Shiota, 1991).

Sacral agenesis may result from a localized defect within the caudal eminence, although it has also been attributed to an exaggeration of the normal process of caudal regression that occurs later in the embryonic period. Complete lack of the caudal eminence would result in cloacal deficiency and consequently an incomplete separation of the two lower limb buds, i.e., symmelia (O'Rahilly and Müller, 1989b).

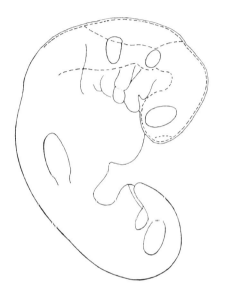

Stage 13: The Closed Neural Tube and the First Appearance of the Cerebellum

Approximately 4–6 mm in Greatest Length
Approximately 32 Postfertilizational Days

Fig. 13-1. Right lateral view of an embryo (CEC 8119) of stage 13 with the brain (CEC 6473) superimposed. From O'Rahilly, Müller, and Bossy (1986).

Normally, at 4 to 5 postfertilizational weeks, in embryos of some 5 mm in length, both neuropores are closed, so that the future ventricular system no longer communicates with the amniotic cavity. The choroid plexuses will not appear for another fortnight, so that the liquid in the neural tube is "ependymal fluid." The terminal-vomeronasal neural crest is arising from the nasal discs, the retinal and lens discs are beginning to develop, and the adenohypophysial pouch is distinct. Three diencephalic neuromeres are present: D1, parencephalon, and synencephalon. The isthmus rhombencephali is visible as a neuromere between M2 and Rh.1. A marginal layer is distinguishable in the wall of the mesencephalon and rhombencephalon. The primordia of various somatic and visceral efferent nuclei, the common afferent tract, and the ganglia of most of the cranial nerves can be discerned. The first indication of the cerebellum appears in Rh.1 during stage 13. Further details: Müller and O'Rahilly (1988a).

105

Fig. 13-2. Right lateral view of the brain (CEC 836). The number of somitic pairs in this extensively studied embryo is now known to have been 32. The mesencephalon is well delimited. The cerebellum is at the alar plate of Rh.1. The roof of the fourth ventricle is translucent. The otic vesicle is closed. The wall of the optic vesicle related to the surface ectoderm becomes flattened and constitutes the retinal disc, and the lens disc becomes distinguishable concomitantly.

The arteries to the head at stage 13 were reconstructed by Padget (1948, Fig. 1), who included the internal carotid and the carotico-basilar anastomoses.

Fig. 13-3. Graphic reconstruction from transverse sections to show a median view of the brain (CEC 836). The asterisk indicates the junction with the spinal cord. Both neuropores are now closed, so that, at approximately 4 to 5 postfertilizational weeks, the cavity of the neural tube is a closed (future ventricular) system, normally no longer in communication with the amniotic cavity. The contained "ependymal fluid" is presumably formed by the lining cells and later, when the choroid plexuses have appeared, will become the cerebrospinal fluid. Once the neural tube has closed, its walls become subject to the pressure of the contained fluid, provided fluid formation is greater than absorption.

The telencephalon is of approximately the same length as D2. The commissural plate is the median area at the level of the nasal plates. The terminal-vomeronasal neural crest is appearing (O'Rahilly, 1965). Cells leave the still convex or flat nasal plates and form cellular buds, which will participate in forming the ganglia of the nervus terminalis and the vomeronasal nerve, as well as in the development of the olfactory nerve.

The roof of D2 bulges slightly at the site of the future synencephalon (Fig. 13-4). The adenohypophysial pouch (Fig. 13-4) and the mamillary region are now distinct. At the transition between D2 and M1, the interstitial nucleus is forming ventrally, and its fibers constitute the uncrossed part of the medial longitudinal fasciculus. The oculomotor and trochlear nuclei are present, the former in M2, the latter in the isthmus.

The isthmus rhombencephali, so named by His, lies between M2 and Rh.1, and is clearly separated from the latter. This is a newly formed neuromere. The rhombencephalon is considerably enlarged dorsoventrally in comparison with stage 12, and the floor of the fourth ventricle is bent in the region of Rh.2. Although the wall of the brain remains histologically simple for the most part, being formed by the pseudostratified epithelium of the ventricular layer, a marginal layer has developed in the mesencephalon and rhombencephalon (Figs. 13-6 and 13-7).

The primordia of the somatic and visceral efferent nuclei of cranial nerves 5, 6, 7, 9–11, and 12 (Fig. 13-6) are present. The common afferent tract is being formed by descending fibers of nerves 5, 7, 9, and 10.

Rhombomeres 2 to 7 are characterized by internal grooves. The first indication of the cerebellum (marked Cbl) can be found in the alar lamina of Rh.1 in most embryos of stage 13. Loosely arranged cells begin to constitute its intermediate layer.

Fig. 13-2.

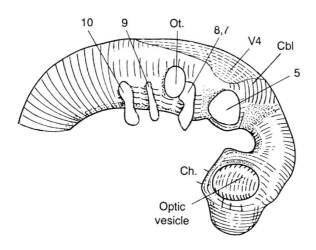

Fig. 13-3.

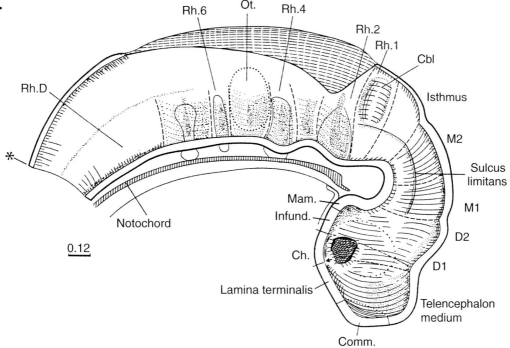

Fig. 13-4. Median section of the brain at stage 13 (CEC 9297). Neuromeres can be distinguished by dorsal and ventral bulges. A portion of the roof of the fourth ventricle is included. The notochord still extends as far rostrally as the caudal wall of the adenohypophysial pouch. The rhombomeres, the mesencephalon, and part of D2 (Syn.) are epinotochordal in position, whereas the rostral part of D2 and D1 are prenotochordal. The epinotochordal portions of the brain possess a floor plate. From Müller and O'Rahilly (1988a).

The levels of the sections in Figures 13-5 to 13-7 are shown in a key adjacent to Figure 13-7. Bars = 0.1 mm.

Precision

Median plane is the correct term, not midsagittal, nor midline. The term parasagittal is superfluous because all planes parallel to the median are simply sagittal.

Fig. 13-5. Silver-impregnated section (CEC 6473) showing ganglion 7/8v containing two long afferent fibers.

Important

The cerebellum begins to develop at this stage

Fig. 13-4.

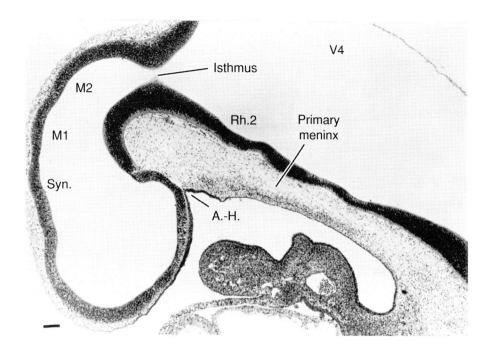

Fig. 13-5.

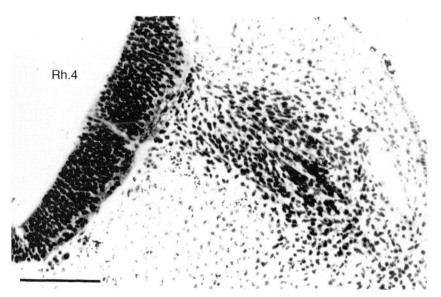

Fig. 13-6. The bilateral hypoglossal nuclei (CEC 6473) are formed by unipolar neurons that at this stage are situated peripherally, being more laterally placed than the visceral efferent nuclei of nerves 5, 7, and 9–11. The extent of the hypoglossal nucleus on the left is indicated by arrowheads. From Müller and O'Rahilly (1988a).

Fig. 13-7. A hypoglossal root (CEC 6473) from the neural tube (at left) to somite 3 (at right). The nerve fibers are accompanied by neural crest cells. The hypoglossal roots are not rigidly segmental, some somites receiving two roots. The cells of the primordial hypoglossal nucleus are relatively lateral in position, but that changes during development, as described with Figure 14-4. From Müller and O'Rahilly (1988a).

The hypoglossal artery participates in the carotico-basilar anastomosis, which is prominent until stage 15 (Fig. 19-17).

Fig. 13-6.

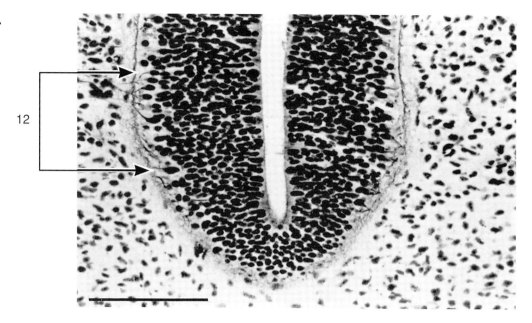

Fig. 13-7.

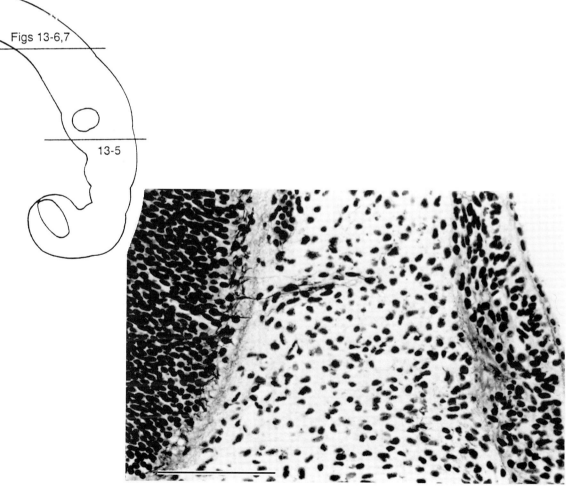

Fig. 13-8. The neuromeres at stage 13, as shown in a graphic reconstruction. D2 now consists of the synencephalon caudally and the parencephalon rostrally, and the isthmus rhombencephali constitutes a distinct neuromere. Bar for key: 0.2 mm.

(A) Sagittal section (CEC 9297) near the median plane to show the rhombomeres (Rh. 2, 4, and 6 having ventral evaginations that are numbered). The mamillary region is distinguishable, and the notochord can be seen to end close to the incipient adenohypophysial pouch.

(B)–(D) The dorsal and ventral eminences that represent the future dorsal and ventral thalami (d and v). The more caudal portions of the sections include the spinal cord (with the sulcus limitans), the dorsal aortae, as well as the truncus arteriosus and pharyngeal arches 1 and 2 (in B), the pharynx (in B and C), and the atria (in C). The bar for A–D represents 0.5 mm.

Fig. 13-8.

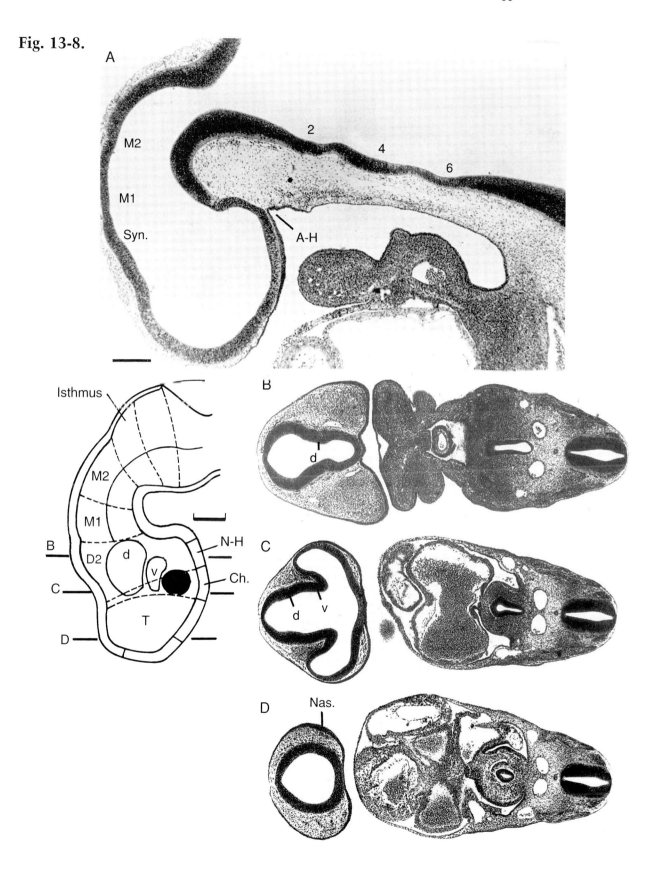

Comments on Neuroteratology (Stage 13)

Cerebral dysraphia, the first phase in the development of anencephaly, has been described in detail in a twin embryo of stage 13, and reconstructions are available (Müller and O'Rahilly, 1984). The neural tube was open over part of the midbrain and forebrain, although the situs neuroporicus (at the locus of the future commissural plate) was closed. Hence, in future anencephaly, fusion at the "terminal lip" of the rostral neuropore to form the embryonic lamina terminalis (Fig. 11-6A) may not be affected. It is possible that a causal relationship exists between neural tube defects and monozygotic twinning.

Communication between the amniotic fluid and the ependymal (future cerebrospinal) fluid is normally eliminated by stage 13 because of neuroporal closure, so that α-fetoprotein no longer diffuses into the amniotic cavity, except in such conditions as anencephaly and spina bifida cystica.

Cebocephaly. Indications of this condition have been found in an embryo (CEC 148) attributed to stage 13. A graphic reconstruction was prepared, from which it could be seen that the notochord did not reach the adenohypophysis, as normally it would. A convergence of the nasal discs indicated a narrow median region of the head. The nasal septum would not develop, and the single nasal cavity would possess a single nostril. Cebocephaly arises earlier than **arhinencephaly,** in which the brain is almost normal except for absence of the olfactory bulbs. It has been found experimentally in the mouse that in cebocephaly little or no tissue from the medial nasal processes is involved in the development of the nose, lips, and palate. The single nostril in cebocephaly ends blindly, and the eyes are closely set. The brain is holoprosencephalic in type and the forebrain septum is absent or reduced. The corpora striata are not separated from each other.

Cerebellar agenesis, although rarely total, could arise as early as stage 13, or even in stage 12. The first part of the cerebellum to develop is material for the hemispheres, whereas the primordium of the vermis becomes defined only at stages 18 and 19.

Abducent-facial palsy (Möbius sequence) presents as a non-specific, commonly bilateral, mask-like facies. The nuclei of cranial nerves 6 and 7 are usually degenerated, but they may be absent. Most of the motor nuclei of the cranial nerves begin to develop at about stage 13. Other cranial nerves may be involved in the sequence, and limb defects are frequent. Some of the variable features, e.g., micrognathia and microglossia, are probably secondary. Moreover, some instances of the sequence are considered either to be caused by involvement of peripheral nerves or as a myopathy. Abnormal torsional and vertical eye movements could be produced by disturbance of the interstitial nucleus (Crawford et al., 1991). That nucleus appears in stage 13 at the ventral transitional area between diencephalon and mesencephalon (Fig. 14-6).

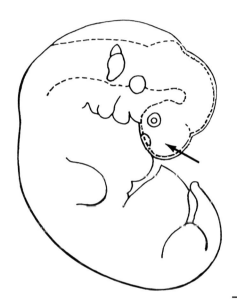

Stage 14: The Future Cerebral Hemispheres

Approximately 5–7 mm in Greatest Length
Approximately 33 Postfertilizational Days

Fig. 14-1. Right lateral view of an embryo (CEC 6502) of stage 14 with the brain superimposed. The arrow indicates the right cerebral hemisphere. From O'Rahilly, Müller, and Bossy (1986).

The future cerebral hemispheres become identifiable during stage 14 and are delimited from the telencephalon medium by the torus hemisphericus internally and by the di-telencephalic sulcus externally. Particularly advanced in the prosencephalon are the hypothalamic, amygdaloid, hippocampal, and olfactory regions. The synencephalon is identifiable. The mesencephalic flexure is less marked and is occupied by the future tentorium cerebelli. The pontine flexure appears. The cerebellum is formed by the alar plate of the isthmus as well as by that of rhombomere 1. Blood vessels now penetrate the wall of the brain. Various bundles (e.g., the medial and lateral longitudinal fasciculi, the common afferent tract) and a number of nuclei of cranial nerves are present. Further details: Müller and O'Rahilly (1988b).

115

Fig. 14-2. Right lateral view of the brain (CEC 2841). The future cerebral hemispheres begin to form during stage 14, but they were not evident in this embryo. The lens pit is present (Fig. 14-7). The synencephalon is recognizable. A minute, dorsal mesencephalic evagination (between M1 and M2) is frequently found: *vergängliche epiphysenähnliche Anlage des Mittelhirndaches* (Hochstetter, 1919). The isthmus participates in the formation of the cerebellum. The hypoglossal roots and/or rootlets begin to unite usually into two trunks.

The arteries to the head of this embryo were reconstructed by Padget (1948, Fig. 2), who showed that the carotico-basilar anastomoses are beginning to regress.

Fig. 14-3. Graphic reconstruction based on transverse sections to show a median view of the brain (CEC 6502). The asterisk indicates the junction with the spinal cord. The dividing line between the telencephalon medium and the future cerebral hemispheres is the torus hemisphericus, in the basal part of which the medial ventricular eminence (Fig. 6-2) develops. Externally, the groove that accompanies the torus is the di-telencephalic sulcus. In the median plane, the borderline between diencephalon and telencephalon extends from the velum transversum to the preoptic recess. The velum transversum is a ridge in the roof of the prosencephalon, situated between D1 and the telencephalon medium. The telencephalon is surrounded by some mesenchyme, even ventrally.

The prosencephalon occupies almost one-quarter of the length of the brain. Four areas are particularly advanced: (1) the hypothalamic region at the level of the chiasmatic plate as well as lateral to it [this is the area of the hypothalamic cell cord, from which the preoptico-hypothalamic tract arises (Fig. 14-4)]; (2) the amygdaloid region of the medial ventricular eminence; (3) the primordium of the hippocampus; and (4) the olfactory region.

Topographically the hypothalamic cell cord corresponds to the "medial zone of the anterior hypothalamus," which participates postnatally in the regulation of sexual comportment.

The mesencephalic flexure has diminished to about 50°, so that only a narrow space (the *Mittelhirnpolster* of Hochstetter) exists between the diencephalon and the rhombencephalon. The contained mesenchyme will form the tentorium cerebelli, the medial part of which now appears and is continuous with the cellular sheath of the notochord. A few extracerebral oculomotor and abducent fibers are present, and intracerebral trochlear fibers are developing. Blood vessels are much more numerous and, for the first time, penetrate the wall of the mesencephalon and rhombencephalon.

The pontine flexure is beginning as a slight bulging of the ventral wall of the hindbrain. The cerebellum, which is the widest part of the brain, is formed by the alar plate of two rhombomeres: the isthmus rostrally, and Rh.1 caudally. An intermediate layer is present in most of the cerebellum, and the future rhombic lip is discernible. The sclerotomes of the four occipital somites form two components near the base of rhombomere D. These will give rise to the basioccipital and exoccipital portions of the skull.

The key drawing shows the torus hemisphericus between the velum transversum and the preoptic recess. The diencephalon, which is thereby delineated from the telencephalon, possesses three elevations: the medial ventricular eminence, and the ventral and dorsal thalami. The entrance into the optic ventricle and the (dotted) outline of the optic cup are included.

Fig. 14-2.

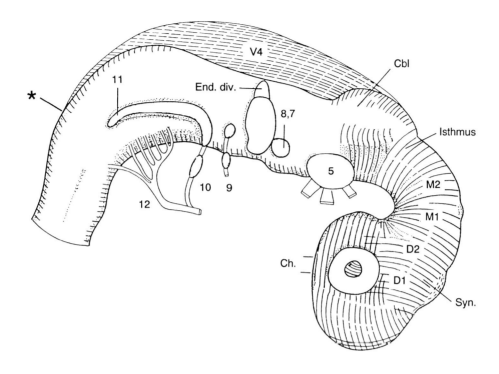

Fig. 14-3.

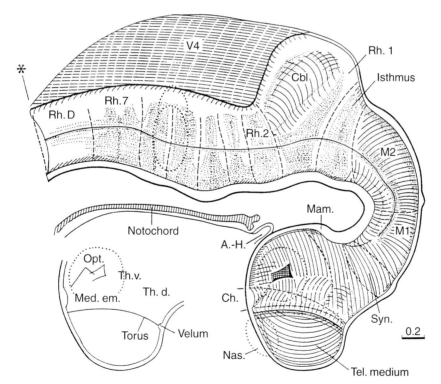

Fig. 14-4. (**A**) Developing fasciculi, nerve exits, and motor nuclei (CEC 6502). The outline of the right optic primordium is indicated by an interrupted line. The preoptico-hypothalamo-tegmental tract (black band indicated by a dagger) and the ventral longitudinal fasciculus are identifiable and could be important in the transportation of monoamines from the locus caeruleus to the forebrain. The former tract, together with fibers from the hypothalamic cell cord, may already reach the tegmentum. The surface overlying the area of the future amygdaloid nuclei possesses tall horizontal cells of the Cajal–Retzius type. This is the first region where a primordial plexiform layer begins to develop. This is not surprising, because the site is adjacent to the diencephalon, and the only possible access for corticipetal fibers into the embryonic cerebral cortex is through the ditelencephalic sulcus (Marín-Padilla, 1988a). The medial longitudinal fasciculus (thick black band) begins in the interstitial nucleus of the prerubral area (Fig. 14-6) and joins the ventral longitudinal fasciculus of the rhombencephalon. The lateral longitudinal fasciculus is indicated by a wide, stippled band. Dorsally, along the sulcus limitans, the common afferent tract (unshaded) contains sensory fibers from the cranial nerves. Present also are the beginnings of the habenulo-interpeduncular and medial tectobulbar tracts, and the mesencephalic tract of the trigeminal nerve. The exits of cranial nerves 3, 6, and 12 are ventral, whereas those of the others are along the sulcus limitans, where all afferent fibers enter. (**B**)–(**D**) Schematic drawings (CEC 8141) to show the development of the motor nuclei: (**B**) the accessory and hypoglossal, (**C**) the vestibulofacial, and (**D**) the trigeminal nuclei. Arrowheads point to the sulcus limitans; m, motor; s, sensory fibers. From Müller and O'Rahilly (1988b).

The original position of the somatic efferent nuclei in a ventrolateral cell column and of the visceral efferent nuclei in a ventromedial column was illustrated and clarified previously (O'Rahilly, Müller, Hutchins, and Moore, 1984). It is not generally appreciated that the position changes considerably during development (Windle, 1970; Müller and O'Rahilly, 1990c, Table 2).

Fig. 14-5. The telencephalon, showing the development of the future cerebral hemispheres in right lateral (1), median (2), and head-on (3) views: (**A**) no indication of cerebral hemispheres is seen; (**B**) hemispheric evagination has begun; (**C**) the future hemispheres are evident (C belongs to stage 15). In column 2, the telencephalon is stippled and the entrance to the left optic stalk is shown in black. In column 3, the telencephalic portion of the third ventricle is marked by horizontal hatching, whereas the lateral ventricles are shown by light stippling. From Müller and O'Rahilly (1988b).

Fig. 14-4.

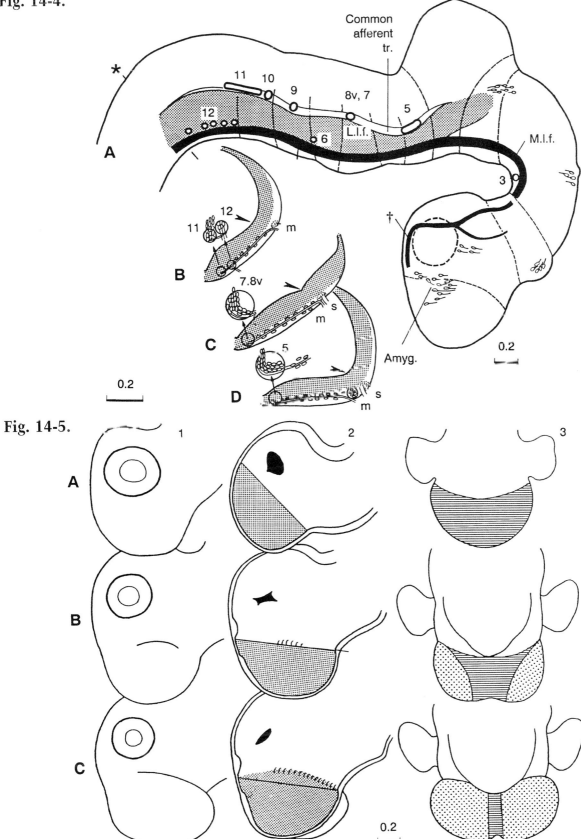

Fig. 14-5.

The levels of the sections in Figures 14-6 to 14-11 are shown in the key drawing above Figure 14-6. The bars represent 0.1 mm.

Fig. 14-6. Section through the midbrain and hypothalamus (CEC 6502). The interstitial nucleus is discernible at the ventral transitional area between diencephalon and mesencephalon. The adenohypophysial pocket is at all times closely related to the diencephalic floor. The mesenchyme adjacent to the brain is becoming looser: this is the primary meninx. From Bartelmez and Dekaban (1962).

Fig. 14-7. Section through the optic stalks and optic cups (CEC 6502). The optic ventricle still communicates with the interval between the retinal layers (where so-called detachment of the retina can occur). From Bartelmez and Dekaban (1962).

The initial appearance of the neuromeres is summarized in Table 14-1.

TABLE 14-1. The Neuromeres of the Human Embryo

Primary neuromeres	Secondary neuromeres
Prosencephalon	Telencephalon (T) ⎫ Diencephalon 1 (D1) ⎬ 10 Diencephalon 2 (D2) ⎭
	Parencephalon rostralis ⎫ 14 Parencephalon caudalis ⎭
	Synencephalon ———— 13
Mesencephalon	Mesencephalon 1 (M1) ⎫ 12 Mesencephalon 2 (M2) ⎭
	Isthmic neuromere ———— 13
Rhombomeres Rh. A Rh. B Rh. C Rh. D	Rhombomeres: Rh. 1, Rh. 2, Rh. 3, Rh. 4, Rh. 5, Rh. 6, Rh. 7, Rh. 8 — 11

(9 for primary)

Note: Stages of appearance are indicated by numbers to the right of the respective columns for the neuromeres.

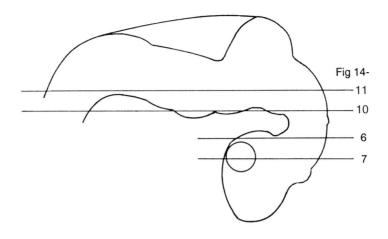

Fig. 14-6.

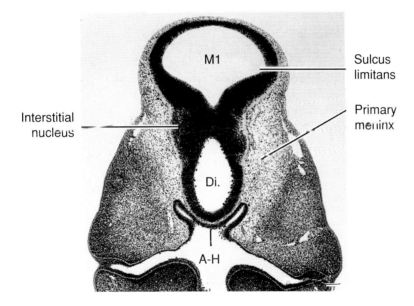

Fig. 14-7.

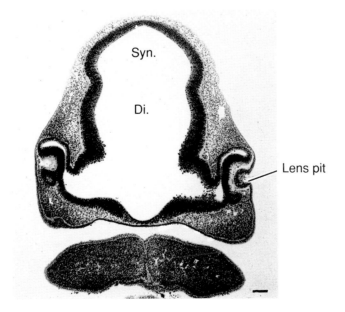

Fig. 14-8. The neuromeres at stage 14 as shown in graphic reconstructions. The distinction that can now be made between the rostral and caudal parts of the parencephalon completes the series of 16 neuromeres (Table 14-1). The rostral parencephalon contains the opening of the optic ventricle on each side and is associated with the infundibular region and the ventral thalamus, whereas the caudal parencephalon presents the dorsal thalamus and the mamillary region. Further details: Müller and O'Rahilly (1997b).

(**A**) Longitudinal section of the brain stem (CEC 8552) at the level indicated in the key. The mesencephalon is joined to the rhombomeres by the isthmus. Bar: 0.25 mm.

(**B**) Section through the forebrain (CEC 6502) along the line B. The cerebral hemispheres are beginning to evaginate. The nasal discs and their neural crest are visible on each side. In the key drawing the asterisks denote the sulcus medius, which separates the dorsal (d) from the ventral (v) thalamus. The hypothalamic cell cord (stippled) indicates longitudinal differentiation in the diencephalon even before the hypothalamic sulcus appears at the next stage. Bar: 0.25 mm.

(**C**) Section through the forebrain (CEC 6502) along the line C. The four compartments separated by horizontal lines are synencephalon, caudal parencephalon, rostral parencephalon, and D1 (immediately above the chiasmatic plate). The sulcus medius is marked by an arrowhead. Portions of the optic stalk and optic cup are visible on the right-hand side of the photomicrograph. Bar: 0.25 mm.

Fig. 14-8.

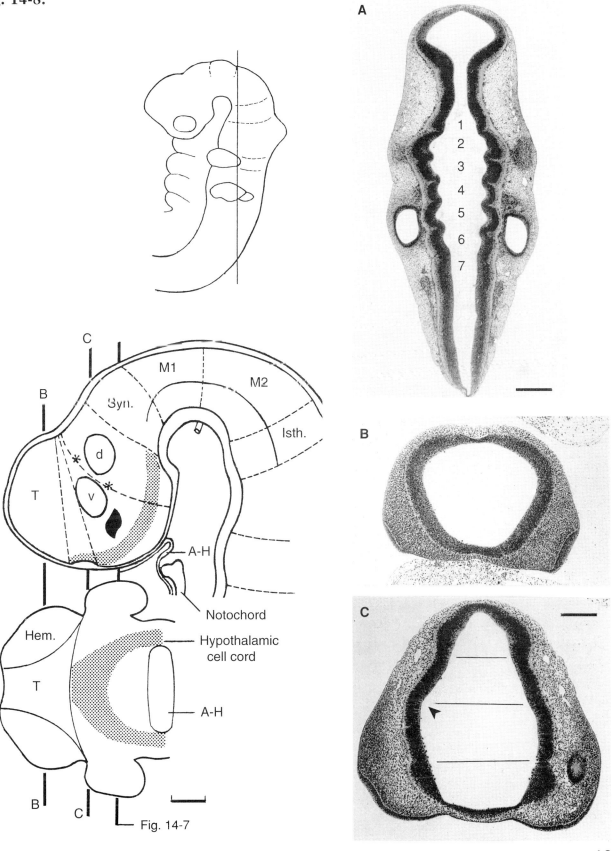

A

B

C

Fig. 14-7

C

M1

Byn.

M2

Isth.

B

d

*

*

v

T

A-H

Notochord

Hem.

Hypothalamic
cell cord

T

A-H

B

C

1
2
3
4
5
6
7

Fig. 14-9. Comparison of the wall of the developing forebrain and that of its derivative, the optic cup, at about $4\frac{1}{2}$ weeks, discloses the following features:

1. The cavities (future third ventricle and temporary optic ventricle) are continuous (Fig. 14-7).
2. Adjacent to the cavities is a terminal bar net, known in the retina as the external limiting membrane (ELM).
3. Germinal or proliferative cells, adjacent to the ventricle.
4. Mantle layer.
5. Marginal layer.
6. The basement membrane is the external limiting membrane of the brain. In the eye, however, because of the invagination that forms the optic cup, it is the internal limiting membrane (ILM) of the retina.

From O'Rahilly and Müller (1996a).

Fig. 14-9.

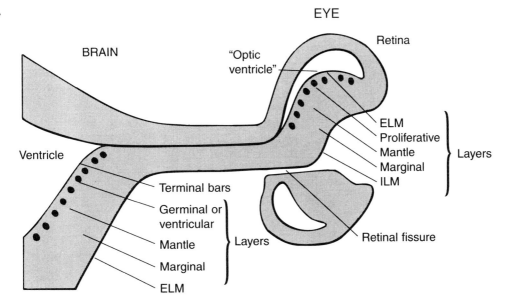

Figures 14-10 and 14-11 are from silver-impregnated sections (D-51).

Fig. 14-10. Section through the trigeminal ganglion. Nerve fibers from the ganglion enter the rhombencephalic wall and form the common afferent tract. It is maintained that the motor fibers of the pharyngeal nerves leave the even-numbered rhombomeres, in which case (in the mouse) the trigeminal fibers that arise in the motor nuclei of Rh.2 and Rh.3 emerge from rhombomere 2.

Fig. 14-11. Section through hypoglossal rootlets, which emerge from the still laterally placed hypoglossal nucleus and traverse the clear marginal layer of the rhombencephalic wall. From Müller and O'Rahilly (1988b).

Fig. 14-10.

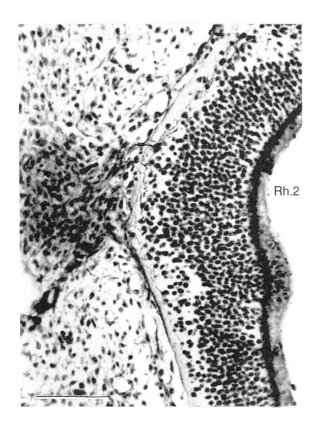

Fig. 14-11.

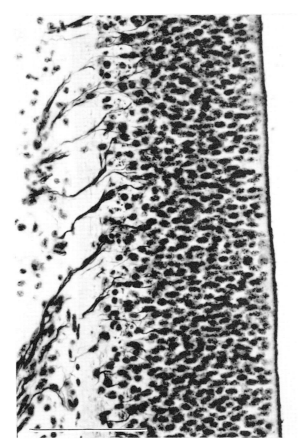

Comments on Neuroteratology (Stage 14)

Holoprosencephaly. Many basal areas of the forebrain that become distinct in stage 14 are absent in holoprosencephaly, e.g., the olfactory region (paleocortex), the optic stalks, and the neurohypophysial area. Hence, holoprosencephaly is more than a mere failure to "diverticulate" into cerebral hemispheres. It involves an even more fundamental event, such as induction, and has an early origin (probably in stage 8). In those rare instances where holoprosencephaly is found independently of synophthalmia and arhinencephaly, the origin is possibly at a later time, but nervertheless not later than stage 13 or 14. The clinical manifestations of holoprosencephaly, together with a survey of holoprosencephalic syndromes and an atlas of 35 cases, can be found in a useful book by Siebert et al. (1990).

Arnold–Chiari Malformation (Chiari Type 2). This obscure condition was first described by Cleland in 1883. Hypoplasia of the tentorium cerebelli is found, and hydrocephaly and myelomeningocele are usual but not invariable accompaniments. Many features are probably secondary rather than primary (Gardner, et al., 1975). A failure of the pontine flexure (stage 14) to form is believed to be an important factor in the abnormal elongation of the hindbrain, but attempts to formulate a unified theory have been singularly unconvincing. The time of origin of the condition lies in the embryonic period proper, perhaps between 3 and 5 weeks. An example at about stage 16 has been described (Ruano Gil, 1965).

Myelomeningocele. Numerous embryos and fetuses with myelomeningocele have been described (Lemire et al., 1975), including an embryo of stage 14 with caudal myeloschisis. It was believed that the lesion occurred before closure of the neural tube; defects in the basement membrane of the neural ectoderm were noted and the condition was considered to have been a forerunner of lumbosacral myelomeningocele (Lemire et al., 1965).

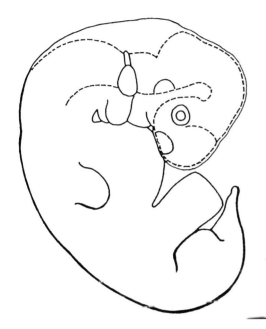

Stage 15: Longitudinal Zoning in the Diencephalon

Approximately 7–9 mm in Greatest Length
Approximately 35 Postfertilizational Days

Fig. 15-1. Right lateral view of an embryo (CEC 3441) of stage 15 with the brain superimposed. From O'Rahilly, Müller, and Bossy (1986).

The neuromeres of the forebrain are still recognizable. Each cerebral hemisphere is limited externally by the di-telencephalic sulcus and internally by the torus hemisphericus. The medial ventricular eminence of the basal nuclei has appeared in the previous stage and it is diencephalic. The lateral ventricular eminence, which now appears, is telencephalic (Fig. 6-2). The amygdaloid region will be derived mainly from the medial eminence. The wall of the diencephalon presents five longitudinal zones: epithalamus, dorsal thalamus, ventral thalamus, subthalamus, and hypothalamus. The primordium of the epiphysis cerebri is beginning. The sulcus limitans ends rostrally at the midbrain (M1) and is not continuous with the hypothalamic sulcus. Hence the alar/basal distinction does not arise in the forebrain. Some new tracts, commissures, and nuclei are appearing. The cerebellum is derived from both the isthmus and rhombomere 1. Most cranial nerves are present. Axodendritic synapses have been detected in the cervical region of the spinal cord, followed by axosomatic synapses early in the fetal period (Okado, 1981). The vertebrae are first clearly defined. Further details: Müller and O'Rahilly (1988c).

Fig. 15-2. Right lateral view of the brain (CEC 3216). The asterisk indicates the junction with the spinal cord. The cerebral hemisphere is demarcated from the diencephalon by the di-telencephalic sulcus. The lens vesicle and the optic cup with its retinal ("choroid") fissure are shown (Fig. 15-7). Still funnel-shaped, the isthmus blends at its wider end with the cerebellar region and narrows towards M2.

Fig. 15-3. Graphic reconstruction prepared from transverse sections (CEC 6506 with some features of CEC 3385 added) to show a median view of the brain. The asterisk indicates the junction with the spinal cord. The cerebral hemisphere is limited from the diencephalon by an internal crest, the torus hemisphericus (Fig. 15-6), which begins at the velum transversum and ends as a basal thickening in the medial ventricular eminence (Table 15-1). In the development of the basal nuclei (Fig. 6-2), the lateral ventricular eminence, which is telencephalic, has appeared (Fig. 15-3, inset). The medial eminence, however, is entirely diencephalic, although it has been misinterpreted by others as the lateral eminence. The chiasmatic plate is well defined and is limited by preoptic and postoptic recesses. The infundibular recess is appearing adjacent to the adenohypophysial pouch. The caudal part of the diencephalon (formerly D2) is the synencephalon, which will give rise to the prerubrum and the pretectum. At this level, the epiphysis cerebri begins as a thickening, but a recess is not yet present.

A characteristic feature of this stage is the appearance of longitudinal zones in the diencephalon (Fig. 15-6 and Table 18-1). For example, the hypothalamic sulcus delineates the hypothalamus from the thalamus. In addition, the hypothalamus comprises subthalamus and hypothalamus *sensu stricto* (separated by a faint sulcus); the thalamus consists of epithalamus, dorsal thalamus, and ventral thalamus (Table 18-1). The dorsal and ventral thalami are incompletely separated in more advanced embryos by the beginning formation of the zona limitans intrathalamica, which is marked on the interior relief by the marginal ridge. Blood vessels begin to penetrate the wall of the diencephalon.

The midbrain consists of two neuromeres: M1 and M2. The sulcus limitans ends at the rostral limit of M1. M2 is joined to the hindbrain by the isthmus. The supramamillary commissure is marked by a dagger. In the hindbrain, the cerebellar plate is distinct and extends over two rhombomeres: the isthmus and Rh.1. The roof of the isthmus forms the superior medullary velum. The locus caeruleus is indicated (Fig. 15-9). The notochord is partly surrounded by sclerotomic material that represents the future basioccipital component of the skull.

The inset drawing shows the contiguity of the torus hemisphericus and the medial ventricular eminence. The lateral eminence is visible in the lateral wall of the (left) cerebral hemisphere.

The boundaries between the major divisions of the brain are listed in Table 15-1 at the end of this chapter.

Fig. 15-2.

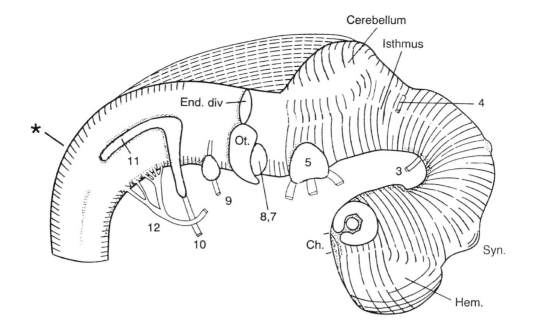

Fig. 15-3.

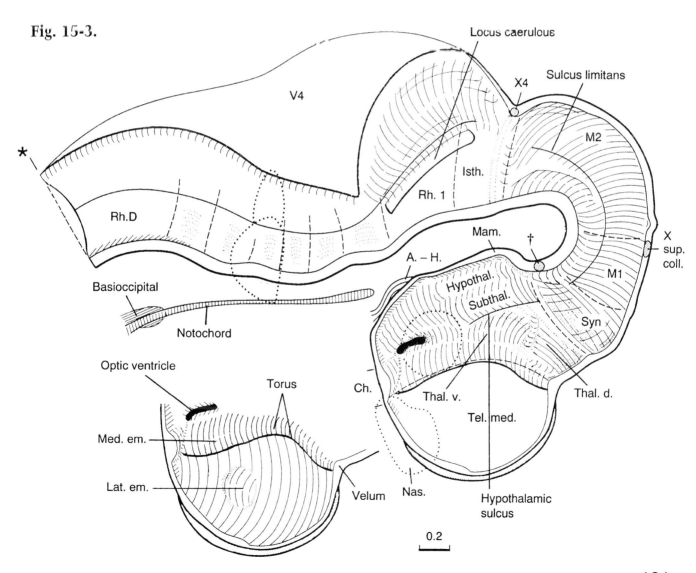

131

Fig. 15-4. A number of tracts (CEC 6505) have appeared in the following order: the lateral longitudinal fasciculus, the spinal tract of the trigeminal nerve (which is a component of the common afferent tract), the medial longitudinal fasciculus, the mesencephalic tract of the trigeminal nerve, and the mamillotegmental tract (dagger). Fibers of the preoptico-hypothalamic tract are present, and precursor fibers of the habenulo-interpeduncular and hypothalamo-thalamic tracts are forming. Fibers of the decussation of the superior colliculi are the precursors of the tectobulbar tract. Fibers from the amygdaloid part of the medial ventricular eminence (future striatosubthalamic tract) constitute a portion of the medial prosencephalic fasciculus. The shifting of the amygdaloid area into a clearly telencephalic position is comparable to the relocation of the globus pallidus from the diencephalon into the corpus striatum.

Fig. 15-5. Right lateral view (CEC 6506) showing some peripheral nerves. All cranial nerves are present except 1, 2, and 8c. (The optic nerve is represented merely by the optic stalk until nerve fibers appear at stage 18.) The least advanced is the abducent, which is found in only one-third of embryos of this stage. Intramural trochlear fibers are indicated by two rows of dots. The vestibular nerve possesses sensory fibers that join the common afferent tract. The hypoglossal nerve has many connections with cervical nerves 1 to 3. The various ganglia of the cranial nerves are identifiable. From Müller and O'Rahilly (1988c).

Pax, En, and *Wnt* genes are involved in the patterning of the mesencephalon and metencephalon (Song et al., 1996), and the mes-rhombencephalic boundary shows *Pax*-5 gene expression (Gérard et al., 1995).

TABLE 15-1. Boundaries Between the Major Divisions of the Brain

Division of brain	Limit at roof	Limit at floor
Telencephalon medium		
	Velum transversum	Preoptic recess
Diencephalon		
	Between posterior commissure and commissure of superior colliculi	Caudal supramamillary commissure
Mesencephalon		
	Rostral commissure of trochlear nerves	Rostral to nuclei of trochlear nerves
Rhombencephalon	End of hypoglossal rhombomere (Rh.D)	
Spinal cord		

Fig. 15-4.

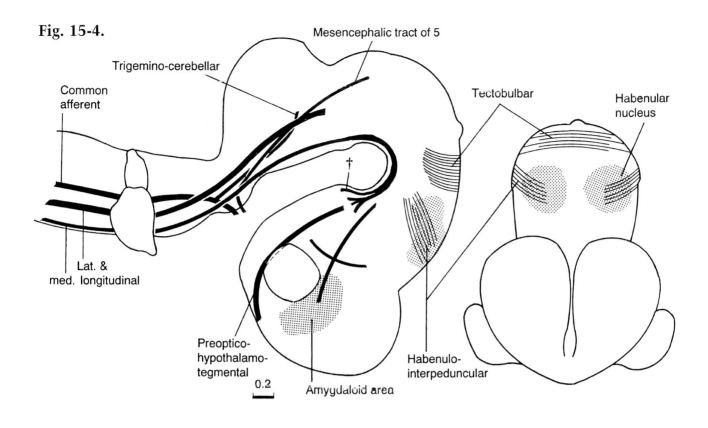

Common afferent

Trigemino-cerebellar

Mesencephalic tract of 5

Tectobulbar

Habenular nucleus

Lat. & med. longitudinal

†

Preoptico-hypothalamo-tegmental

0.2

Amygdaloid area

Habenulo-interpeduncular

Fig. 15-5.

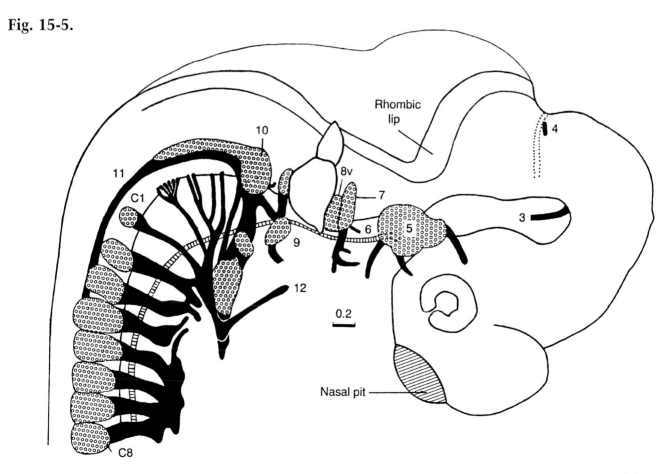

Rhombic lip

10

11

C1

8v

7

4

6

5

3

9

12

0.2

C8

Nasal pit

Figures 15-6 to 15-9. These four photomicrographs are from the same embryo (CEC 8997) and their planes of section are shown in a key drawing adjacent to Figure 15-9. Bars: 0.15 mm.

Fig. 15-6. Section through the forebrain and isthmus rhombencephali showing various features of the prosencephalon. The hippocampal thickening is distinct on each side of the lamina terminalis. From Müller and O'Rahilly (1988c).

Fig. 15-7. Section through the diencephalon and rhombencephalon showing the optic cup and the cerebellar plate on each side. The lens vesicles are closed from the surface. The optic stalk on the right-hand side of the photomicrograph shows the continuity between the third ventricle and the temporary optic ventricle. From Müller and O'Rahilly (1988c).

Important

By this stage all five major subdivisions of the brain are present: myelencephalon, metencephalon, mesencephalon, diencephalon, and telencephalon (the future cerebral hemispheres as well as the telencephalon medium).

Fig. 15-6.

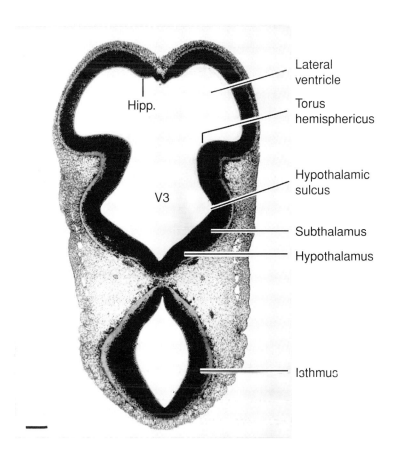

Lateral
ventricle

Torus
hemisphericus

Hipp.

Hypothalamic
sulcus

V3

Subthalamus

Hypothalamus

Isthmus

Fig. 15-7.

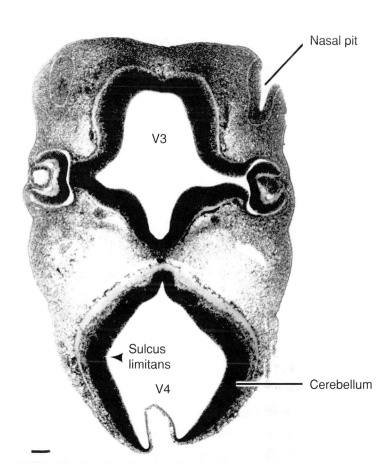

Nasal pit

V3

Sulcus
limitans

V4

Cerebellum

135

Fig. 15-8. Section through the hypothalamus and adenohypophysial pouch, showing a part of the optic chiasma.

Fig. 15-9. Section through the cerebellar region at Rh.1 showing the locus caeruleus. From Müller and O'Rahilly (1988c).

The cells of the future locus caeruleus are present early (stage 13) and are situated in the intermediate layer of rhombomeres 1 and 2, ventral to the sulcus limitans. Later (at about stages 19 and 20), brightly fluorescent processes have been traced into the telencephalic wall (Zecevic and Verney, 1995), and dopamine and adrenergic fibers reach the tectum.

Fig. 15-8.

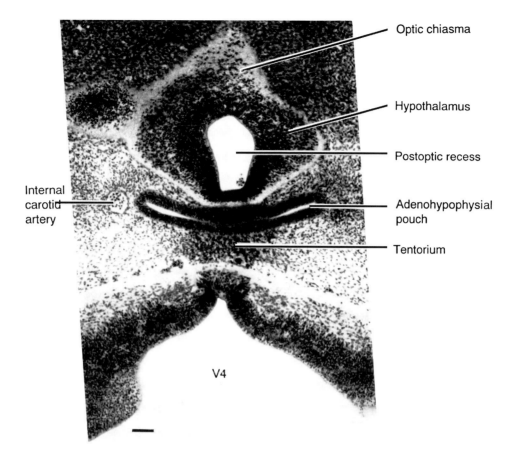

Optic chiasma

Hypothalamus

Postoptic recess

Adenohypophysial pouch

Tentorium

Internal carotid artery

V4

Fig. 15-9.

Sulcus limitans

Locus caeruleus

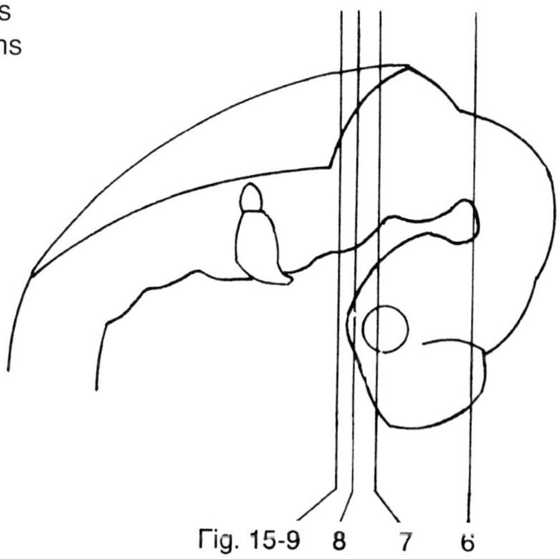

Fig. 15-9   8   7   6

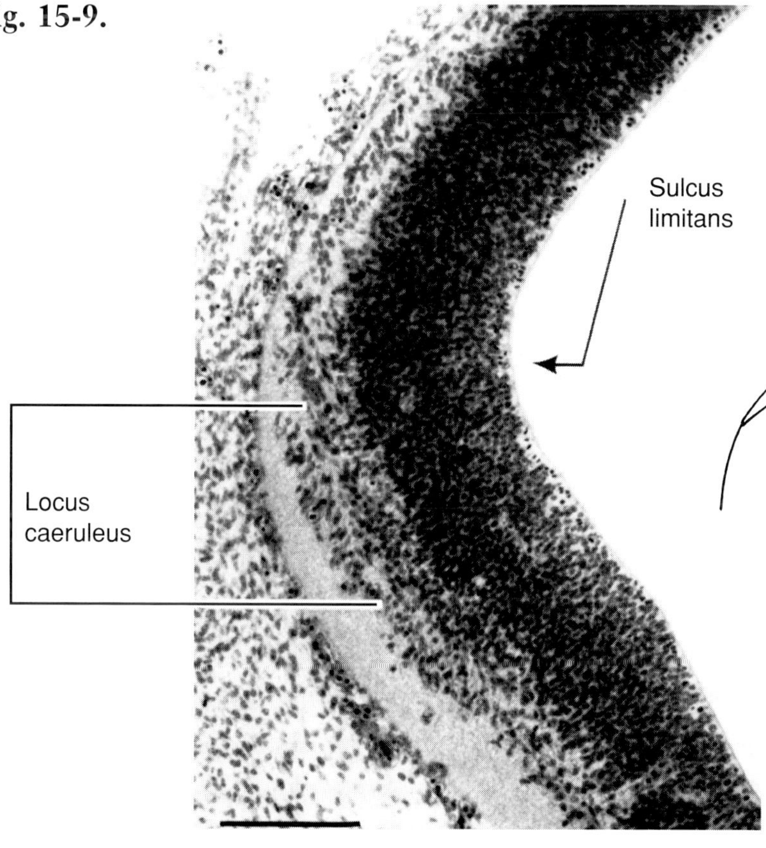

Comments on Neuroteratology (Stage 15)

Spina bifida occulta is possible from the first sign of the appearance of vertebrae at stage 15 until completion of the neural arches early in fetal life. Postnatally a radiologically detectable failure in the completion of one or more neural arches may be merely a lack of ossification dorsomedially, especially in the lumbosacral region. This is a normal finding in children of 2 years of age and also in one-fifth of adults.

Meningocele probably arises late in the embryonic period (e.g., stages 18–23) or early in the fetal period. The timing of various anomalies, however, is tentative and the retrospective use of embryological timetables for ascertainment of origin and causes of congenital malformations is hazardous, as frequently stressed by Warkany.

Caudal Aplasia. The caudal tip of the trunk appears particularly tapered at 5 weeks because it contains merely neural tube, but it is in no sense a future vertebrated "tail."

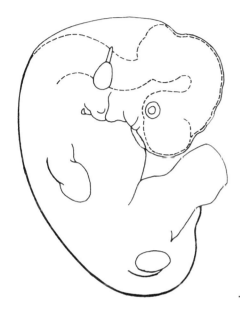

Stage 16: Evagination of the Neurohypophysis

Approximately 8–11 mm in Greatest Length
Approximately 37 Postfertilizational Days

Fig. 16-1. Right lateral view of an embryo (CEC 6517) of stage 16 with the brain (CEC 792) superimposed. From O'Rahilly, Müller, and Bossy (1986).

The presence of the hippocampal thickening and various histological features makes possible a distinction among the main, future cortical areas: archipallium, paleopallium, and neopallium. The most advanced differentiation is in the cortex of the future temporal pole at the periphery of the amygdaloid area, in which the primordial plexiform layer can be discerned. Olfactory fibers enter the wall of the brain at the site of the future olfactory bulb, and the future olfactory tubercle is detectable. The olfactory tubercle is the earliest component of the prosencephalic septum to appear. The marginal ridge separates the dorsal from the ventral thalamus. The neurohypophysial outgrowth is now becoming distinct. A number of important pathways are beginning, e.g., olfactory and vestibulocerebellar. The cochlear nerve has suddenly appeared. Asymmetry of the cerebral hemispheres has been recorded in one embryo. Further details: Müller and O'Rahilly (1989a).

139

Fig. 16-2. Right lateral view of the brain (CEC 792). The inset is an end-on view showing the cerebellar plates, mesencephalon, epiphysis cerebri, diencephalon and optic cups, and cerebral hemispheres. In one embryo (CEC 6510) the cerebral hemispheres were strikingly asymmetrical, the left hemisphere being smaller than the right (as confirmed by a Born reconstruction). Such an early cerebral asymmetry does not seem to have been recorded previously.

In the eye, the retinal (so-called choroid) fissure closes during stages 16 and 17. The polygonal outline of the (future iridial) rim of the optic cup is characteristic. Photomicrographs of the embryonic eye at each stage have been published (O'Rahilly, 1966), as well as a comparison of the wall of the neural tube and that of the optic cup (ibid., Fig. 8). In addition, the main events of optic development have been summarized (O'Rahilly, 1983).

Fig. 16-3. Graphic reconstruction prepared from transverse sections (of D1, an unlisted embryo) to show a median view of the brain. The asterisk indicates the junction with the spinal cord. The outgrowth of the infundibulum is now becoming marked; i.e., the evagination of the neurohypophysis is becoming distinct (Table 16-1). The rhombencephalon has become flatter and broader, and the isthmus, which has become clearer, now shows an enlargement ventrally. The change in shape of the isthmus was appreciated by Hochstetter (1919), who described this region as funnel-shaped (at stage 15). The pontine flexure is deeper. The rhombomeres are no longer clearly visible on the external surface. Amoeboid cells that may be precursors of microglial cells have been detected histochemically in the cerebral wall at about stage 16 (Fujimoto, et al., 1989). Furthermore, glial cells can be distinguished immunologically from neurons at about this time.

TABLE 16-1. Development and Components of the Hypophysis Cerebri

The adenohypophysial (A–H) and the neurohypophysial (N–H) primordia (upper left-hand corner) are in contact from their first appearance. Hence the adenohypophysial pouch and the neurohypophysial evagination are also in contact and result in the adult pituitary gland (rectangle). The terminology in the adult is that of Rioch, Wislocki, and O'Leary Res. Publ. Ass. Nerv. Ment. Dis. 20:3, 1940. The variously defined terms "anterior" and "posterior" lobes are best avoided.

Fig. 16-2.

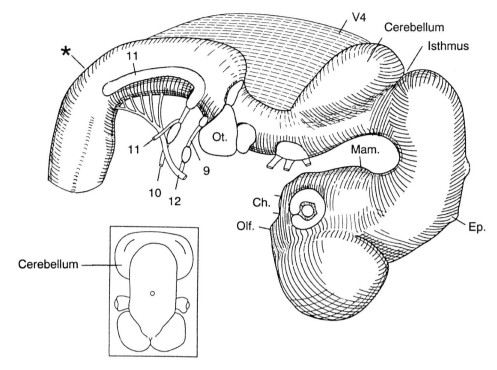

Fig. 16-3.

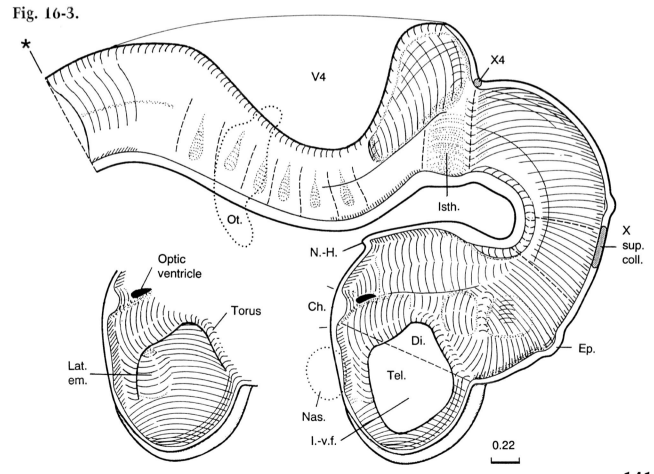

Figs. 16-4 and 16-5. Cranial nerves and tracts. The cochlear nerve appears suddenly, and all the cranial nerves are now visible. The hypoglossal nerve, which now reaches the apex of the tongue, is joined by fibers of cervical nerves 2 and 3, presumably the precursors of the ansa cervicalis and its roots (O'Rahilly and Müller, 1984b). Most motor nuclei of the cranial nerves have developed during stages 12 to 14. An examination of first-class material shows that it is not possible to distinguish the nucleus ambiguus at stage 16 or earlier, as has been claimed (Brown, 1990). Fibers ascending to the cerebellum are situated mainly along the sulcus limitans and are not clearly seen to penetrate that organ. Vestibulocerebellar and trigeminocerebellar fibers proceed towards the basal part of the cerebellar plate. The diencephalic subthalamic nucleus is present and includes fibers proceeding to the supramamillary commissure. The preoptico-hypothalamotegmental tract is marked by a dagger (Fig. 16-5). From Müller and O'Rahilly (1989a).

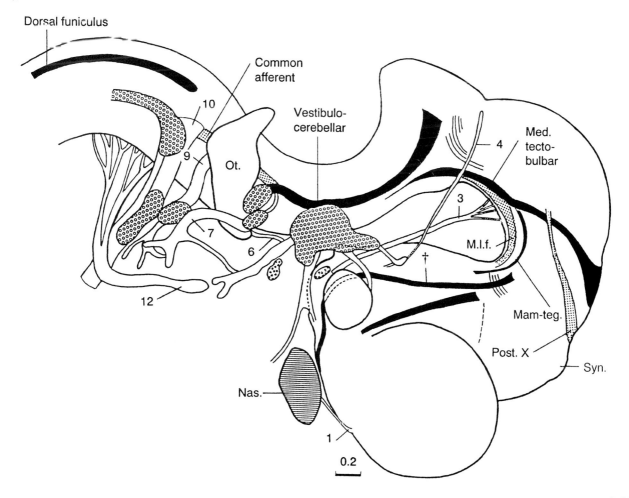

Fig. 16-4. Dorsal funiculus · Mesencephalic tract of 5 · Common aff. · Vestibulo-cerebellar · 4 · Ot. · 3 · 11 · 9 · X sup. coll. · 7 · 6 · 5 · Opt. · 10 · Syn. · 12 · Med. pros. fasc. · Habenulo-interpeduncular · 1

Fig. 16-5. Dorsal funiculus · Common afferent · Vestibulo-cerebellar · 10 · 9 · Ot. · Med. tecto-bulbar · 4 · 3 · M.l.f. · 7 · 6 · Mam-teg. · 12 · Post. X · Syn. · Nas. · 1 · 0.2

Fig. 16-6. Arterial development and the tentorium cerebelli (CEC 6510). The cellular sheath of the notochord, which is anchored to the adenohypophysis (Fig. 15-8), is continuous with the medial part of the future tentorium cerebelli. The space between the hypothalamus and the rhombencephalon becomes increasingly compressed, resulting in a mesenchymal condensation (the *Mittelhirnpolster* of Hochstetter) between the diencephalic floor and the basilar artery. The notochord lies either ventral to or, in the more advanced embryos, within the notochordal cellular sheath. The latter and the sclerotomic material will form the basioccipital part of the skull.

Most of the components of the future circulus arteriosus (of Willis) are now present: the basilar and the paired posterior communicating arteries, as well as the internal carotid vessels on both sides. An anterior communicating artery has not yet developed but will do so during stage 19 (Padget, 1948, Fig. 7b). The posterior communicating represents the original caudal division of the internal carotid artery (Fig. 19-17) and provides carotid supply to the embryonic hindbrain (Padget, 1948). The adult stem of origin of the posterior cerebral is at first the distal end of the original posterior communicating artery (Padget, 1948). Penetrating capillaries can be observed in most parts of the surface of the brain, except in the future archipallial and neopallial components of the telencephalon. They enter as deeply as the ventricular layer. From Müller and O'Rahilly (1989a).

The posterior communicating artery, a very important embryonic vessel that develops from stages 14 to 16, was also reconstructed by Padget (1948, Fig. 4). The posterior communicating is the vessel through which the internal carotid artery supplies the embryonic hindbrain. Although present and illustrated, the posterior cerebral artery was not named in Padget's figure.

Fig. 16-7. (**A**) lateral, (**B**) dorsal, (**C**) medial, and (**D**) ventral views of the telencephalon (CEC 6510). The archipallium (stippled), paleopallium (horizontal lines), and neopallium (unshaded) are distinguishable on the basis of histological differences. The archistriatum (amygdaloid nuclei, Fig. 6-2) is indicated by cross-hatching, and the paleostriatum by interrupted horizontal lines at the interior surface in C. This is the area to which the globus pallidus externus moves during stages 22 and 23 (Figs 23-16 and 23-23). The most advanced differentiation is in the future temporal pole (gamma) at the periphery of the amygdaloid nuclei. Here presumed Cajal–Retzius cells and fibers were already present in stage 15. These horizontally arranged cells in the "marginal" (Fig. 6-3) layer are more developed than the cells of the ventricular layer (Fig. 17-8). The "marginal" layer in this region constitutes the primordial plexiform layer, the "pallial Anlage," which is believed to be functional by stage 20 (Marín-Padilla and Marín-Padilla, 1982). Olfactory fibers enter the wall of the brain at the site of the future olfactory bulb, and cellular islands indicate the future olfactory tubercle.

Up to stage 16 the amygdaloid region, which is derived almost exclusively from the medial ventricular eminence, is recognizable by the advanced differentiation of its primordial plexiform layer. Neurogenesis in the amygdaloid complex of the rhesus monkey begins at a comparable time, and the cells have been considered to be the earliest postmitotic neurons in the telencephalon. Amygdaloid nuclei can be distinguished, in

Fig. 16-6.

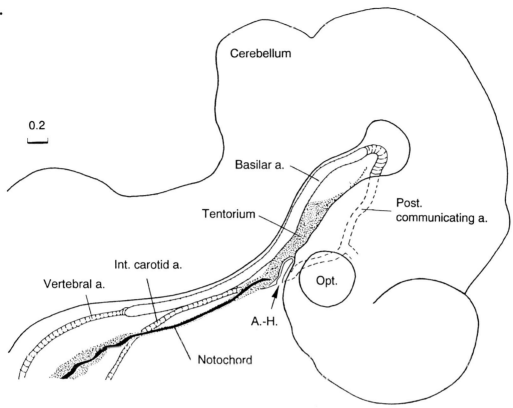

Fig. 16-7.

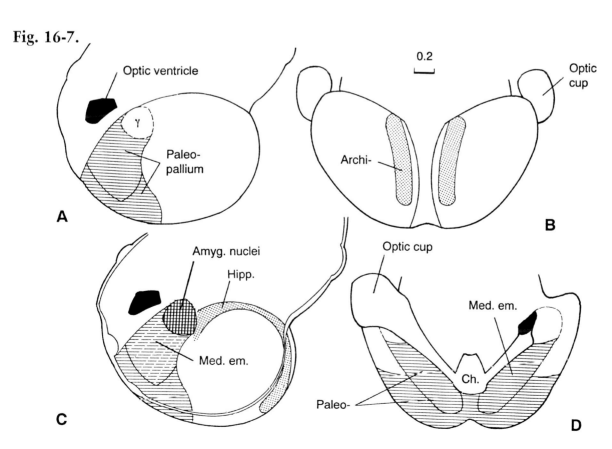

145

the human, only at stage 17 (one or two nuclei) and stage 18 (four nuclei: Fig. 18-5).

Whatever the pros and cons of the tripartite brain hypothesis (so-called reptilian, paleomammalian, and neomammalian regions), scant support for it is apparent in human embryology, any more than for the outmoded "biogenetic law" of "recapitulation." It would be very difficult (with present methods) to attempt to distinguish archi-, paleo-, and neopallial regions before histological differentiation has begun. The recorded appearance of synapses in the neopallium at stage 17 and later, however, serves to emphasize that that region is clearly more advanced than either the hippocampus or the olfactory bulb at the same stage. In other words, there seems to be no evidence that the development of the (human) brain follows a phylogenetic pattern from archi- to paleo- to neocortical structures.

Figures 16-8 to 16-13. Six sections of the brain (CEC 6510). From Bartelmez and Dekaban (1962).

Fig. 16-8.   The olfactory area and the lamina terminalis.

Fig. 16-9.   The medial ventricular eminence forms the basal part of the torus hemisphericus.

Fig. 16-10.   The optic stalk and the hypothalamic cell cord of the two sides of the brain.

Fig. 16-11.   Section at the level of the adenohypophysis.

Fig. 16-12.   The dorsal and ventral thalami, and the hypothalamic sulcus. Both ventral and dorsal thalami possess a thick ventricular layer and a beginning intermediate layer.

Fig. 16-13.   Section at the level of the epiphysis cerebri (pineal body, Table 16-2). The marginal ridge (future zona limitans intrathalamica) can be discerned and separates the ventral from the doral thalamus.

TABLE 16-2.   Development of the Epiphysis Cerebri

Features	*Stadium* of Turkewitsch	Carnegie stage
Site of future epiphysis may be distinguishable		15
Epiphysis detectable in diencephalic roof	I	16
Cellular migration in an external direction begins	II	17
Continuing cellular migration forms a *Vorderlappen* with "follicles"	III	18
The *Vorderlappen* shows a characteristic step and wedge appearance	IV	19
The habenular commissure appears	V	23
Hinterlappen, "ducts," etc.	VI–X	Fetal period

Source: Based on Turkewitsch (1933) on O'Rahilly (1983).

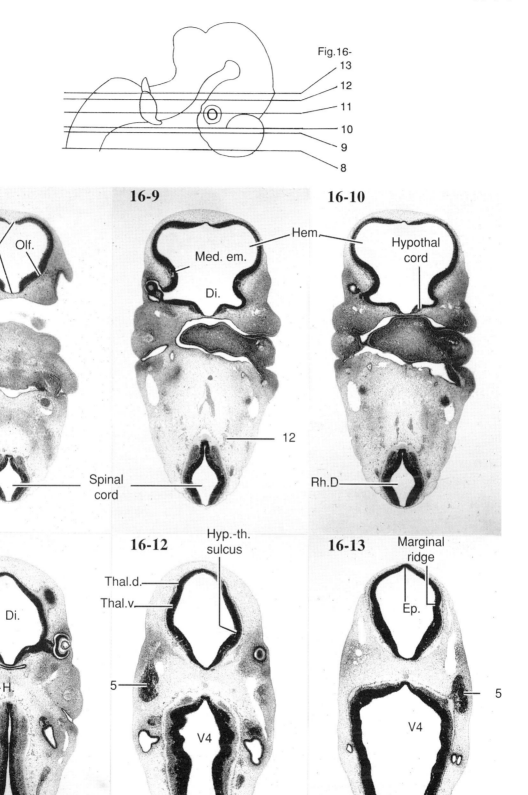

Fig.16-
13
12
11
10
9
8

Fig. 16-8

L.t. Olf.

Spinal cord

16-9

Hem
Med. em.
Di.
12
Spinal cord

16-10

Hypothal cord
Rh.D

Fig. 16-11

Di.
A.-H.
Ot.
10
11
Rh.

16-12

Hyp.-th. sulcus
Thal.d.
Thal.v.
5
V4
Rh.

16-13

Marginal ridge
Ep.
5
V4
Rh.

Figures 16-14 to 16-17. Four sections of the cerebral hemisphere (CEC 6510).

Fig. 16-14. Cerebral hemisphere showing the loose distribution of the superficial cells at the periphery. Up to and including stage 16 the neocortical part of the cerebral hemispheres is avascular (Larroche and Jardin, 1985), although it is already surrounded by a prominent "perineural" vascular process (Streeter, 1919; Padget, 1948; Marín-Padilla, 1978, 1988a,b). Bar: 0.2 mm.

Fig. 16-15. Some two sections more deeply, the surface of the cerebral hemisphere presents widely dispersed cells, indicating progressive differentiation. Bar: 0.2 mm.

The cell columns of the ventricular layer of the diencephalon in Figures 16-15 and 16-16 are high and are penetrated by blood vessels. The cells of the intermediate layer are not as tightly packed as in the telencephalic area shown in Figure 16-17, and this is a clear difference. Peripheral to the intermediate layer, nerve fibers and scattered cells give an impression of a primordial plexiform layer.

Fig. 16-16. The subthalamus, ventral to (below) the hypothalamic sulcus, showing fibers in the marginal layer and capillaries that have penetrated the cerebral wall. Such diencephalic blood vessels are present in most embryos of this stage. Bar: 0.1 mm. From Müller and O'Rahilly (1989a).

Fig. 16-17. The hippocampal area, characterized by a marginal layer and a discrete ventricular thickening. Bar: 0.1 mm. From Müller and O'Rahilly (1989a).

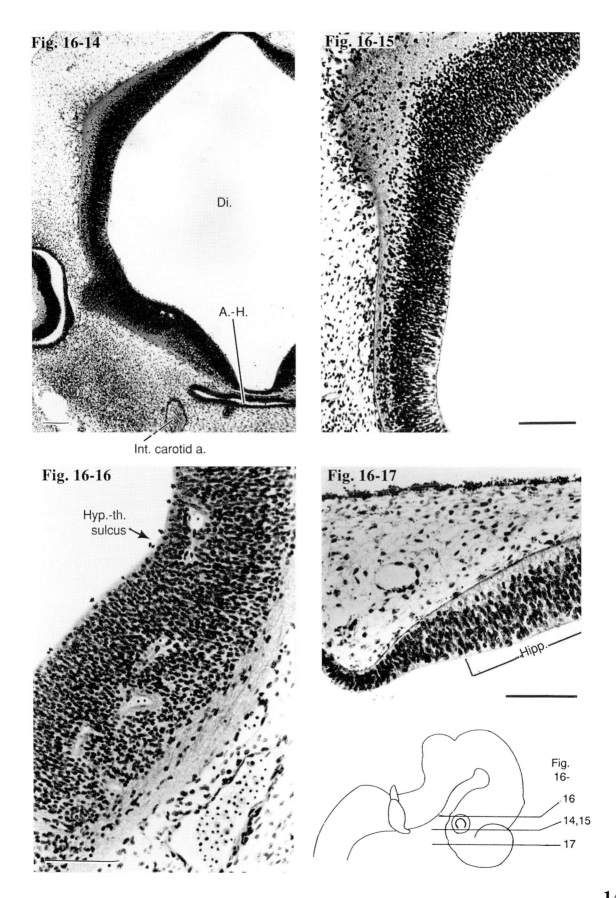

Fig. 16-14

Di.

A.-H.

Int. carotid a.

Fig. 16-15

Fig. 16-16

Hyp.-th. sulcus

Fig. 16-17

Hipp.

Fig. 16-

16

14,15

17

Fig. 16-18. The arterial system at about 4 to 5 postfertilizational weeks. The internal carotid artery is shown in black, and the basilar by horizontal hatching. These four drawings are simplified versions of the graphic reconstructions made by Padget (1948), whose work should be studied for further details. The venous system at stages 14 and 16 has been illustrated by Padget (1957, Figs. 2 and 3).

(**A**) and (**B**) The arteries at stage 13 (CEC 588, with the heart of CEC 836 added in A). Bilateral longitudinal arteries are present and are connected with the internal carotid vessels by the temporary trigeminal and otic arteries (visible ventral to their corresponding ganglia in A), and hypoglossal (marked 12) arteries.

(**C**) The arteries at stage 14 (CEC 2841). The posterior communicating artery can be identified and at this time is the major supply of carotid blood to the hindbrain. Anastomotic channels unite the two longitudinal arteries, thereby initiating the formation of the basilar artery. Aortic arch 2 supplies the hyoid artery, which in turn will give rise to the stapedial artery.

(**D**) The arteries at stage 16 (CEC 617). The two longitudinal vessels have now united to form the basilar artery, and the vertebral arteries are evident.

150

Fig. 16-18.

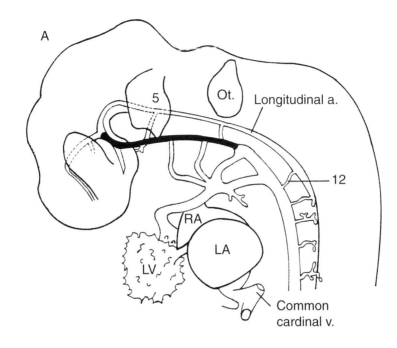

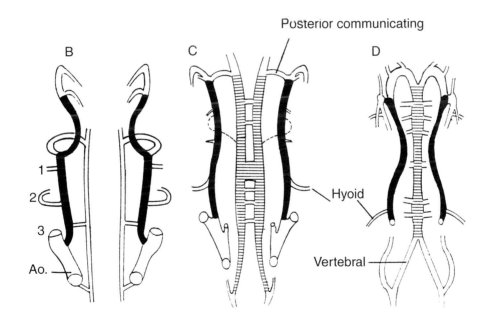

Fig. 16-19. Holoprosencephaly.

(**A**) and (**B**) The normal telencephalon and diencephalon at 5 weeks (stage 16).

(**C–F**) The development of holoprosencephaly.

(**D**) A ventral view in which shading indicates the basal part of the brain that is missing.

(**E**) and (**F**) Dorsal views that show a single telencephalic ventricle. In E the optic cups are partially separated, whereas F has only a single optic cup.

(**G**) Alobar holoprosencephaly in an infant presenting cebocephaly, slight hypotelorism, and median cleft lip and palate.

(**H**) Dorsal view of another example of alobar prosencephaly after removal of the scalp and skull. The single telencephalic ventricle is evident. A to F are based on personal reconstructions, G and H on photographs in Siebert et al. (1990) and in DeMyer (1975), respectively.

From O'Rahilly and Müller (1996a).

Fig. 16-19.

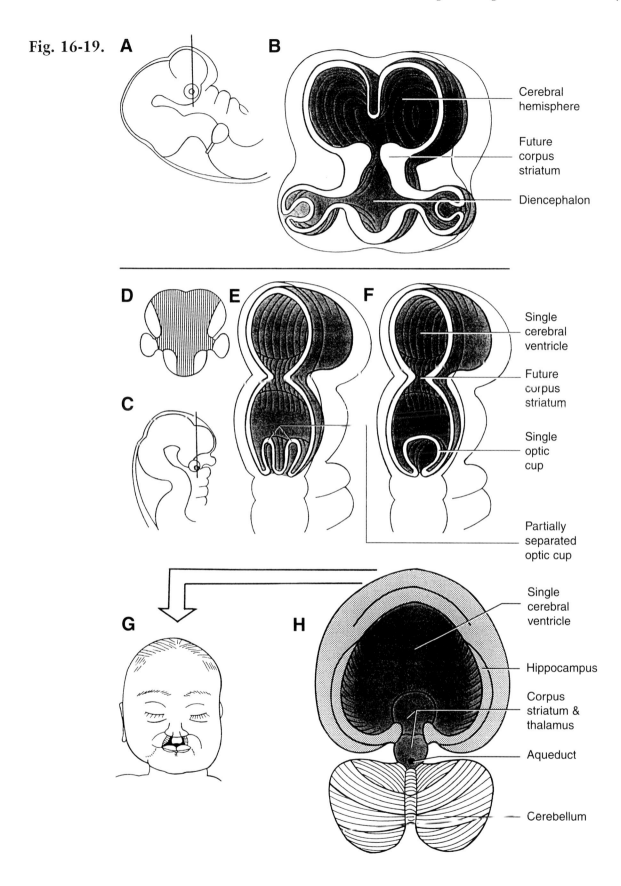

A

B

Cerebral hemisphere

Future corpus striatum

Diencephalon

D

C

E

F

Single cerebral ventricle

Future corpus striatum

Single optic cup

Partially separated optic cup

G

H

Single cerebral ventricle

Hippocampus

Corpus striatum & thalamus

Aqueduct

Cerebellum

153

Comments on Neuroteratology (Stage 16)

Synophthalmia. For an unknown reason, several embryos of this stage showing this variety of cyclopia have been available, and they have been described (Müller and O'Rahilly, 1989c).

Cerebral Asymmetry. A slight asymmetry of the left and right cerebral hemispheres is well documented in the adult and dates back to at least the fetal period (Bossy et al., 1976). It is entirely possible, if not indeed likely, that the asymmetry begins during the embryonic period proper, perhaps even as early as stage 16. Hence some of the problems in lateralization discussed by Geschwind and Galaburda (1985) may have a very early origin.

Holoprosencephaly. The development of this condition was illustrated in Figure 16-19.

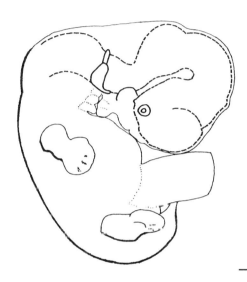

Stage 17: The Future Olfactory Bulb and the First Amygdaloid Nuclei

Approximately 11–14 mm in Greatest Length
Approximately 40 Postfertilizational Days

Fig. 17-1. Right lateral view of an embryo (CEC 6520) of stage 17 with the brain superimposed. From O'Rahilly, Müller, and Bossy (1986).

Rostral and caudodorsal growth of the cerebral hemispheres results in deepening of the longitudinal fissure, in which the vessels of the future choroid plexus develop. The olfactory bulb and tubercle become outlined. The amygdaloid area, which is related to the medial ventricular eminence, contains one or two nuclei. The first indication of a septal nucleus is recognizable. The hemispheric stalk unites the cerebral hemispheres with the ventral thalamus and with the diencephalic part of the medial ventricular eminence. The di-mesencephalic boundary passes between the posterior commissure and the commissure of the superior colliculi (Table 15-1). Gustatory fibers are beginning to separate from the common afferent tract. Further details: Müller and O'Rahilly (1989b).

Fig. 17-2. The various parts of the brain are clearly visible not only in reconstructions but even through the translucent tissues of the intact embryo (CEC 6347). The pontine flexure is now deeper, and the interval between the hypothalamus and the rhombencephalon has become narrow. The future frontal and temporal poles are marked α and γ in the key drawing. A three-dimensional reconstruction, prepared ultrasonically, of the ventricles *in vivo* in an embryo of 13 mm is illustrated by Blaas et al. (1995).

Fig. 17-2.

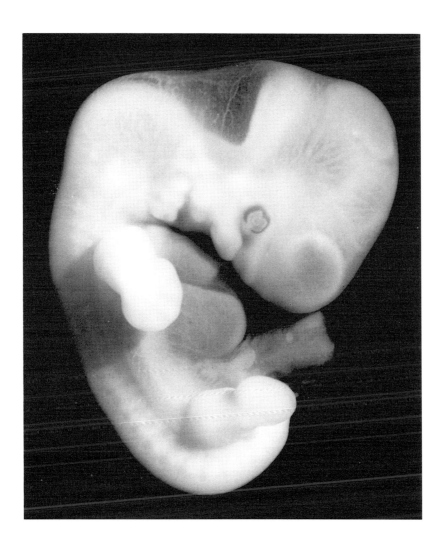

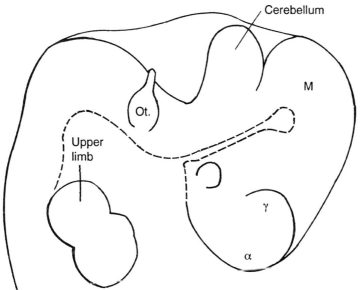

Fig. 17-3. Solid (Born) reconstruction (CEC 6520) and key. The growth of the cerebral hemispheres initiates the appearance of the longitudinal fissure. The telencephalon begins to overlap the diencephalon.

Fig. 17-3.

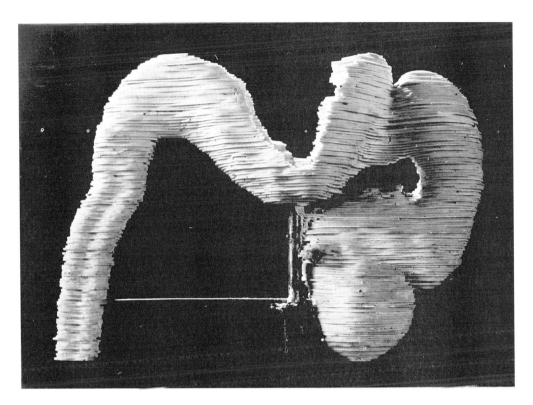

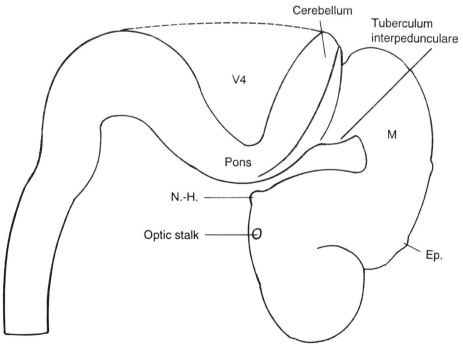

Fig. 17-4. Lateral view (reversed) of the brain (CEC 6258), drawn by Mary M. Cope from a reconstruction and published by Gilbert (1957). An end-on view has been added. The cerebellum has a marginal layer that extends to, although not into, the clearly marked rhombic lip. The lip is a proliferative area in which mitotic figures have become numerous at this stage, as also in the more caudal parts of the rhombencephalon. The cerebellar plate is as wide as the combined width of the two cerebral hemispheres. The inferior cerebellar peduncle is present already, the superior is distinguishable at the next stage, and the middle peduncle develops during the fetal period. The posterolateral fissure delimits the external cerebellar swelling. Included in this figure are the oculomotor and trochlear nerves, the trigeminal ganglion, the three divisions of the trigeminal nerve, and the optic cup.

Fig. 17-5. Graphic reconstruction prepared from transverse sections to show a median view of the brain (CEC 6520). The asterisk indicates the junction with the spinal cord. The medial surface of each cerebral hemisphere has greatly increased and a hemispheric stalk can be identified. This is the junctional area between the telencephalon and the diencephalon. The stalk has been studied by Sharp (1959).

Shown here are the boundaries between the different parts of the brain, the newly developed recesses (arrows), the commissures, the sulci, and the entrance into the optic ventricle (black dot in the diencephalon). Four small arrows indicate the isthmic, supramamillary, inframamillary, and infundibular recesses. The boundaries are summarized in Table 15-1.

The posterior commissure has suddenly appeared and consists of two subcommissures: the posterior commissure *sensu stricto* with fibers of the medial longitudinal bundle, and the commissure of the superior colliculi. Other commissures are the supraoptic in the caudal part of the chiasmatic plate, the supramamillary (dagger), and the commissure of the oculomotor nerves. The ventral commissure of the rhombencephalon, which consists of fibers that cross throughout the length of the floorplate, has not been indicated here. The commissural plate itself does not yet contain crossing fibers.

The sulcus limitans separates the alar and basal laminae of the rhombencephalon and mesencephalon. However, it does not continue into the diencephalon. The hypothalamic sulcus of the diencephalon separates the thalamus *sensu lato* from the hypothalamus *sensu lato* (Table 18-1).

In the inset, features of the medial aspect of the lateral wall of the left cerebral hemisphere have been superimposed on the median reconstruction. The interventricular foramen is surrounded by the hippocampal area of the telencephalon and by the medial ventricular eminence of the diencephalon, as well as by the ventral thalamus. The medial eminence is invading telencephalic territory and is penetrated by blood vessels. The lateral ventricular eminence (Fig. 6-2) is visible in the left hemispheric wall. The internal cerebellar swelling lies between the sulcus limitans and the rhombic lip. Reconstructions from a different embryo (CEC 940) were published by Hines (1922).

Fig. 17-4.

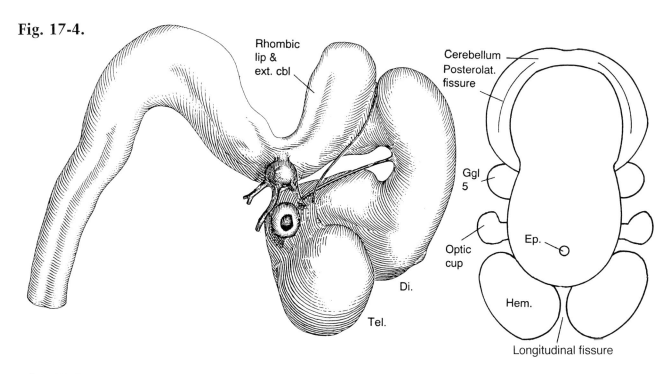

Fig. 17-5.

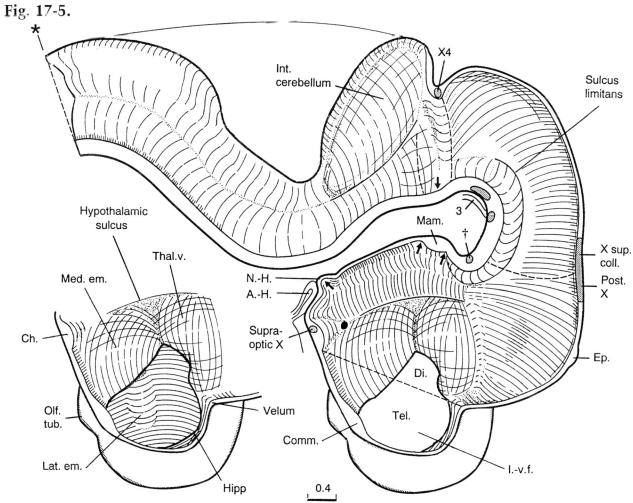

Fig. 17-6. Median section (CEC 8789). All mesenchymal components of the head have increased greatly. Many skeletal elements can already be reconstructed: the stapes, the styloid process, the cartilage (Meckel's) of pharyngeal arch 1, the thyroid laminae, and the cricoid cartilage. The primordia of the so-called hypophysial cartilages (trabeculae; polar cartilages) are present in the area of the future hypophysial fossa. The brain sits on a firm basal condensation of mesenchyme, which, in its rostral part, represents the future nasal septum. This restrains the growth of the cerebral hemispheres in a basal direction. Bar: 1 mm.

The mesenchyme is beginning to form the future dural limiting layer, especially in basal areas, and, beginning at the rostral tip of the notochord, it continues to spread between the diencephalon and the rhombencephalon, i.e., at the site of the mesencephalic flexure. The condensed mesenchyme at the flexure is the primordium of the tentorium cerebelli, which is compressed between the basilar artery and the hypothalamus (Fig. 16-6). The dural limiting layer already contains openings (pori durales) for cranial nerves 3, 4, 5, and 12.

The presence of the dural limiting layer between the pia mater and the skeletogenous sheath initiates the formation of the subarachnoid space. The subarachnoid space clearly begins its development before the presence of choroid plexuses. The roof of the fourth ventricle is very thin. Two areas are beginning to become the areae membranaceae rostralis et caudalis. They are formed by flattened ependymal cells, and their position is indicated by two arrows. Such areas (in the adult mouse) are thought to permit the passage of cerebrospinal fluid containing macromolecules, by way of interependymal cellular clefts. The "ependymal fluid" within the ventricles is believed to be produced by the lining cells that will develop later into ependymal and choroid plexus cells.

Already in the previous stage, the vertebral arteries join the basilar, and an anastomosis is present between the basilar and the internal carotid arteries. An anterior choroid artery is now developing and was reconstructed by Padget (1948, Fig. 5). The main cerebral arteries are now well established. Three dural plexuses (Streeter, 1915, 1918), anterior, middle, and posterior, drain into the primary head sinus and ultimately into the jugular veins (Padget, 1957).

The caudal part of the spinal cord, which forms by secondary neurulation, reaches the caudal tip of the body. The definitive number of somites (usually 39 pairs) seems to be present at this and the next stage. The normal regression of the caudalmost part of the spinal cord may begin at approximately this time.

The key shows the position of the sulcus limitans and the extent of the alar and basal laminae (cf Fig. 6-4). In addition, the median features (recesses and plates) are listed in caudorostral sequence. The neurohypophysis (characterized by folded walls) and the infundibular recess are present in all embryos of this stage.

Cartilage appears in the occipital sclerotomes 1-4, and the hypoglossal foramen has formed in sclerotome 4. The sclerotomic mass is shown in the key.

Fig. 17-6.

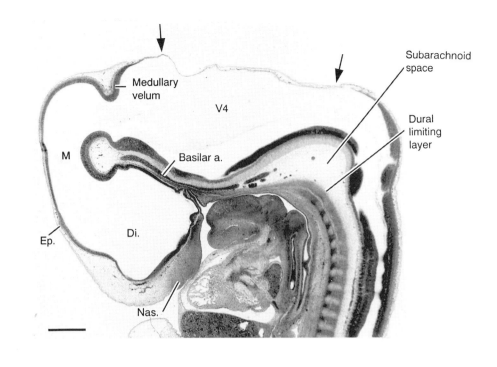

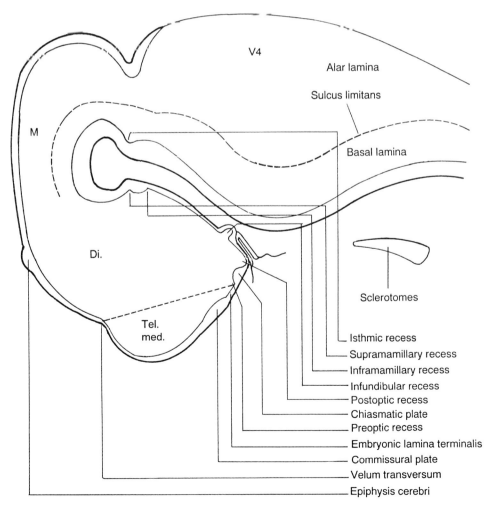

Fig. 17-7. The cranial nerves and tracts (CEC 6520). All cranial nerves have been present since the previous stage. The last of the regular cranial nerves to appear are the abducent and the cochlear, at stage 16. The olfactory fibers, however, become clear in the present stage. Two bundles of nerve fibers, a lateral and a medial, can be distinguished, and at the site of their entrance into the hemispheres, the olfactory bulb will develop in the next stage. The hypoglossal nerve emerges from the occipital sclerotomic mass as either one (as seen here) or two trunks. The ventral ramus of the first cervical nerve joins the hypoglossal. Cervical nerves 1 and 2 unite to form the inferior root of the ansa cervicalis, and the loop is completed by the superior root, which descends from the hypoglossal nerve. Ganglia are indicated by small circles.

Many tracts have appeared during the previous week (from stage 14 onwards). The order of their appearance as determined from graphic reconstructions is: lateral longitudinal fasciculus, common afferent tract, medial longitudinal fasciculus, dorsal funiculus, preopticohypothalamotegmental tract, mesencephalic tract of the trigeminal nerve, medial prosencephalic fasciculus, medial tectobulbar tract, and mamillotegmental and habenulo-interpeduncular tracts. The medial prosencephalic fasciculus contains mainly descending fibers with origin in the amygdaloid and preoptic regions. The habenulo-interpeduncular tract (fasciculus retroflexus) delineates the synencephalon rostrally. Some of the nuclei and areas of loose intermediate layer are indicated by stippling. The term "nucleus" refers here to zones of lower cellular density and slightly larger cellular size. The amygdaloid nuclei form the most histologically advanced area of the cerebral hemispheres. The amygdaloid region is related to the medial ventricular eminence (Fig. 6-2). The subthalamic nucleus, red nucleus, interstitial nucleus, nucleus of the posterior commissure, and nucleus of the mesencephalic tract of the trigeminal nerve, and the locus caeruleus (asterisk) are recognizable. The cells of the locus caeruleus occupy the isthmus and rhombomere 1. Its tall cells, twice the size of ordinary neurons, lie at the innermost aspect of the intermediate layer, ventral to the sulcus limitans. The interstitial nucleus is indicated by a dagger. The gustatory fibers begin to separate from the common afferent tract as the tractus solitarius.

The tectal area of the mesencephalon, shown in stippling, has developed an intermediate layer.

In the cerebellum, cells of the rhombic lip participate in the formation of the dentate and isthmic nuclei, and later (stage 23) in the development of the external germinal layer.

Modified from O'Rahilly, Müller, Hutchins, and Moore (1987).

Fig. 17-8. Photomicrograph showing the periphery of the amygdaloid area (the cortex of the future temporal pole), which contains multiple tall cells with long fibers (CEC 8114); rostral is to the left-hand side of the page. The neurons for the amygdaloid complex belong to the earliest postmitotic neurons. An initial burst of cell formation for the septal nuclei is believed to occur at about this time. Bar: 0.1 mm.

Fig. 17-7.

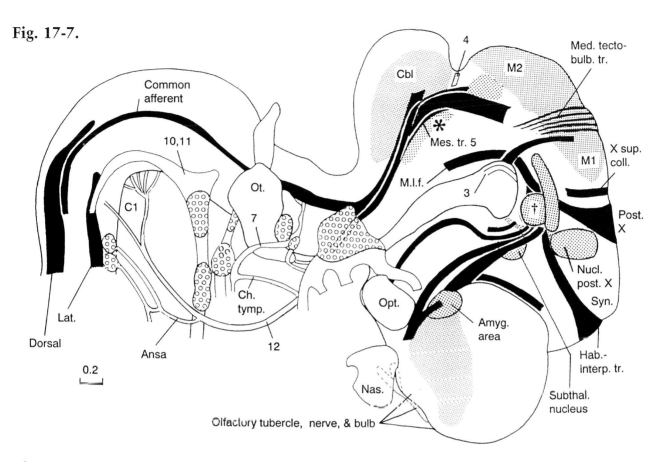

Common afferent

Cbl

4

M2

Med. tecto-bulb. tr.

*

Mes. tr. 5

M.l.f.

3

M1

X sup. coll.

Post. X

10,11

Ot.

C1

7

Ch. tymp.

Opt.

Amyg. area

Nucl. post. X

Syn.

Lat.

Hab.-interp. tr.

Dorsal

Ansa

12

Nas.

Subthal. nucleus

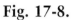

0.2

Olfactory tubercle, nerve, & bulb

Fig. 17-8.

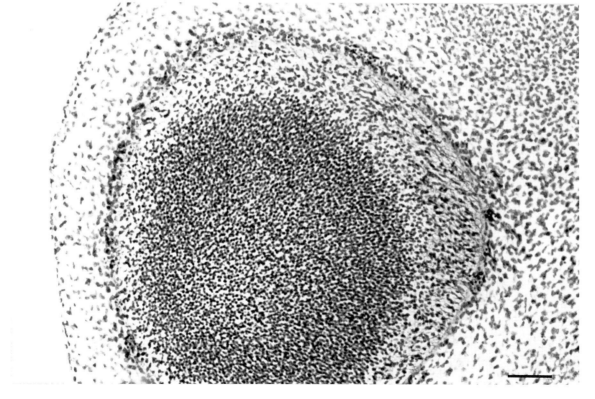

165

Figures 17-9 to 17-13. Horizontal sections through the brain (CEC 6520). The levels of the horizontal sections are indicated in the key drawing. The sections are not quite symmetrical, the left side of the photomicrographs being at a slightly more rostral level than the right. Figures 17-10 to 17-12 were used by Bartelmez and Dekaban (1962). Bars: 0.5 mm.

Fig. 17-9.   The rostralmost section shows only the telencephalic area: the paired cerebral hemispheres, and between them the telencephalon medium. A slight swelling represents the lateral ventricular eminence. The longitudinal cerebral fissure is filled with loose mesenchyme. Here, and elsewhere in the mesenchyme adjacent to the brain, thin-walled blood vessels are numerous, and the anterior choroid artery has appeared. The continuity between the nostril and the nasal sac is visible at the left side. The two nasal sacs are separated by dense mesenchyme that represents the future nasal septum.

Fig. 17-10.   The second section shows the interventricular foramina, which begin their development at about this time. They become relatively narrower as the medial surface of each cerebral hemisphere develops and as the medial ventricular eminence grows.

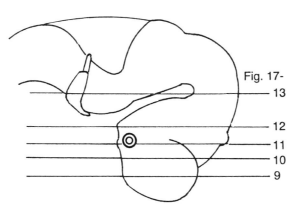

Fig. 17-
13
12
11
10
9

Fig. 17-9.

Fig. 17-10.

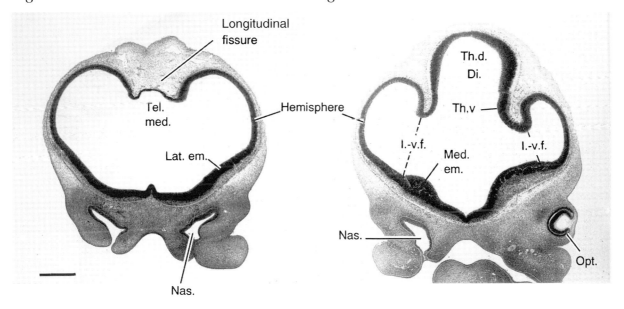

Longitudinal fissure

Tel. med.

Lat. em.

Hemisphere

Nas.

Th.d.
Di.

Th.v

l.-v.f.

Med. em.

l.-v.f.

Nas.

Opt.

Fig. 17-11.   The diencephalon is visible and the dorsal thalamus can be distinguished from the ventral. The two are separated by the marginal ridge (zona limitans intrathalamica of Kuhlenbeck) and are delineated towards the hypothalamus *sensu lato* by the hypothalamic sulcus (Table 18-1). The ventral thalamus (which possesses an intermediate layer) is more advanced than the dorsal thalamus. In the mouse, the zona limitans intrathalamica has been found to be clearly delineated by gene expression. The optic cup is surrounded by condensed material that represents the primordia of the orbital muscles. The retinal ("choroid") fissure of the optic cup is closing. Its continuation on the optic stalk, however, is still open and allows the ingrowth of optic fibers, which begin to develop in this stage. A hyaloid vessel can be seen in the optic stalk. The part of the hemisphere shown contains the amygdaloid area. This figure closely resembles illustrations in various articles (Sidman and Rakic, 1982, Fig. 1-41) and textbooks in which the interpretation is incorrect: a section that includes all five parts of the diencephalon as well as the eyes cannot also pass through the mesencephalon.

Fig. 17-12.   The neurohypophysis and the adenohypophysis are in close apposition, as they are from the beginning of their development, although this is frequently not appreciated. The primordium of the tentorium is attached at the surface of the adenohypophysis.

Fig. 17-13.   The sulcus limitans in the mesencephalon separates the tectum from the tegmentum. The area of the oculomotor nucleus belongs to M2 (future inferior collicular region). Rhombomeres can still be recognized by ventricular grooves. Thinnings appear in the wall of the otic vesicle; the thicker areas represent the future semicircular ducts.

168

Fig. 17-11.

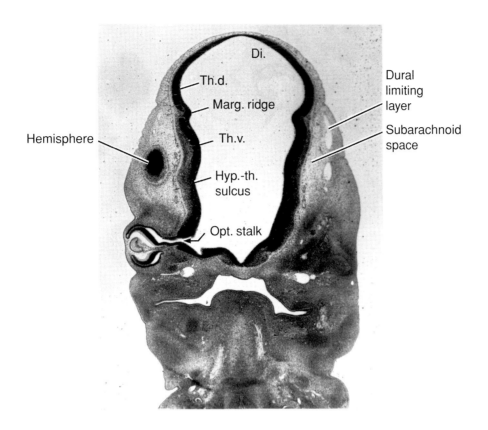

Di.

Th.d.

Marg. ridge

Hemisphere

Th.v.

Hyp.-th. sulcus

Opt. stalk

Dural limiting layer

Subarachnoid space

Fig. 17-12.

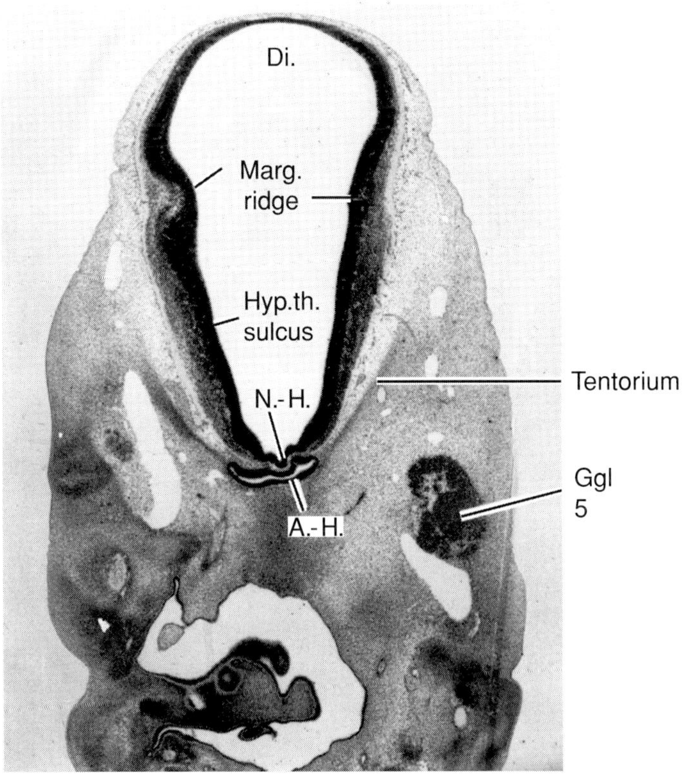

Di.

Marg. ridge

Hyp.th. sulcus

N.-H.

A.-H.

Tentorium

Ggl 5

Fig. 17-13.

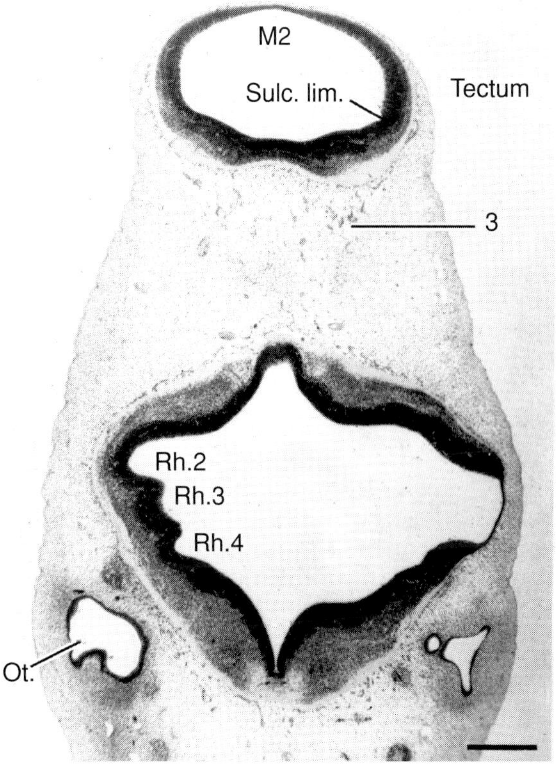

M2

Sulc. lim.

Tectum

3

Rh.2
Rh.3
Rh.4

Ot.

169

Fig. 17-14. The primordial plexiform layer.

(**A**) The earliest afferent (probably catecholamine) fibers in the human embryo can be detected in the primordial plexiform layer of the future temporal cortex at 6 weeks (stage 17; CEC 8114). This is the cortex overlying the primordium of the amygdaloid region. Catecholamine fibers may perhaps participate in early synaptogenesis in the subplate of the human embryo (Larroche, 1981). Axodendritic and axosomatic synapses have been found in the cerebral hemispheres before the appearance of the cortical plate (Choi, 1988). Abbreviations: v, ventricular layer; i, intermediate layer; p, primordial plexiform layer with large neurons. Bar: 20 μm.

(**B**) Epon section (1 μm) of the telencephalic wall of an unstaged human embryo of 6 weeks. The primordial plexiform layer contains scattered Cajal–Retzius cells. The pia mater is visible at the top of the photomicrograph. ×128.

(**C**) Higher-power view of the primordial plexiform layer showing Cajal–Retzius (CR) cells. A glial barrier (the glia limitans, GL) is formed by cell processes at the pial (PM) surface. The glial barrier and the basement membrane are thought to be critical to the migration and final positioning of the neurons and to the differentiation of the laminar cortical pattern within the developing neopallium (Choi, 1994). ×697.

(**D**) Another higher-power view showing Cajal–Retzius cells with ovoid nuclei, prominent nucleoli, and abundant cytoplasm. A mitotic figure is evident in the lower left-hand corner. ×697. B, C, and D are reproduced by courtesy of Ben H. Choi, M.D., Ph.D., University of California, Irvine.

170

Fig. 17-14.

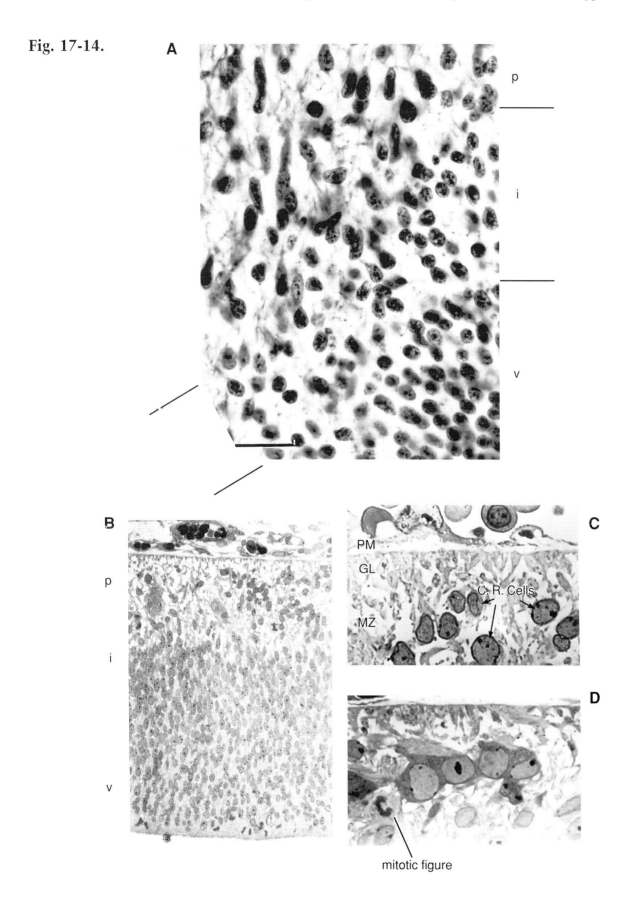

Comments on Neuroteratology (Stage 17)

Dandy–Walker Syndrome. This ill-understood complex includes dysgenesis of the vermis, cystic dilatation of the fourth ventricle, a high tentorium, and hydrocephaly. It is different from the Arnold–Chiari malformation (Gardner, et al., 1975). Lack of patency of one or more of the apertures in the roof of the fourth ventricle is frequent. A number of features are probably secondary rather than primary. Maldevelopment of the ventricular roof (the rostral membranous area) is believed to be an important factor in the development of the abnormality. The time of origin of the condition is probably in the embryonic period proper, likely later than that of the Arnold–Chiari malformation, perhaps 6 to 8 weeks.

Diagnostic studies and clinical experiences can be found in a treatise by Raimondi, et al. (1984).

Dysgenesis of the Optic Nerve. The optic nerves are elaborations of the optic stalks and their persistence depends on the ingrowth of optic nerve fibers. In the absence of such an ingrowth (e.g., because of premature closure of the fissure in the stalk), the optic nerve does not develop.

Neuronal Ectopia. Disruption of the pia–glial barrier may lead to the migration of neurons and glial cells into the subarachnoid space (Choi, 1987).

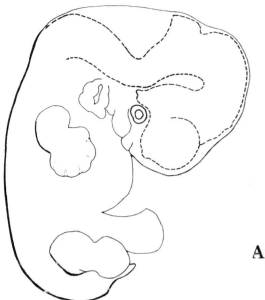

Stage 18: The Future Corpus Striatum, the Inferior Cerebellar Peduncle, and the Dentate Nucleus

Approximately 13–17 mm in Greatest Length
Approximately 42 Postfertilizational Days

Fig. 18-1. Right lateral view of an embryo (CEC 8101) of stage 18 with the brain (D-7924) superimposed. The head is noticeably more compact than in the previous stage. From O'Rahilly, Müller, and Bossy (1986).

The head is now more compact and the cerebral hemispheres are slightly flattened in the future insular region. The olfactory bulb and tubercle are separated by a sulcus. The C-shaped hippocampus, accompanied by the area dentata, reaches the olfactory region. The lateral ventricular eminence of the future corpus striatum (Fig. 6-2) is distinct. Four amygdaloid nuclei are present in the region of the medial ventricular eminence, so that the archistriatum is now identifiable. The interventricular foramina are relatively narrower. The prosencephalic septum is recognizable. Optic fibers form, although they do not yet enter the chiasmatic plate. The red nucleus is present and the substantia nigra is beginning to develop. The external cerebellar swellings represent the flocculi. The internal cerebellar swellings contain the dentate nuclei. The inferior cerebellar peduncles reach the region of these nuclei. The primary sensory nuclei of the rhombencephalon are now present. Choroid plexuses develop in the lateral as well as in the fourth ventricle, so that the production of cerebrospinal fluid *sensu stricto* can now begin. The vomeronasal organ, nerve, and ganglion have appeared. At least two semicircular ducts are isolated. Further details: Müller and O'Rahilly (1990a).

173

Fig. 18-2. Right lateral view of the brain (CEC 492). The cerebral hemispheres are slightly flattened in the area overlying the corpus striatum, i.e., in the future insular region. Frontal and temporal poles are indicated in the key by α and γ respectively. The optic cups are assuming a more ventral position.

The pontine flexure is deep, in association with shortening of the head. The bilateral cerebellar swellings (*äusserer Kleinhirnwulst* of Hochstetter, 1929) represent the flocculi, which are delineated by the posterolateral fissure. The rhombic lip is part of the external cerebellar swelling and is characterized by "non-surface mitotic" figures, which are found also in the otic region, where the rhombic lip seems to participate in the formation of the cochlear nuclei. The ventral outpocketing of the isthmus was named *Isthmushöcker* and *Tuberculum interpedunculare* (dagger) by Hochstetter (1919). It is identified also in the key to Figure 17-3. It serves as an important landmark for the localization of the interpeduncular nucleus, because dopaminergic cells develop rostral to this ventral projection. The semicircular ducts are becoming isolated one from another, and at least two are distinct, which is typical for this stage. The main events in the development of the ear have been summarized elsewhere (O'Rahilly, 1983).

The inset is an end-on view showing the cerebellar plate, mesencephalon, epiphysis cerebri, diencephalon, and cerebral hemispheres.

The cerebellar plate is still slightly wider than the combined cerebral hemispheres. The posterolateral or dorsolateral fissure (Larsell, 1947) or sulcus transitorius (Hochstetter, 1929) is marking off the rhombencephalic lip, including the anlage of the flocculus (Larsell, 1947), whereas according to Hochstetter this area represents the external cerebellar swelling and is more than the primordium of the flocculus. Comparison between Hochstetter's figures and the reconstructions of the present authors would suggest that only the most lateral part of the external cerebellar bulge is the primodium of the flocculus, and that it probably corresponds to the *Randstreifen*, which gives rise also to the nodule and to the inferior medullary velum.

Fig. 18-2.

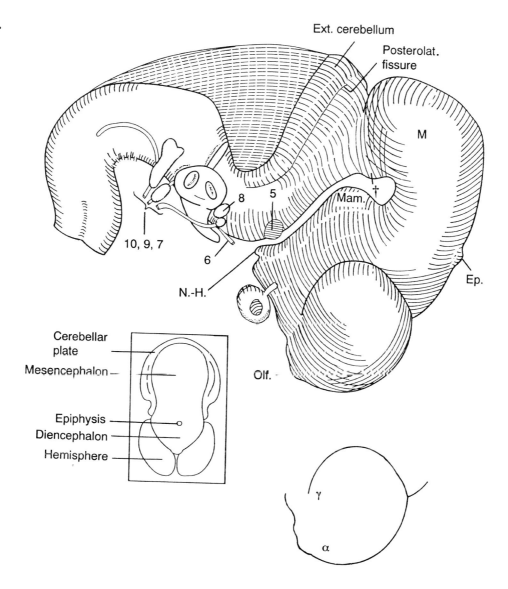

Ext. cerebellum

Posterolat. fissure

M

10, 9, 7

8

5

6

Mam.

+

N.-H.

Ep.

Cerebellar plate

Mesencephalon

Epiphysis

Diencephalon

Hemisphere

Olf.

γ

α

Fig. 18-3. Graphic reconstruction prepared from transverse sections to show a median view of the brain (D-7924). The asterisk indicates the junction with the spinal cord. The olfactory bulb is separated from the olfactory tubercle by a groove, the sulcus circularis rhinencephali (Fig. 18-9). The bulb shows a recess, and the olfactory ventricle is forming.

In the inset, the medial wall of the left hemisphere is shown as if transparent, so that the C-shaped hippocampus can be seen to reach the olfactory region. It is accompanied by a small rim of area dentata, adjacent to which the area epithelialis is visible. In the future corpus striatum, a groove (the "intereminential" sulcus) separates the medial from the lateral ventricular eminence. The interventricular foramina become relatively narrower, chiefly because of the enormous growth of the medial ventricular eminence. Each foramen is bounded rostroventrally by the commissural plate and the medial ventricular eminence (Fig. 6-2), and dorsocaudally by the ventral thalamus. The medial eminence continues to invade telencephalic territory, as seen rostral to the interrupted line that extends from the preoptic recess to the velum transversum.

The prosencephalic (forebrain) septum is the area between the embryonic lamina terminalis and the olfactory bulb. It can be regarded as a junctional region where hippocampal, amygdaloid, and olfactory germinal matrices meet. What has been termed the septum verum (Andy and Stephan, 1968) is the basal part of the medial walls of the hemispheres. Hence it is formed when the hemispheres expand beyond the lamina terminalis, beginning at stage 17. The fibers of the supraoptic commissure, which are fine and pale, can readily be distinguished from the optic fibers, which appear coarse and black. Although optic fibers are present in about half the embryos of stage 18, they do not yet enter the chiasmatic plate. The adenohypophysial pouch is now closed off from the pharynx, with which it is connected by a solid epithelial cord.

The caudodorsal part of the midbrain is wide, presaging the appearance of a cul-de-sac (*hinterer Mittelhirnblindsack* of Turkewitsch, 1935). The midventral proliferative area participates in the formation of the red nucleus and the substantia nigra. The latter has been stated to develop in the monkey at a time that would correspond to human stages 18–21.

The internal cerebellar swelling of Rh.1 is more prominent than the tegmentum. It contains the dentate nucleus (reconstructed by O'Rahilly, Müller, Hutchins, and Moore, 1988), the site of which is shown here by an interrupted line.

Choroid folds are present bilaterally in the fourth ventricle of nearly half of the embryos, and their villi present cylindrical cells characterized by protrusions into the ventricular cavity.

A photomicrograph of a median section has been published (Müller and O'Rahilly, 1990a, Fig. 1B).

176

Fig. 18-3.

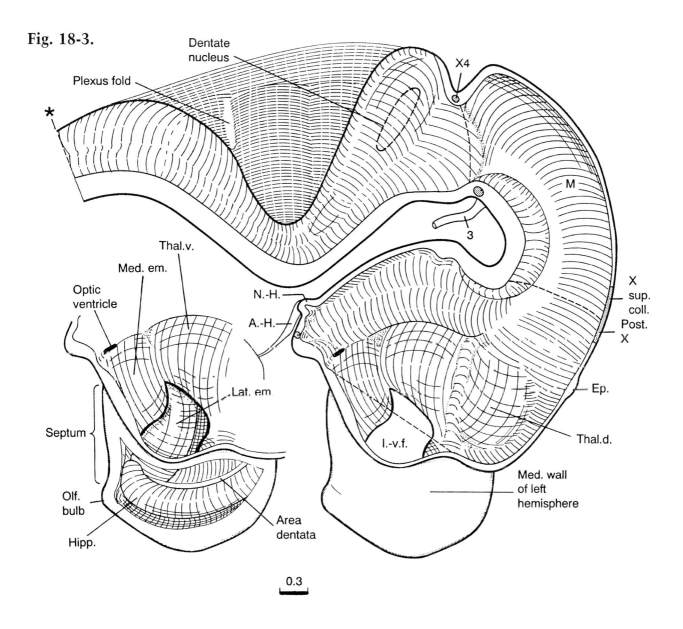

0.3

Fig. 18-4. The cerebral hemispheres and relationships between the diencephalon and the telencephalon. The di-telencephalic border (arrowheads) is shown in (A)–(C). The primordial plexiform layer extends over most of the cerebral hemispheres. It contains horizontally branching corticipetal fibers, vertical cytoplasmic prolongations of the neuroepithelial cells, and occasional neurons (Marín-Padilla, 1978).

(**A**) Ventral view showing olfactory and optic areas (G-15.5). The adenohypophysis, neurohypophysis, nasal sacs, and medial and lateral ventricular eminences (interrputed lines) are projected onto the ventral surface, and the chiasmatic plate is marked. The supraoptic commissure is formed by fibers of the preoptico-hypothalamic tract (dagger).

(**B**) Dorsal view from the same embryo. The di-telencephalic border passes caudal to the paraphysis. Newly arisen nuclei in the dorsal thalamus are marked by asterisks. The sites of medial and lateral ventricular eminences are indicated by interrupted lines. The longitudinal fissure occupies approximately a third of the cerebral hemispheres.

(**C**) Frontoventral view (D-7924) showing the relationship between the olfactory and amygdaloid areas. (This view appears foreshortened in comparison with A because of its different angle of projection.) The optic nerves reach the diencephalon lateral to the rostral part of the chiasmatic plate.

(**D**) The future temporal pole with the projected amygdaloid nuclei (hatched) of the right cerebral hemisphere (D-7310) and the future insula. The future insula is the flat area overlying the region of the lateral ventricular eminence, i.e., the future corpus striatum (interrupted line).

Fig. 18-4.

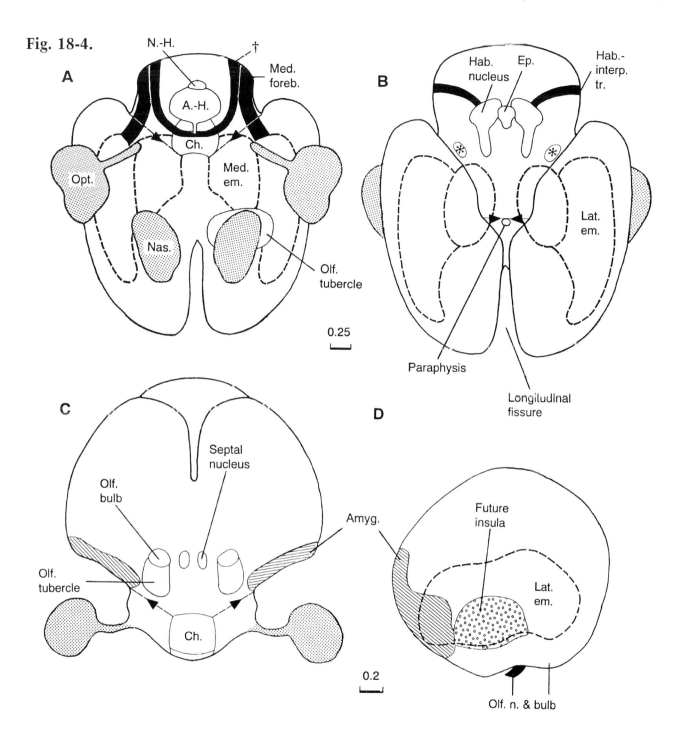

Fig. 18-5. The future amygdaloid body indicates the developing temporal pole (D-7924). Three blocks through the ventricular eminences are presented, as shown in the key (D). The di-telencephalic sulcus is marked by a long black arrow. The small arrow points to the hypothalamic sulcus.

(**A**) The lateral ventricular eminence, which is visible adjacent to the roof of the interventricular foramen.

(**B**) Four amygdaloid nuclei, which are arising almost entirely from the medial ventricular eminence. The nuclei present at this stage are cortical (1), anterior (2), basolateral (3), and medial (4). The medial ventricular eminences are clearly visible. Humphrey (1968) provided the only detailed study of the development of the human amygdaloid body, but did not make reconstructions. Her claim that the human amygdaloid body is derived exclusively from the telencephalon is incorrect. The lateral and particularly the medial eminence at stages 18–20 contain large cavities that were observed by earlier investigators.

(**C**) The basal part of the cerebral hemispheres, showing the ventral thalami. The optic stalk enters at the rostral part of the chiasmatic plate.

(**D**) The right cerebral hemisphere and the ventricular eminences are projected onto a median section. The asterisk indicates the site of the future temporal pole. From Müller and O'Rahilly (1990a).

Fig. 18-5.

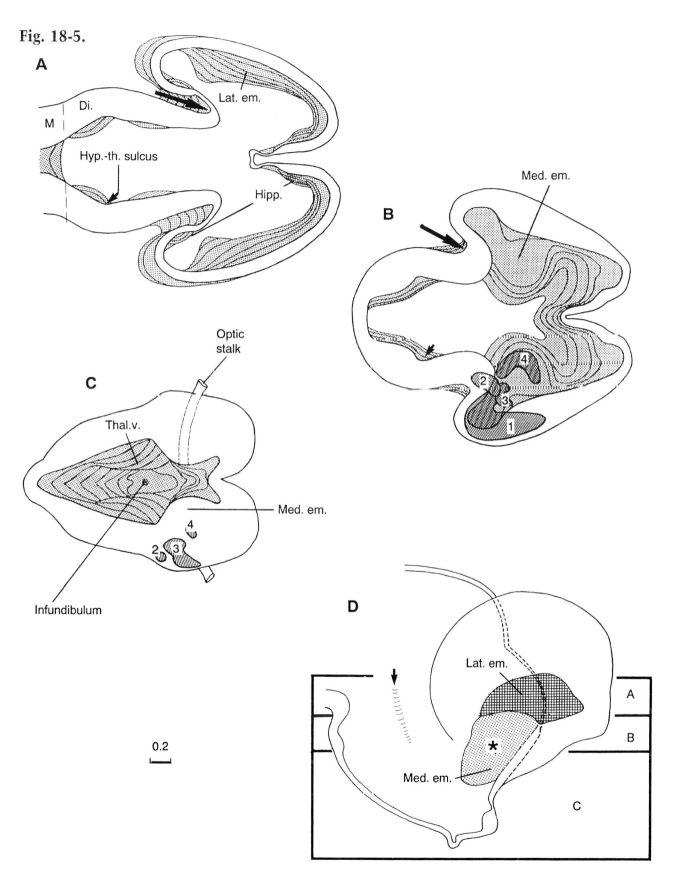

Figures 18-6 to 18-13. The bars represent 0.2 mm.

Fig. 18-6. The di-telencephalic transition (CEC 7707) showing the zona limitans intrathalamica, ventral thalamus, subthalamus, and hypothalamus. Two amygdaloid nuclei (the medial, No. 4, and the basolateral, No. 3) are identifiable.

The five subdivisions of the diencephalon (Table 18-1) are based on the comportment of their matrix zones, as elucidated by Kahle (1956), adopted by Richter (1965), and confirmed by Müller and O'Rahilly (1988c). The subdivision of dorsal and ventral thalami used by Bartelmez and Dekaban (1962) and Kuhlenbeck (1978) is similar, although based on different grounds. The dorsal and ventral thalami are separated by the sulcus medius, which is adjacent to the marginal ridge that overlies the zona limitans intrathalamica. This last is the precursor of the lamina medullaris externa. Hochstetter (1919) marked the marginal ridge by *"Leiste"* and generally by an asterisk. His S.M. (Sulcus Monroi, hypothalamic sulcus) has been incorrectly taken by many writers to be the sulcus medius.

Fig. 18-7. A section from the same embryo (CEC 7707) to show the interventricular foramen, the medial ventricular eminence, and the amygdaloid area. The medial prosencephalic (forebrain) bundle is indicated by an arrowhead. The optic stalk and a portion of the eye are visible below. The ventricular eminences show a distinct subventricular layer. In addition to their separation by the sulcus medius, the ventral thalamus is distinguishable by its possession of a distinct intermediate layer, whereas the dorsal thalamus has only ventricular and marginal layers. Intramural capillaries penetrate the ventricular layers, but the vessels in the subarachnoid space are not yet distinguishable histologically as arteries and veins.

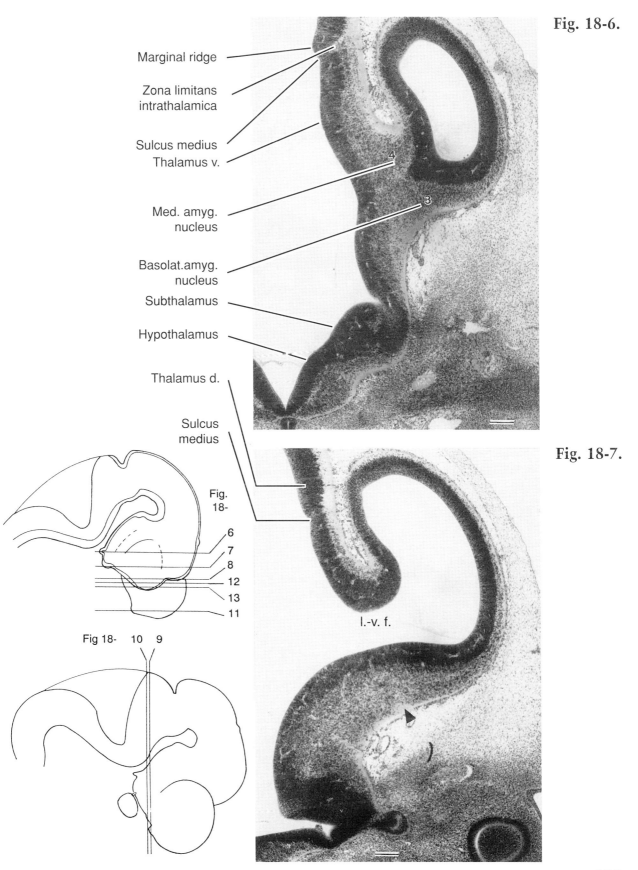

Fig. 18-6.

Marginal ridge

Zona limitans
intrathalamica

Sulcus medius
Thalamus v.

Med. amyg.
nucleus

Basolat.amyg.
nucleus

Subthalamus

Hypothalamus

Thalamus d.

Sulcus
medius

Fig.
18-

6
7
8
12
13
11

Fig 18-   10   9

Fig. 18-7.

l.-v. f.

The levels of the sections in Figures 18-8 to 18-13 are given in key drawings adjacent to Figure 18-7.

Fig. 18-8.   The rostral area (CEC 6529) showing the lateral ventricular eminences, the paraphysis in the roof between the hemispheres, and beginning vacuoles in the subdural space. The roof of the telencephalon medium and the lamina epithelialis of the lateral ventricle form a choroid fold that is lined by a relatively thick epithelial layer of four to five nuclear rows. The nasal sacs are evident, as well as related mesenchymal condensations, especially that of the nasal septum.

The neocortical differentiation of an embryo of stage 18 was illustrated by Marín-Padilla (1983, 1988a).

Fig. 18-9.   The olfactory bulbs (CEC 492), separated from the septal area by the sulcus circularis (arrowhead). The longitudinal fissure, filled with mesenchyme, can be seen between the hemispheres below.

Fig. 18-10.   The prosencephalic septum and the olfactory tubercles (CEC 492). The arrowheads point to cellular islands. The light area marked by an asterisk is the olfactory nerve.

Fig. 18-11.   The cerebral hemispheres and the olfactory nerves (CEC 7707). The arrowhead points to the intermediate layer along the lateral ventricular eminence, the primordium of the future caudate nucleus. The dark cells between the olfactory bulbs and the nasal sacs (visible also in Figs. 18-12 and 18-13) are neural crest and ganglionic cells. The olfactory bulb is indicated, and the numeral 1 marks the olfactory nerve.

Fig. 18-12.   The caudal part of the nasal sacs (G-13.5). The oronasal membrane (arrowhead) has almost regressed on the other side.

Fig. 18-13.   The vomeronasal ganglion (v-n), the nerve fibers of which begin in the wall of the vomeronasal organ (G-13.5), which appears bilaterally as an epithelial pocket in the nasal septum. Further details: O'Rahilly and Müller (1987a). The organ continues to enlarge during prenatal life, and measurements have been published (Smith et al., 1997). Its involution postnatally has been queried.

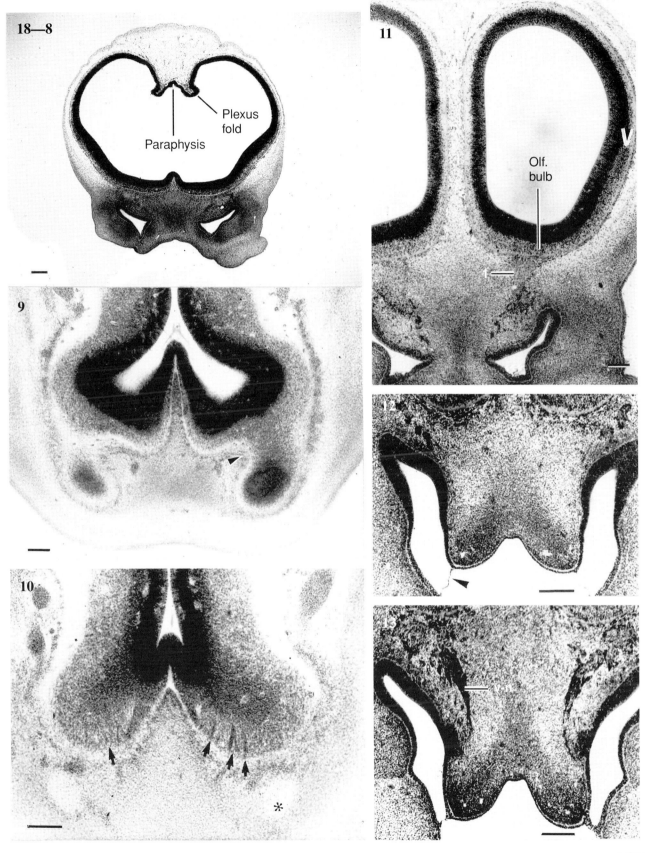

Fig. 18-14. Hypophysis and epiphysis.

(**A**) A transverse section at stage 18 (CEC 7707) to show the hypophysis. The adenohypophysis and the neurohypophysis are in close apposition; mesenchyme has not yet infiltrated between them. In contrast, vascular mesenchyme has penetrated between the adenohypophysis and the hypothalamic floor. The folded wall of the neurohypophysis seems to be characteristic at this time. Various extensions of the lumen of the adenohypophysial pouch have been described (Conklin, 1968). × 133.

(**B**) A transverse section of the same embryo to show the epiphysis, which now appears as a dorsal evagination of the synencephalon. One so-called follicle is visible. The adjacent part of the diencephalic roof is a portion of the habenular region. The epiphysis is now at *Stadium III* of Turkewitsch (1933). × 214.

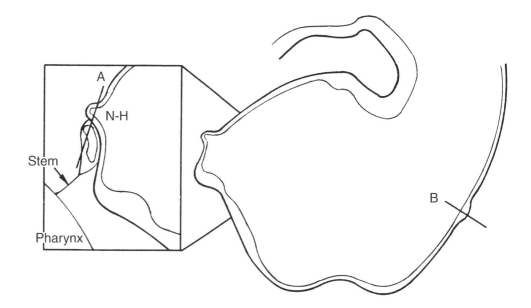

Fig. 18-14. A

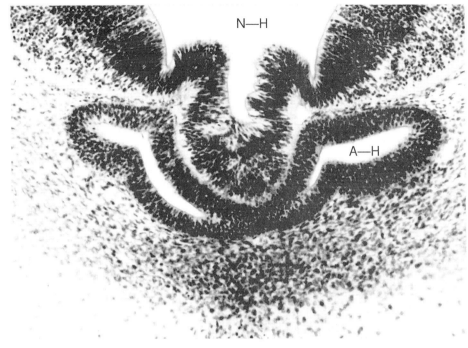

B

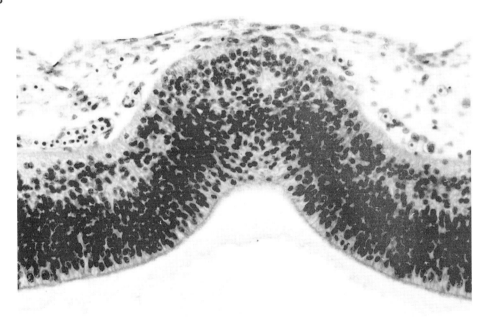

Fig. 18-15. The cerebellar plate at stage 18.

(**A**) Medial view of the right half of the brain, indicating the right part of the cerebellar plate shown in B.

(**B**) Medial view, as seen from the ventricular cavity, to show the internal cerebellar swelling. The cerebellar primordium is formed not only by rhombomere 1 but also by a part of the isthmus.

(**C**) Left lateral view of the brain, indicating the portion shown in D.

(**D**) Left lateral view to show the external cerebellar swelling. Cranial nerve 8 is in close proximity and vestibular fibers from it already reach the flocculus.

(**E**) A block of tissue shown in F and G has been removed from D.

(**F**) The posterolateral fissure delimits the rhombic lip and the primordium of the flocculus from the remainder of the alar lamina. The fibers to and from the cerebellum are arranged in two strata, internal and external; the latter is the marginal layer. The fibers to the primordium of the flocculus are mostly vestibulocerebellar (shown by small black arrows at the level of the external cerebellar swelling).

(**G**) To clarify the two sources of the cells that build up the cerebellum: (1) radially migrating cells produced by the ventricular layer, and (2) tangentially migrating cells from the rhombic lip. The two streams intermingle. The open (white) arrow marks the direction of the afferent fibers to the cerebellum. (F) and (G) from Müller and O'Rahilly (1990a).

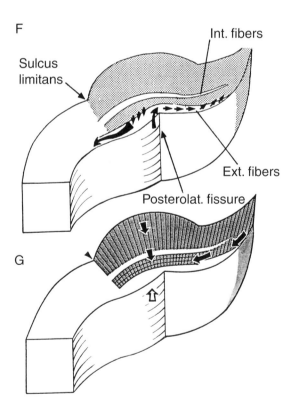

Fig. 18-15.

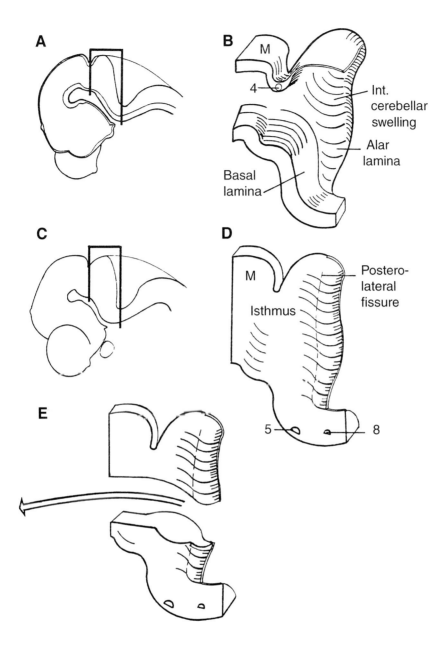

Fig. 18-16. Transverse sections through the cerebellum (CEC 7707).

(**A**) A laterally situated band of cells that represents the region of the future flocculus. The internal cerebellar swelling (i) faces the fourth ventricle.

(**B**) The transitional region between the internal (above) and external (below) cerebellar swellings (e). Two streams of cellular migration can be recognized and are indicated by arrows in the upper inset drawing: (1) radially oriented cells produced in the ventricular layer form the main cellular mass, and (2) tangentially oriented cells produced by the rhombic lip form a peripheral band. A layer of nerve fibers is present internal to that band, and another external to it.

Fig. 18-16.

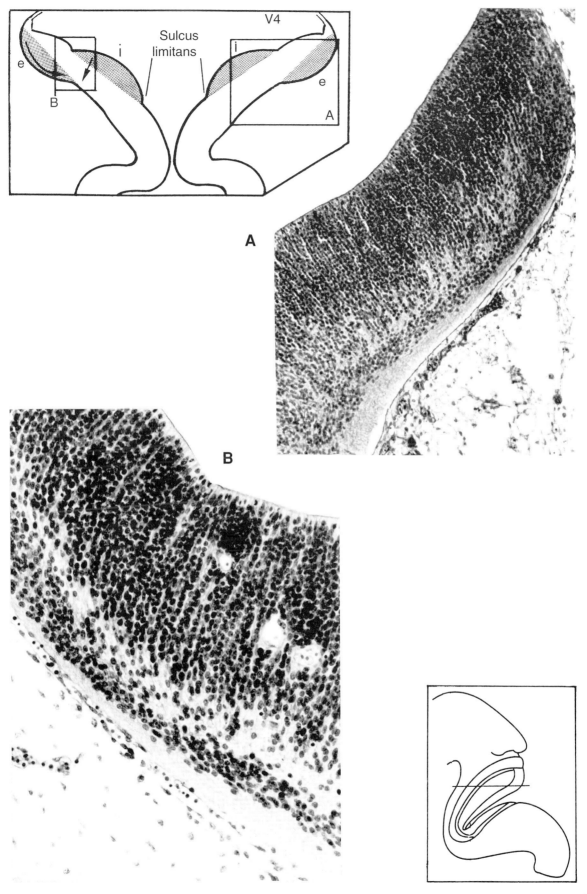

Fig. 18-17. The nuclei of the cranial nerves (D-7924). The visceral efferent, ventromedial cell column and the nuclei derived from it are hatched. The somatic efferent nuclei and the reticular formation are stippled. The afferent nuclei are marked by dots. Comments on the original site of the nuclei and their migration were included in the legend of Figure 14-4.

(**A**) The oculomotor nucleus lies lateral to the midventral proliferative area and the interpeduncular nucleus. The material of the interpeduncular nucleus has been identifiable since stage 15.

(**B**) The trochlear nucleus in the isthmus has a more medial position than the oculomotor nucleus.

(**C**) and (**D**) The trigeminal area is continuous with the cerebellar plate. An afferent trigeminal nucleus has appeared.

(**E**) The dorsal nucleus of the trapezoid body or superior olivary nucleus (dagger) is lateral to the reticular formation. The medial cell column for the facial nerve is still voluminous. Only a few fibers of the genu cross the rostral part of the abducent nucleus.

(**F**) Fibers of the cochlear nerve with the basal and dorsal cochlear nuclei. Also recognizable is the vestibular zone with fibers to the medial longitudinal fasciculus. The nuclei of the abducent (6) and (in G and H) hypoglossal (12) nerves are in a similar position, but are not continuous.

(**G**) The glossopharyngeal nerve with its motor and sensory components, and the cell mass derived from the rhombic lip.

(**H**) The nucleus ambiguus of the vagus.

Abbreviations: m and s (after the numeral of a cranial nerve, motor and sensory components, respectively. From Müller and O'Rahilly (1990a).

Tracts present at stage 18 include the stria medullaris thalami, mamillothalamic tract, medial and lateral tectobulbar, dentatorubral, and the tractus solitarius. The inferior cerebellar peduncles have been reconstructed (O'Rahilly, Müller, Hutchins, and Moore 1988). They contain vestibulocerebellar and trigeminocerebellar fibers, and they reach the region of the dentate nuclei (Fig. 18-3). Collateral vestibular fibers run to the flocculus. The tracts mentioned will be illustrated with the next stage.

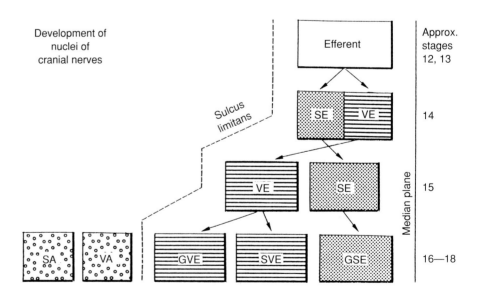

Fig. 18-17.

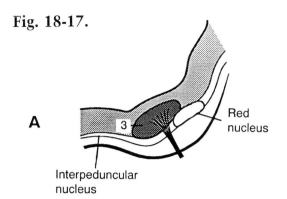

A

Red
nucleus

Interpeduncular
nucleus

3

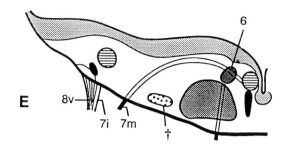

E

6

8v

7i 7m

†

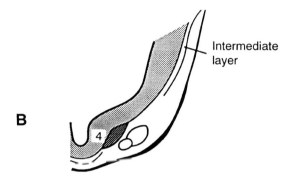

B

Intermediate
layer

4

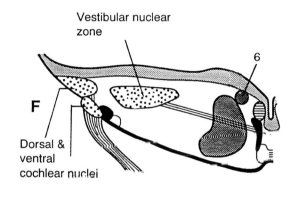

F

Vestibular nuclear
zone

6

Dorsal &
ventral
cochlear nuclei

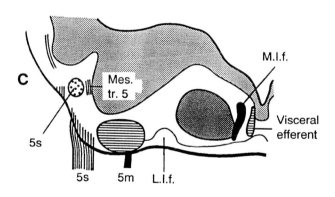

C

Mes.
tr. 5

M.l.f.

Visceral
efferent

5s

5s   5m   L.l.f.

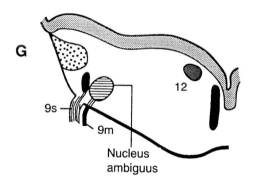

G

12

9s

9m

Nucleus
ambiguus

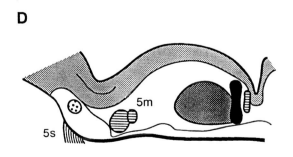

D

5m

5s

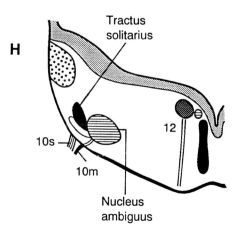

H

Tractus
solitarius

10s

10m

12

Nucleus
ambiguus

193

TABLE 18-1.   **Longitudinal Zones of the Diencephalon**

	Zone	Fig.*	Sulcus
			Di-telencephalic sulcus
Thalamus	1. Epithalamus		
	2. Dorsal thalamus	16-12 17-10 18-6	
		17-11 18-6 18-7	Sulcus medius, marginal ridge, zona limitans intrathalamica
	3. Ventral thalamus	16-12 18-6	
			Hypothalamic sulcus
Hypothalamus *sensu lato*	4. Subthalamus	18-6	
			Faint, unnamed sulcus
	5. Hypothalamus *sensu stricto*	18-6	

* The figure references are to photomicrographs. Further details are given in Table 20-1.

Stage 19: The Choroid Plexus of the Fourth Ventricle and the Medial Accessory Olivary Nucleus

---

**Approximately 16–18 mm in Greatest Length
Approximately 44 Postfertilizational Days**

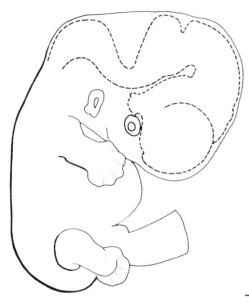

Fig. 19-1. Right lateral view of an embryo (CEC 4501) of stage 19 with the brain (D-203) superimposed. From O'Rahilly, Müller, and Bossy (1986).

Caution needs to be exercised in assigning an embryo to stages 19–23, and details of internal structure are particularly important here. The embryo (which is human since the time of fertilization) now has a recognizably human face (Padget, 1957).

The olfactory nerve, bulb, and tubercle are well developed. The nucleus accumbens appears. The cerebral hemispheres have grown rostrally, so that the prosencephalic septum has become larger. A paraphysis may be present and is telencephalic. Optic fibers arrive in the chiasmatic plate. The globus pallidus externus has developed in the diencephalon. The dorsal and ventral thalami are demarcated by the marginal ridge, and the dorsal thalamus shows an intermediate layer. The habenular region and its connections are well formed. Many bundles are identifiable, including the thalamostriatal and the stria medullaris thalami. The fourth ventricle possesses lateral recesses and a choroid fold. Cerebellar connections are increasing. The medial accessory olivary nucleus is beginning to form. Electrical activity can be detected in the brain stem at about stages 18 and 19 (Borkowski and Bernstine, 1955). Three semicircular ducts are isolated. The basicranium comprises occipital and sphenoidal parts. Further details: Müller and O'Rahilly (1990a).

195

Fig. 19-2. Lateral view (reversed) of the brain (CEC 5609), drawn by Mary M. Cope from a reconstruction and published by Gilbert (1957). For the first time, an occipital pole can be indicated (β in the key drawing). The olfactory bulb and tubercle are visible. The well-developed olfactory nerve, although not shown here, can be seen in Figure 19-10. The roof of the fourth ventricle is shown intact. Because of the pronounced pontine flexure in this embryo, the roof represents mostly the area of the lateral recess. The inset (end-on view) demonstrates that the cerebellar plates are still wide and that their width equals that of the cerebral hemispheres. Cranial nerves 2 to 5 have been included. The insular region was identified by Rager (1972, Fig. 7) in an intact embryo of 17 mm. The cerebellar plate is "vertical" and at almost a right angle to the longitudinal axis of the rest of the rhombencephalon.

Fig. 19-2.

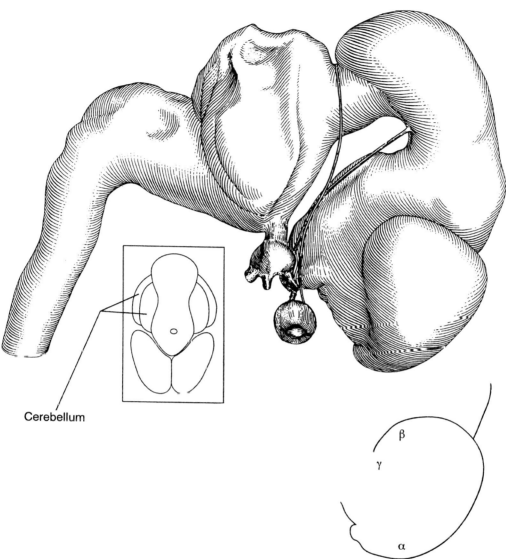

Cerebellum

Fig. 19-3. Graphic reconstruction prepared from transverse sections to show a median view of the brain (D-9588). The asterisk indicates the junction with the spinal cord. Clearly the cerebral hemispheres have grown rostrally, and hence the prosencephalic septum (inset) has increased in size. The nuclei in the septum will be discussed with the next stage. The interventricular foramen is narrow and is bounded mainly by the ventral thalamus (dorsally), the medial ventricular eminence (ventrally), and the hippocampal region (rostrally). Some embryos possess a paraphysis, which opens into the telencephalic part of the third ventricle. The choroid plexus becomes visible by ultrasonography *in vivo* at 7 postovulatory (9 menstrual) weeks.

The di-telencephalic borderline is indicated by an interrupted line between the velum transversum and the preoptic sulcus. The first optic fibers arrive in the chiasmatic plate but do not yet cross to the opposite side. The commissure shown is formed by supraoptic fibers. The epiphysis cerebri is adjacent to the posterior commissure and contains several follicles. At stages 19–21 it corresponds in general to *Stadium IV* of Turkewitsch (1933), as pointed out by O'Rahilly (1968). The globus pallidus externus has developed in the subthalamus. The dorsal and ventral thalami are well separated from each other by the marginal ridge associated with the sulcus medius at the ventricular side and with the zona limitans intrathalamica (Fig. 18-6). The dorsal thalamus possesses an intermediate layer. The epithalamus is well delimited, and its habenular nucleus (Fig. 19-9) has sent fibers (the habenulo-interpeduncular tract) to the midbrain since stage 17. The fibers arriving in the habenular area constitute the stria medullaris thalami, and arise mostly in the nucleus ovalis of the diencephalon (Figs. 19-7 and 19-16). Medial and lateral ventricular eminences, seen partly by transparency, are shown in the inset.

The isthmic groove between the mesencephalon and the cerebellum is indicated by a short arrow. The lateral recess and choroid fold of the fourth ventricle are shown. The floor of the rhombencephalon is thickened, and this will become more pronounced with the addition of further fibers in subsequent stages. The medial accessory olivary nucleus (Fig. 19-4) is beginning to form in between the roots of the hypoglossal nerve, and its site is indicated schematically by a projection onto the median plane. The lemniscal decussation is visible.

The characteristic hairpin bend of the mesencephalic flexure is formed by the metencephalon and the diencephalon, and indicates the site of the future pontine and interpeduncular cisterns of the subarachnoid space. The apex of the flexure marks the exit of the oculomotor nerves. The pontine flexure is eliminated later, so that the medulla and pons are in a straight line postnatally.

198

Fig. 19-3.

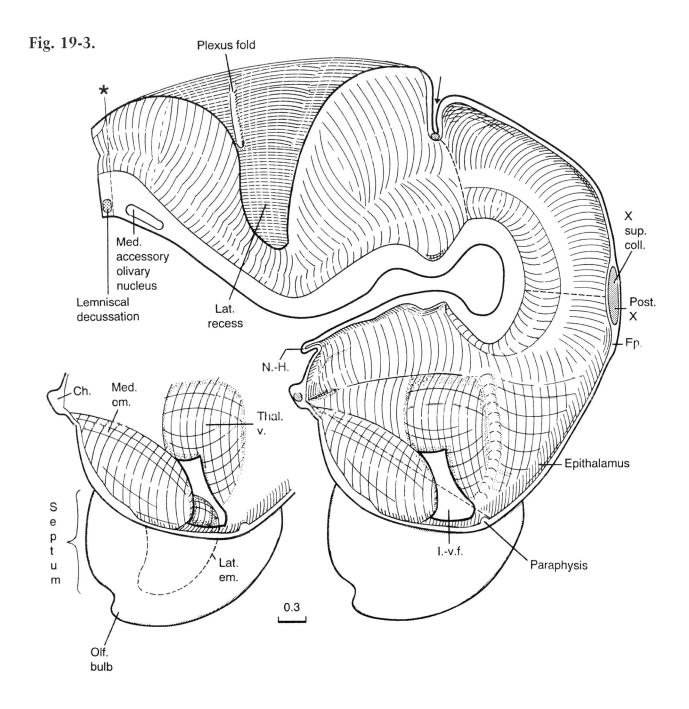

Plexus fold

*

Med.
accessory
olivary
nucleus

Lemniscal
decussation

Lat.
recess

N.-H.

Ch.

Med.
om.

Thal.
v.

S
e
p
t
u
m

Lat.
em.

Olf.
bulb

0.3

l.-v.f.

Paraphysis

Epithalamus

X
sup.
coll.

Post.
X

Fp.

199

Fig. 19-4. Median section of the brain and the related cartilaginous skeleton (CEC 390). The chiasmatic and commissural plates are important landmarks. The choroid fold of the fourth ventricle is evident, and the subdural mesenchyme is a fluid-filled meshwork. Among the injected arteries, the basilar is especially well visible. Fine vessels can be seen in the area of the future falx cerebri. The dorsal funiculus appears as a thick bundle in the spinal cord. The median raphe (His, 1890), known as the *septum medullae rhombencephali,* consists of sagittally arranged fibers derived from the embryonic floor plate and representing the adult floor plate (Sidman and Rakic, 1982). In the photomicrograph, it is clearly visible above the basilar artery.

The basicranium (reconstructed by O'Rahilly and Müller, 1984) now consists of an occipital part (developed from sclerotomes 1–4) and a sphenoidal part, which has grown rostrally to reach the adenohypophysis. Although not visible here, the orbital wing of the sphenoid (mainly the postoptic root) is forming. From Müller and O'Rahilly (1990a).

Fig. 19-4.

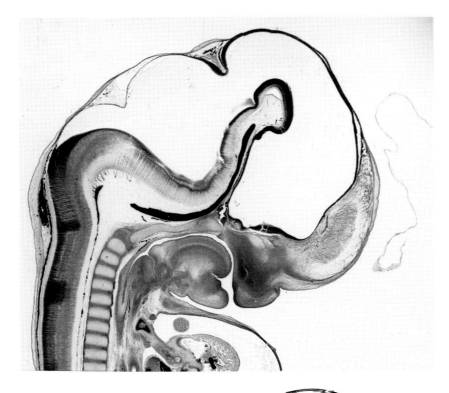

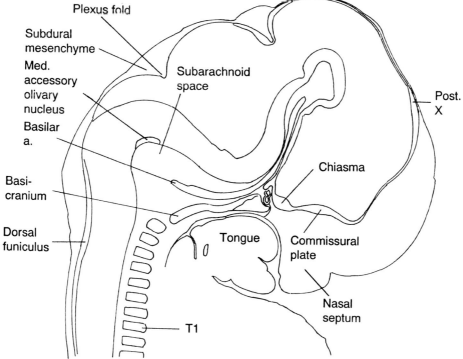

Fig. 19-5. Reconstruction of the developing basal nuclei (D-15, transitional between stages 18 and 19).

(**A**) Medial view of the right half of the forebrain, in which the medial wall of the right cerebral hemisphere is shown as if transparent.

(**B**) Dorsal view of the cerebral hemispheres, with the right hemisphere opened to illustrate its basal aspect from the interior. The medial ventricular eminence has almost completely invaded telencephalic territory (cf. Fig. 19-3). The lateral eminence represents the main primordium of the future corpus striatum (Fig. 6-2). From O'Rahilly, Müller, Hutchins, and Moore (1988).

The medial ventricular eminence has been found in the rat to resemble the globus pallidus histochemically far more than it does the lateral eminence, and it is connected to the dopamine pathway that leads from the ventral tegmental region of the midbrain to the forebrain.

The nucleus accumbens develops as a separate entity far earlier than in rodents, and projects as a thickening into the ventricular cavity. It was shown by Hewitt (1958, Fig. 3) in an early human fetus, where it appeared as the elevation known as the "paraterminal body." It is regarded by various authors as a ventromedial extension of the caudato-putamen complex. Its superficial component includes the nucleus of the diagonal band (Kuhlenbeck, 1973). The nucleus accumbens has been shown in the human to contain dopamine, and it resembles the caudato-putamen complex in its histochemical development (Brana et al., 1995).

Fig. 19-5.

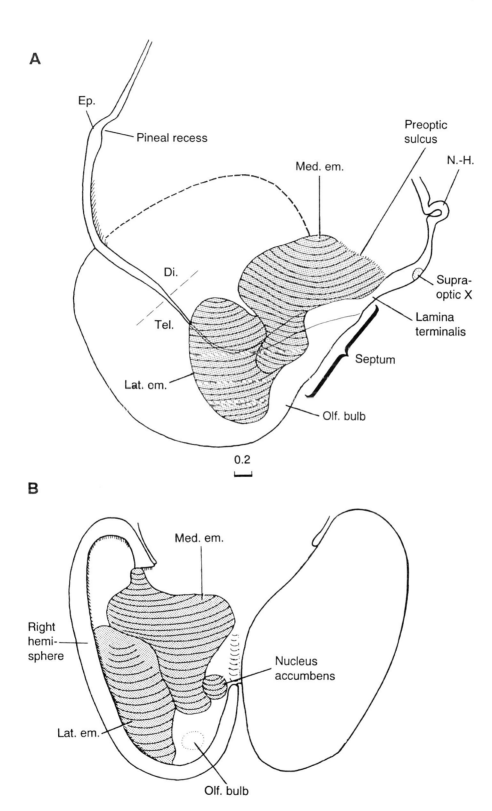

Figures 19-6 to 19-11 show neocortical areas and choroid plexuses. Figures 19-6 to 19-8 are from Müller and O'Rahilly (1990a). The bars represent 0.1 mm.

Fig. 19-6. Sagittal section (D-203) showing cerebral hemisphere, choroid plexus (rectangle), medial prosencephalic (forebrain) bundle (arrowhead), and dorsal and ventral thalami. Connections between the amygdaloid nuclei in the medial eminence and the diencephalon belong mostly to the medial prosencephalic bundle, which is the main pathway for longitudinal connections in the hypothalamus (Fig. 19-16). The lateral ventricle is invaded by the choroid fold, which, thicker than that of the fourth ventricle, consists of a multilayered epithelium and a mesenchymal core with thin-walled blood vessels.

Fig. 19-7. Another section, to show the olfactory bulb and tubercle, and the medial ventricular eminence. The stria medullaris thalami (arrowhead at right) arises in the diencephalon from the nucleus taeniae or ovalis (Fig. 19-15), although minor contributions come from the lateral prosencephalic bundle. The choroid fissure is visible (arrowhead at left).

Fig. 19-8. Still another section, to show the medial ventricular eminence and the ventral thalamus. Preoptico-hypothalamic (lower arrowhead) and mamillotegmental (upper arrowhead) tracts are identifiable.

Fig. 19-6.

Fig. 19-7.

Fig. 19-8.

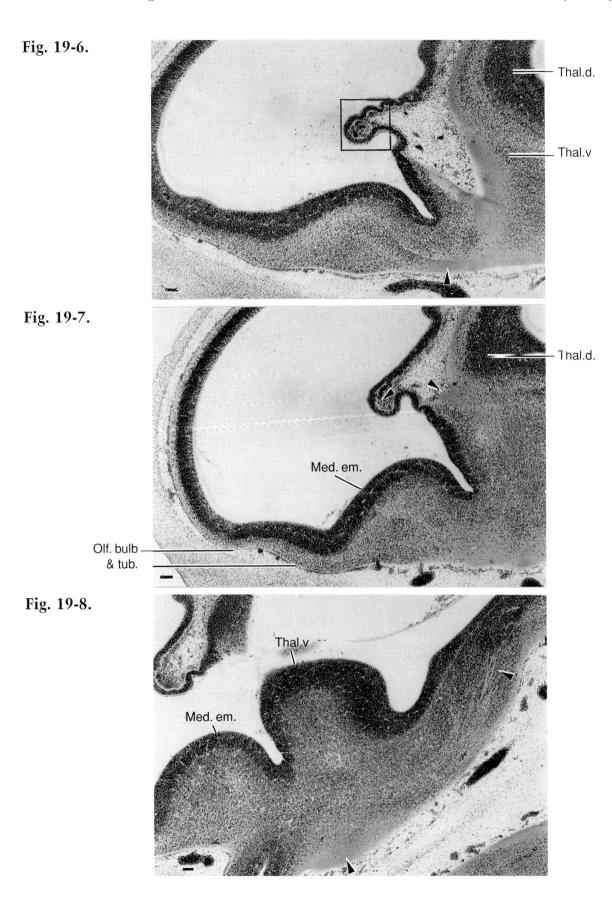

Fig. 19-9. The lateral habenular nucleus in a sagittal section (D-38), an example of a far-advanced epithalamic area. The arriving fibers are of the stria medullaris thalami, the leaving fibers form the habenulo-interpeduncular tract (Fig. 19-16).

Fig. 19-10. Relationships of olfactory tubercle and bulb, showing the entry of the nervus terminalis into the olfactory tubercle, and of the olfactory nerve fibers (marked 1) into the olfactory bulb (D-38). The olfactory ventricle is evident. Both tubercle and bulb possess an intermediate layer, and multiple nerve fibers are present in the tubercle. The sulcus circularis is marked by an arrowhead. The neural crest of earlier stages had developed into vomeronasal and terminal ganglia, but only after a certain degree of development of the central structures (tubercle and bulb). Both ganglia are medial, but the terminalis is more rostral, although its nerve fibers enter the brain caudal to the sulcus circularis. The ganglion of the nervus terminalis, although not yet present in the previous stage, is almost constantly present in stage 19. The fibers of the nervus terminalis appear later than the ganglion, as described in a fetus of 38 mm by Pearson (1941).

Fig. 19-11. The isthmic nucleus and the commissure of the trochlear nerves (D-9588). The level of this coronal section is shown in the key drawing. The bilateral isthmic nuclei are ventrolateral and rostral to the trochlear decussation (X4). Details have been provided by O'Rahilly, Müller, Hutchins, and Moore (1988).

Important

The isthmus contains the trochlear decussation and its alar lamina contributes to the cerebellum and the rostral medullary velum. Its site in the adult is indicated by the trochlear nerves

---

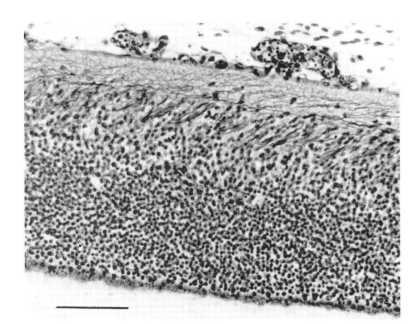

Fig. 19-9

Stria medullaris
thalami

Habenulo-interpeduncular
tract

Lateral habenular
nucleus

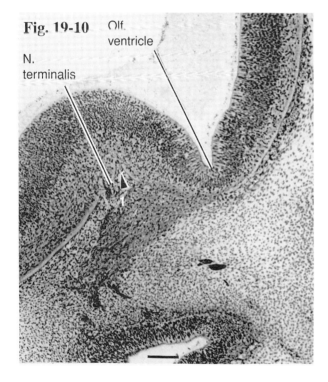

Fig. 19-10 Olf.
ventricle

N.
terminalis

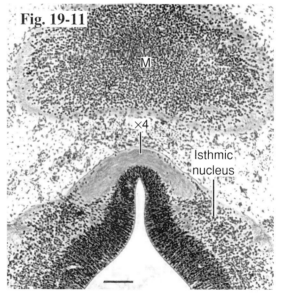

Fig. 19-11

M

×4

Isthmic
nucleus

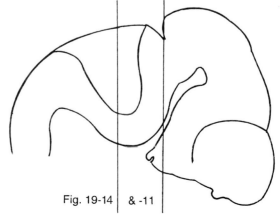

Fig. 19-14 | & -11

207

Fig. 19-12. The hypophysis and the epiphysis. (**A**) A median section at stage 19 (D-203) to show the hypophysis. Mesenchyme has now penetrated between the adjacent parts of the adenohypophysis and the neurohypophysis. The wall of the neurohypophysis is characteristically folded. The stem of the adenohypophysis, which is now solid, is embedded in the chondrocranium. Commissural fibers in the chiasmatic plate are marked by an arrowhead. Bar: 0.1 mm.

(**B**) A sagittal section of the same embryo to show the epiphysis, which is now a rostrally directed outgrowth of the roof of the synencephalon. This is the *Vorderlappen* of *Stadium IV* of Turkewitsch (1933). It projects towards the left side of the photomicrograph and forms a characteristic "step" (*Stufe*). Two so-called follicles are visible, as observed also by Hochstetter (1923). The site of the epiphysial evagination is marked by the pineal recess. Bar: 0.05 mm.

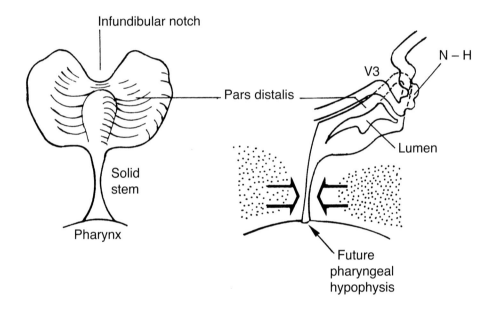

Fig. 19-12.

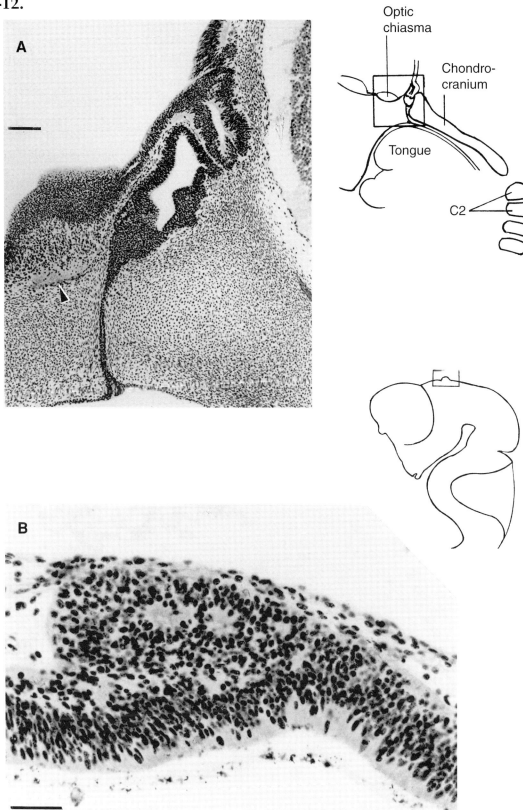

Fig. 19-13. The area of the pontine flexure with cranial nerves 5, 7, 8, 9, and 10 (D-38, silver-impregnated). Many tracts are identifiable, e.g., the mesencephalic tract of the trigeminal nerve, the trigeminospinal tract, and the tractus solitarius. Among the cerebellar connections are found the inferior cerebellar peduncle (vestibulocerebellar and trigeminocerebellar fibers) and even components of the superior peduncle (dentatorubral fibers, which pass lateral to the nucleus isthmi). The *porus duralis* of the trigeminal nerve is visible. The internal carotid artery, sectioned below the trigeminal ganglion, is filled with blood and possesses a thick arterial wall. Bar: 0.2 mm. From Müller and O'Rahilly (1990a).

In monkeys at a comparable stage, cerebellar neuronal production is at a peak. Two migratory waves participate in the formation of the cerebellum: from the rhombic lip, the migrating cells being at the surface, to which their nuclei are parallel; and from the ventricular layer, the cells lying at a right angle to the surface of the cerebellum. The cells of the two migrations become partly mixed, as is true in the dentate nucleus.

Parasympathetic ganglia appear in the head between stages 15 and 19 (Woźniak and O'Rahilly, 1980).

Fig. 19-14. The cochlear nerve and nuclei (D-9588). The level of this coronal section is shown in the key drawing below Figure 19-11. The cochlear nerve has a spiral, pattern like a rope from stage 19 onwards. It pierces a dense mass of cells (the ventral cochlear nucleus), where it enters the rhombencephalon. Both cochlear nuclei are lateral to the inferior cerebellar peduncle, whereas the vestibular nuclei are medial. An asterisk indicates the tractus solitarius in the key. Bar: 0.1 mm.

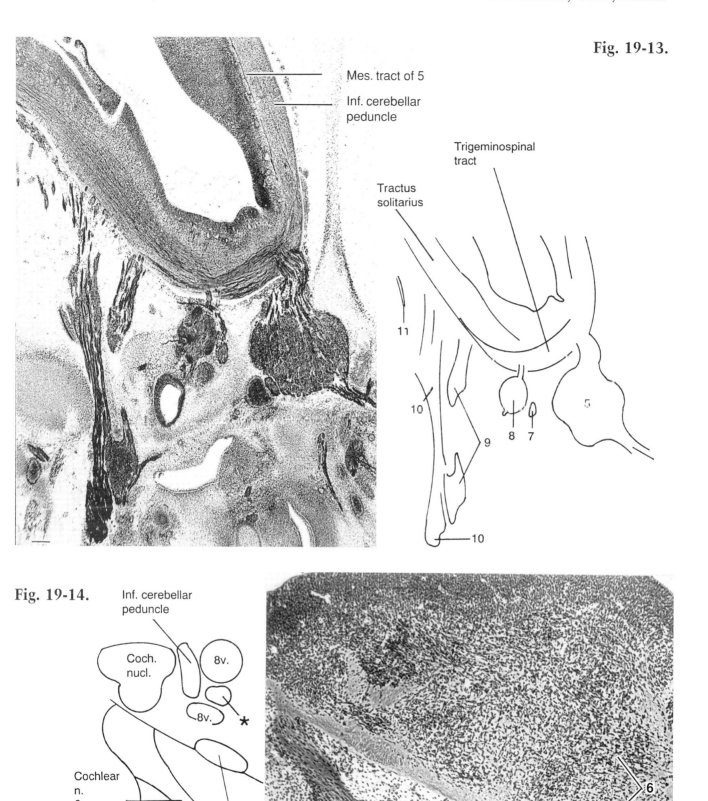

Fig. 19-13.

Mes. tract of 5

Inf. cerebellar peduncle

Trigeminospinal tract

Tractus solitarius

11

10

9

8 7

10

5

Fig. 19-14.

Inf. cerebellar peduncle

Coch. nucl.

8v.

8v.

*

Cochlear n. & ganglion

Trigemino-spinal tr.

6

211

Figs. 19-15 and 19-16. Tracts of the forebrain (D-38) in a median and a right lateral view, respectively. Some of the nuclei are shown as stippled areas, and superficially situated tracts are also stippled. New tracts in stage 19 include the thalamostriatal tract (*Stammbündel* of His or lateral prosencephalic fasciculus), around which the internal capsule continues to develop (but does not yet reach the pallium), the stria medullaris thalami, the fibers of the zona intrathalamica, and the amygdalo-habenular tract. The tract of the zona limitans intrathalamica later becomes the lamina medullaris externa. The sequence of appearance of the tracts is given in Appendix 3. From O'Rahilly, Müller, Hutchins, and Moore (1988).

The fibers of the catecholamine neurons seem to penetrate no further than the ventricular eminences (Zecevic et al., 1995). At about this stage it has been found in the rat that septohippocampal projections reach the hippocampus, and that they are preceded by hippocamposeptal projections.

Fig. 19-15.

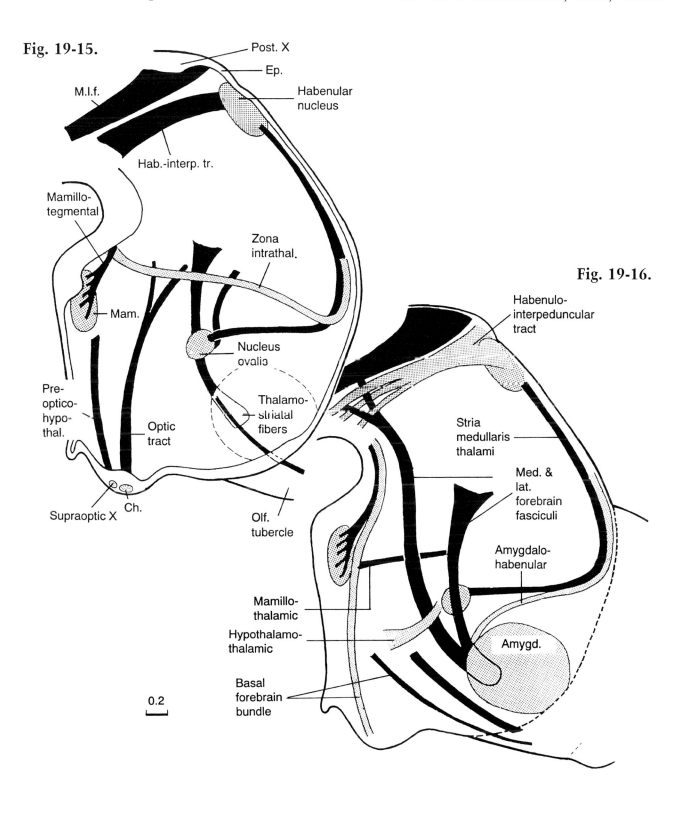

Fig. 19-16.

Fig. 19-17. Simplified scheme of the origin of the various cerebral arteries, based mostly on the data of Padget (1948). The circulus arteriosus, which is visible in a reconstruction by Padget (1948, Fig. 7) is completed in the period from stage 19 to stage 21. Abbreviations: AICA, anterior inferior cerebellar artery; c, caudal division of internal carotid artery; PICA, posterior inferior cerebellar artery; r, rostral division of internal carotid artery; 1, 2, 3, aortic arches.

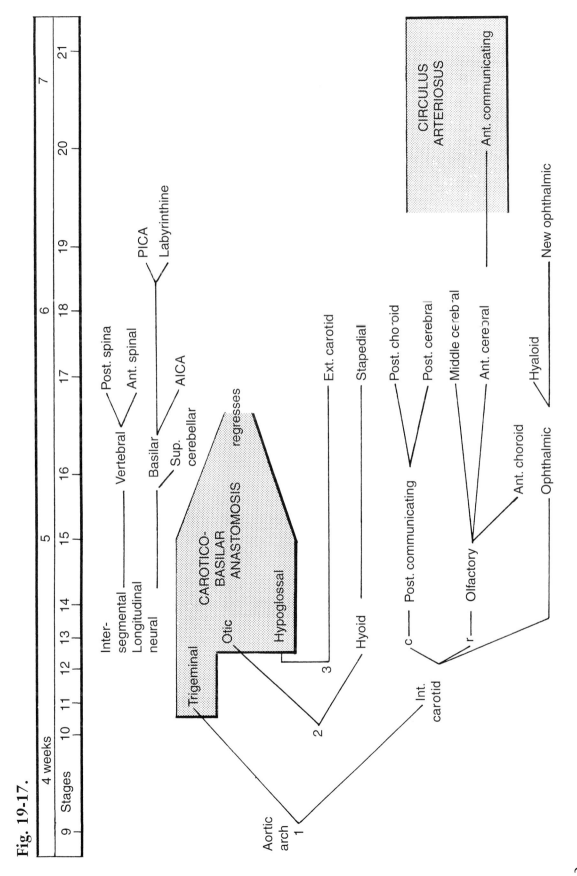

Fig. 19-17.

Stage 20: The Choroid Plexus of the Lateral Ventricles, the Optic and Habenular Commissures, and the Interpeduncular and Septal Nuclei

Approximately 18–22 mm in Greatest Length
Approximately 47 Postfertilizational Days

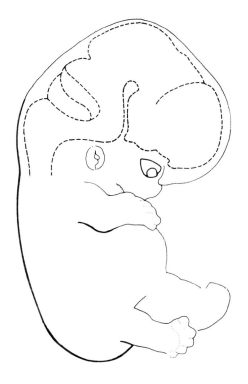

Fig. 20-1. Right lateral view of an embryo (CEC 8157) of stage 20 with the brain (D-7959) superimposed. From O'Rahilly, Müller, and Bossy (1986).

The globus pallidus externus is distinct in the subthalamic area. The optic commissure is present, and crossing fibers begin to form in the future habenular commissure. The medial septal nucleus and the nucleus of the diagonal band are differentiating, and fiber connections with the hippocampus and the medial prosencephalic fasciculus are present. Important fiber connections of the olfactory system are now identifiable: from the olfactory bulb to the olfactory tubercle, to the septal nuclei, to the amygdaloid nuclei and via the stria medullaris thalami to the habenular nuclei; then from there via the habenulo-interpeduncular tract to the interpeduncular nucleus. Connections exist also from the septal nuclei, via the olfactory tubercle and amygdaloid nuclei, to the medial prosencephalic fasciculus, and from there to the tegmentum of the mesencephalon. The choroid plexuses of the lateral ventricles at stage 20 are at the "club-shaped" phase. Cuneate and gracile decussating fibers are present. Histological differences are now apparent between perimural arteries and veins (although not in the intramural vessels until trimester 2). Further details: Müller and O'Rahilly (1990a,b).

Fig. 20-2. Right lateral view of the brain (CEC 966). The frontal, occipital, and temporal poles are indicated (by α, β, γ). The tuberculum interpedunculare (of Hochstetter), which faces the mamillary region, is particularly evident in this embryo (dagger). The roof of the fourth ventricle leaves a part of the cerebellum free (*äusserer Kleinhirnwulst* of Hochstetter, 1929). The ventricular cavity between the internal cerebellar swelling and the caudal part of the rhombencephalon has become very narrow. The cranial nerves have been cut short. A mesencephalic *Blindsack* (the site of the future inferior colliculus) is visible on each side of the mesencephalon and almost touches the cerebellum.

In the left-hand inset (a dorsal view), the cerebellar hemispheres are seen to be separated from each other. Dorsally, the left and right halves of the cerebellum are joined only in the area of the rostral (superior) medullary velum.

The right-hand inset is an end-on view showing the cerebral hemispheres, part of the diencephalon with the epiphysis, and the mesencephalon.

The neocortical development of an embryo belonging to stage 20 was illustrated by Marín-Padilla (1983, 1988a). At this stage the intrinsic vascularization of the neocortex begins. "It evolves from perforating capillaries of the pia-vascular plexus, and progressively advances in ventro–dorso–lateral and antero–posterior [rostrocaudal] gradients, paralleling the differentiation and maturation of the neocortex" (Marín-Padilla, 1988a). The intraneural vascular territories of the cerebral cortex in the embryo and in the adult are quite similar. Both are characterized by a short-link anastomotic network of intracortical capillaries established between adjacent perforating vessels (Marín-Padilla, 1988b). Certain portions of the primordial plexiform layer are considered to be functionally active in the embryo by this stage (Marín-Padilla and Marín-Padilla, 1982).

Is has been found in the cat that corticipetal and some corticofugal fibers are present prior to the appearance of the cortical plate.

218

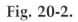

Fig. 20-2.

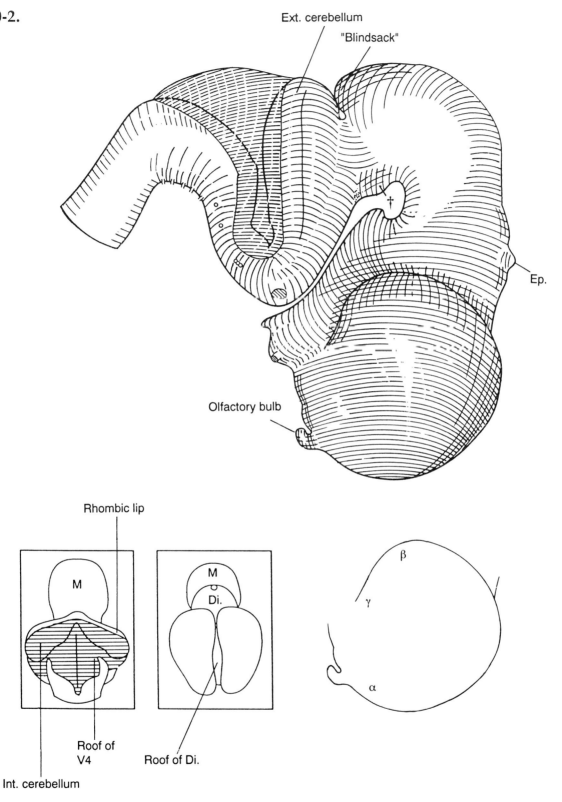

Fig. 20-3. Graphic reconstruction prepared from coronal sections to show a median view of the brain (D-7959 combined with features of G-21). The asterisk indicates the junction with the spinal cord.

The choroid plexuses of the lateral ventricles at stage 20 are at the "club-shaped" phase described by Shuangshoti and Netsky (1966). In the diencephalon, the position of the marginal ridge no longer corresponds to that of earlier stages. A ventral shift has occurred, whereby the dorsal thalamus has become larger towards the interventricular foramen. The earliest part of the globus pallidus, the globus pallidus externus, appears at the surface of the subthalamus in this and in the previous stage. Subsequently it moves into the hemispheric stalk. The optic chiasma lies rostroventral to the decussating fibers of the preoptico-hypothalamotegmental tract, and these form the supraoptic commissure. In most embryos of this stage, the epiphysis cerebri is immediately rostral to the posterior commissure. The caudal shift is probably caused by a growth gradient. It is likely that the habenular commissure, containing a few fibers, is present in most embryos of this stage. The habenulo-interpeduncular tract is no longer at the surface but runs between the ventricular and intermediate layers of the diencephalon and arrives in the mesencephalon lateral to the interpeduncular nucleus (Fig. 20-9).

The commissural fibers of the oculomotor nerves (dagger) are joined by the crossing fibers of the dentatorubral tract. This is the beginning of the decussation of the superior cerebellar peduncles.

The basal plate of the rhombencephalon has increased greatly in thickness, especially in its caudal part. The lateral portions of the rhombencephalon are depressed in the region of the pontine flexure and hence are not visible in this view. The cerebellar hemispheres are conspicuous. The villi of the choroid plexus of the fourth ventricle extend from the choroid fold into the wall of the lateral recesses. The septum medullare (median raphe of His, 1890) begins at the isthmic recess. It is derived from the rhombencephalic floor plate and is important in the production of neurotransmitters.

Cuneate and gracile decussating fibers are present at the transition from rhombencephalon to spinal cord.

Fig. 20-3.

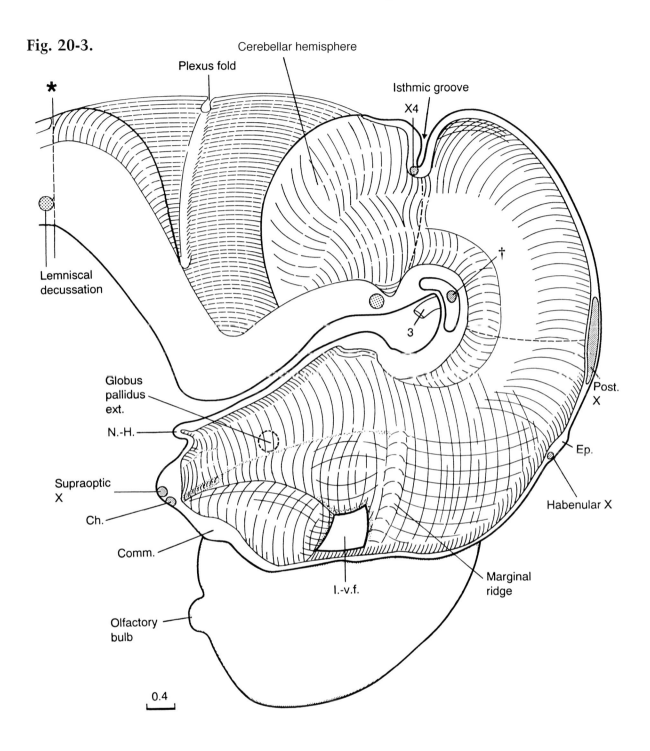

✱

Plexus fold

Cerebellar hemisphere

Isthmic groove

X4

Lemniscal
decussation

†

3

Globus
pallidus
ext.

N.-H.

Post.
X

Supraoptic
X

Ep.

Ch.

Habenular X

Comm.

Marginal
ridge

l.-v.f.

Olfactory
bulb

0.4

Fig. 20-4. Sections through the prosencephalon (CEC 462).

(**A**) A portion of the wall of the brain from the rectangle indicated in B. The ventricular layer gives origin to the ventricular ependyma (that lining the ventricle) and to the choroidal ependyma (of the choroid plexus), and the two are continuous with each other. The choroid plexus consists of choroidal ependyma and tela choroidea; the latter is a vascularized pia mater.

(**B**) Transverse section showing that the interventricular foramina are now narrow. The choroid plexus extends into the lateral ventricle on each side, and its line of invagination is the choroid fissure. The ependyma of the plexus is continuous with the medial wall of the lateral ventricle.

(**C**) An enlargement of a portion of the choroid plexus (D-203 at stage 19) from the rectangle indicated in B. The epithelium is the choroidal ependyma, the layers of which enclose the vascular pia mater known as the tela choroidea. Bar: 0.05 mm.

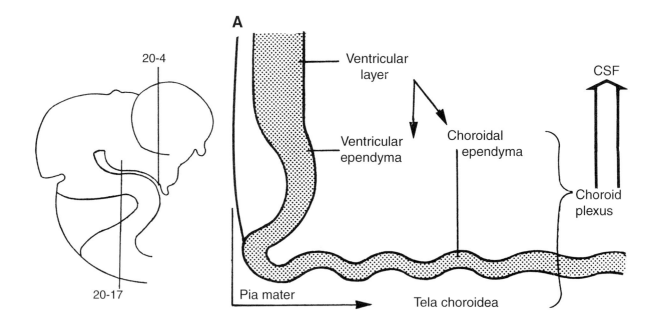

Fig. 20-4.

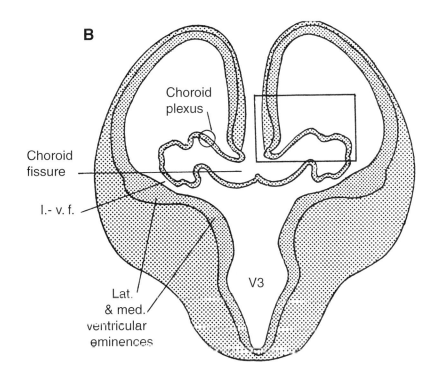

B

Choroid
plexus

Choroid
fissure

l.- v. f.

Lat.
& med.
ventricular
eminences

V3

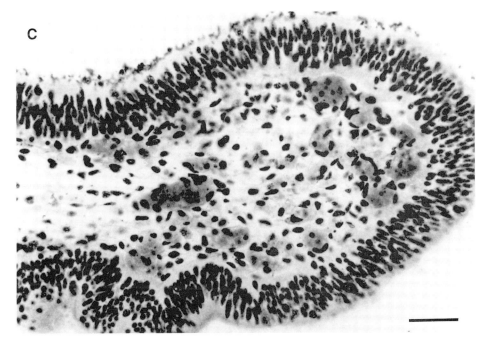

C

Figures 20-5 to 20-9 show the development of the interpeduncular nucleus from 5 to 7 weeks. This nucleus is important for neural grafts as a possible treatment for Parkinson disease (Freeman et al., 1991; Freed et al., 1992). The levels of Figures 20-8 and 20-9 are shown in the key drawing beside Figure 20-16. The bars represent 0.1 mm.

Catecholaminergic cell groups have been detected at as early as 5 weeks in the rhombencephalon and mesencephalon, and at 6 weeks (ca. stage 17) in the hypothalamus (Verney et al., 1991). A band of densely packed cells that corresponds to the primordium of the dopaminergic substantia nigra and ventral tegmental region has been recorded at 7 weeks (Verney et al., 1991). Nigrostriatal fibers develop at this time and extend initially to the subventricular zone of the lateral ventricular eminence (Freeman et al., 1995).

Fig. 20-5. At stage 15 (CEC 6506) a ventral proliferative area of the mesencephalon, between the right and left oculomotor nuclei, is already visible (arrowheads).

Fig. 20-6. At stage 16 (CEC 8773) the loose material between the oculomotor nuclei has increased to several rows of cells.

Fig. 20-7. At stage 17 (D-8996) transverse fibers ventral to the proliferative area represent the commissure of the oculomotor nerves. From Müller and O'Rahilly (1989b).

Fig. 20-5.

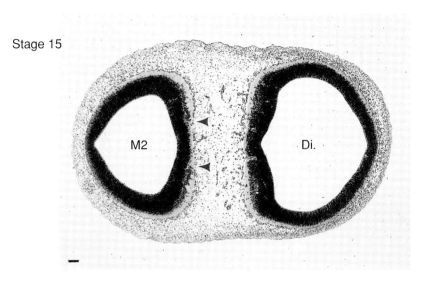

Stage 15

M2

Di.

Fig. 20-6.

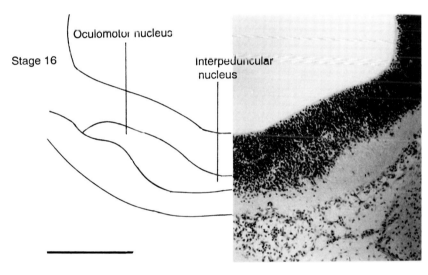

Oculomotor nucleus

Stage 16

Interpeduncular nucleus

Fig. 20-7.

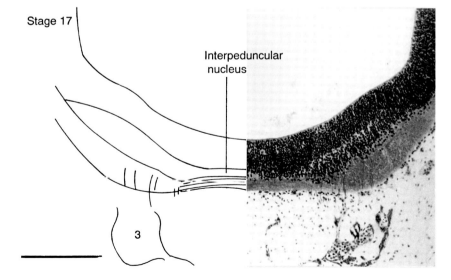

Stage 17

Interpeduncular nucleus

3

Fig. 20-8. At stage 20 (D-7959) the fibers passing through the tegmentum of the mesencephalon have increased to such an extent that the cerebral peduncles and the interpeduncular groove have begun to appear. The interpeduncular nucleus is visible, and the nucleus niger is lateral to it. The neurons of the substantia nigra are believed to be generated (in the rat) in the region of the isthmus rhombencephali. Transverse fibers, which are beginning to penetrate the loose cellular sheath, probably are rubrocerebellar fibers belonging to the superior cerebellar peduncles (Cooper, 1946a). The oculomotor nuclei are visible. From Müller and O'Rahilly (1990b).

Fig. 20-9. At stage 21 (CEC 8553) habenulo-interpeduncular fibers are seen to arrive in the lateral part of the interpeduncular nucleus. The substantia nigra is lateral to those fibers. The commissure of the superior colliculi is visible dorsally in the roof. Mesencephalic dopaminergic neurons have been detected at approximately this stage (Freeman et al., 1991). The red nucleus, which is already distinguishable at stage 17, is lateral and slightly dorsal to the oculomotor nucleus. The ventral tegmental region is dorsal to the interpeduncular nucleus, and its fibers ascend in the medial forebrain bundle. From Müller and O'Rahilly (1990b).

Fig. 20-8.   Stage 20

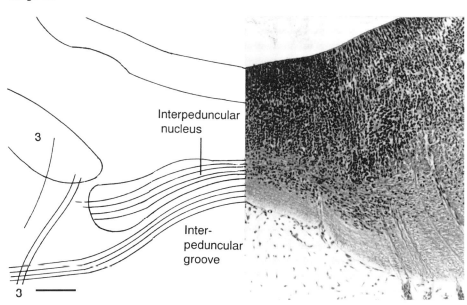

Interpeduncular
nucleus

Inter-
peduncular
groove

3

3

Fig. 20-9.

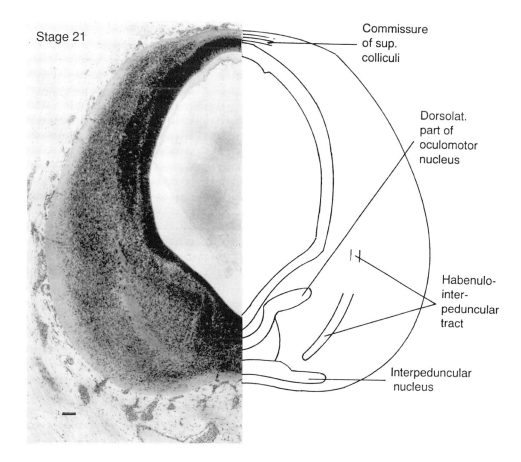

Stage 21

Commissure
of sup.
colliculi

Dorsolat.
part of
oculomotor
nucleus

Habenulo-
inter-
peduncular
tract

Interpeduncular
nucleus

Figures 20-10 to 20-14 show the nuclei of the prosencephalic septum. The septal nuclei are cellular agglomerations at the periphery of the intermediate layer. The cholinergic neurons of the nuclei at the base of the forebrain are believed to be important in the degenerative processes leading to Alzheimer disease. Septo-hippocampal cholinergic fibers reach their target (in the rat) at what would correspond to stage 19.

The basal part of the medial telencephalic wall (the septum verum) forms as the cerebral hemispheres expand beyond the lamina terminalis, and it extends between the commissural plate and the olfactory bulb. From Müller and O'Rahilly (1990a).

Fig. 20-10. A graphic reconstruction and two transverse sections (G-21). The medial septal nucleus is near the hippocampus and includes two separate portions, X and Y. The nucleus of the diagonal band is ventrocaudal and occupies the middle third of the septum. Nerve fibers are present between the nucleus and the hippocampus.

The nucleus of the diagonal band is identified by its projecting fibers (b) to the hippocampus. The caudalmost part of this area, however, is less clear. In the monkey (studied by thymidine marking), the production of cells of the septal nuclei (medial and nucleus of the diagonal band) is almost simultaneous with that of the nucleus basalis (of Meynert). This would correspond approximately to Carnegie stage 14, followed by a second wave between stages 18 and 22. The three functional cholinergic groups of the basal forebrain (medial septal, nucleus of the diagonal band, and nucleus basalis) "are the most outstanding sets of neurons regulating cortical functions. Each group specifically ends in a part of the cortex," and their number and function are "statistically diminished in AD {Alzheimer disease} patients" (Toledano, 1992).

Fig. 20-11. A graphic reconstruction (D-7959). The medial septal nucleus consists of one separate mass in this specimen. Two additional fiber bundles are shown: a, between the olfactory bulb and the medial septal nucleus, and b, between the rostral and caudal septal areas.

Fig. 20-10.

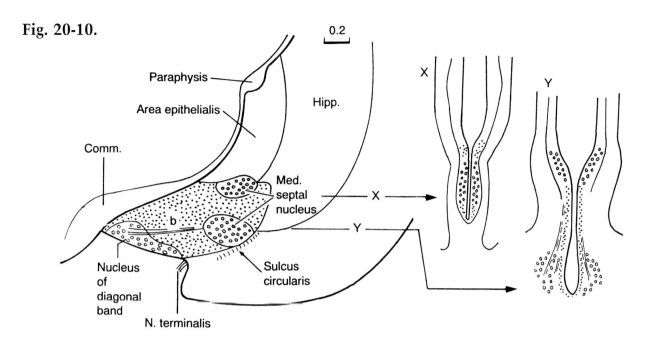

Fig. 20-11.

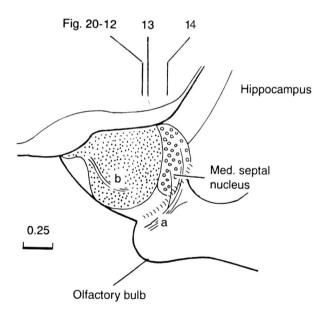

Figures 20-12 to 20-14. Sections (D-7959) at the levels indicated in Figure 20-11. The bars represent 0.1 mm.

Fig. 20-12. Detail of the septal area of the right hemisphere in a coronal section. The cellular agglomeration at the periphery of the intermediate layer of the medial wall of the telencephalon represents the primordium of a septal nucleus.

Fig. 20-13. A more rostral section showing the right and left sides of the septal area. The connection is the commissural plate, which at this time consists mainly of ventricular layer. The cellular agglomeration in the septal area is evident.

Fig. 20-14. A coronal section at the level of the olfactory bulbs. Fibers from the developing external fibrous layer of the olfactory bulb ascend (arrowheads) to the medial septal nucleus.

Fig. 20-12.

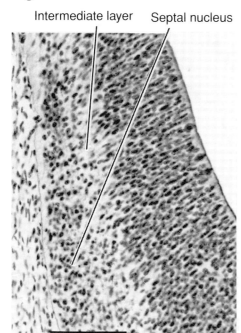

Fig. 20-13.

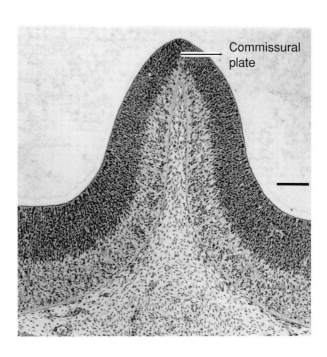

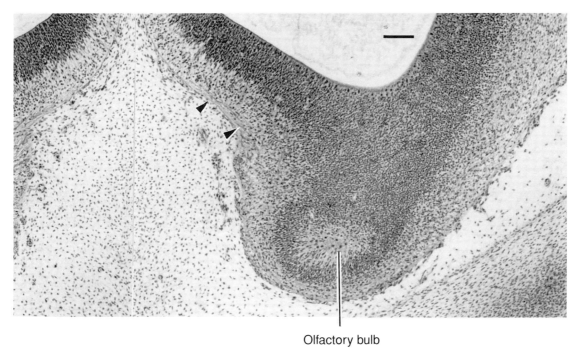

Fig. 20-14.

231

Fig. 20-15. A coronal section through the rhombencephalon (D-7959) in the region of the facial nucleus. The septum medullae, which is a part of the floor plate, is present in the epinotochordal region and extends as far rostrally as the diencephalon (to the boundary between caudal and rostral parencephalon). The septum is a specialized grid formed by intersecting sagittal and transverse fibers, between which are migrating cells from the floor plate. These cells form the raphe nuclei, which, because of their neurotransmitters, are essential for the development of the brain. Moreoever, they are related to the locus caeruleus, the substantia nigra, the red nucleus, and (after stage 20) to the cortical plate. Bar: 0.1 mm.

At their first appearance the visceromotor nuclei are ventromedial in position (stage 13). Subsequently, the neurons of cranial nerves 5 and 9–11 migrate laterally. The facial nucleus, however, remains medially and is now also dorsal in position. Migration of the facial neurons laterally and rostrally occurs relatively late (Windle, 1970): in the late embryonic or early in the fetal period. The facial nucleus becomes better defined at the beginning of the fetal period (Pearson, 1946; Jacobs, 1970).

The migration of the facial nucleus and the unexpected course of its fibers around the abducent nucleus are an example of neurobiotaxis, a term introduced in 1907 by C. U. Ariëns Kappers (1932) for the retention of a neuron as close as practicable to its main source of stimulation, and the migration that may occur in the direction from which the greatest density of stimuli arises, achieved by elongation of the axon. The mechanism of this phenomenon remains obscure. Another example is provided by the nucleus ambiguus.

Precision

A common ventromedial efferent column appears early and gives rise to somatic efferent (SE) and visceral efferent (VE) cellular groups. Unlike the adult arrangement, however, and contrary to most accounts, the VE column is at first medial to the SE column. The VE cells then migrate laterally (an example of neurobiotaxis), allowing the SE cells to remain nearer to the median plane.

Fig. 20-15.

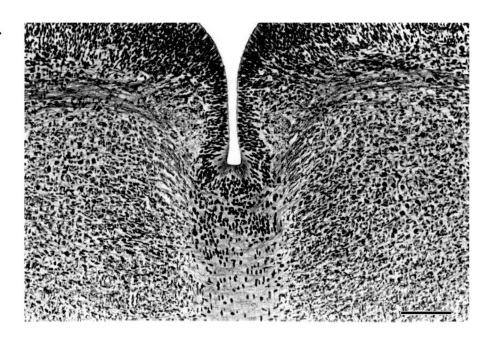

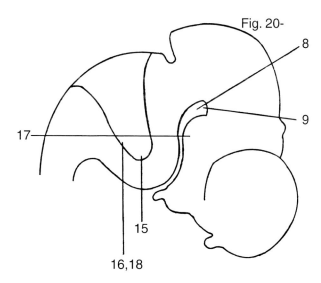

Fig. 20-16. A coronal section of the rhombencephalon (D-7959). The medial accessory olivary nucleus arises between the hypoglossal roots of the two sides. This nucleus is the first of five (Müller and O'Rahilly, 1990c) that will be present by the beginning of the fetal period (Fig. 24-4). The hypoglossal nucleus is visible dorsally. Migratory material has accumulated at the ventral surface of the section. The migratory material arises in the rhombic lip and was first described in the human embryo by Essick (1912). His term "olivo-arcuate migration" is unsatisfactory, however, because it has since been shown (in the monkey) that the olivary nuclei arise mainly from the ventricular layer. Tall cells present in the raphe are contacted by fibers from the nuclei of nearby cranial nerves, and are important in the production of neurotransmitters. Bar: 0.2 mm. From Müller and O'Rahilly (1990a).

Fig. 20-16.

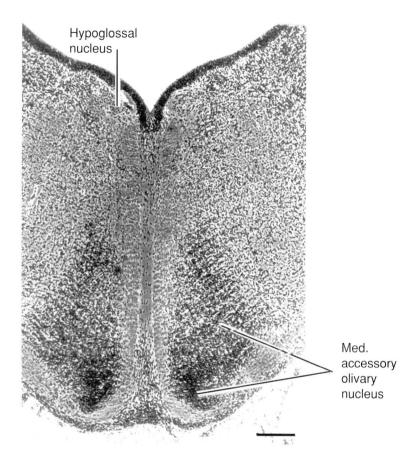

Hypoglossal
nucleus

Med.
accessory
olivary
nucleus

Fig. 20-17. A transverse section through the hindbrain (CEC 462) showing the internal cerebellar swellings. The alar and basal laminae, which are lateral and medial in this region, are separated from each other on their ventricular surface by the sulcus limitans. The rhombic lip on one side is indicated by a circle.

Fig. 20-18. A coronal section (D-7959) a short distance caudal to that in Figure 20-15. The region of the beginning medial olivary nucleus and two roots of the accessory nerve are visible. The sulcus limitans is not sharply defined at this level, but the rhombic lip and the choroid plexus are distinct on each side. × 36. Bar: 0.3 mm.

Fig. 20-17.

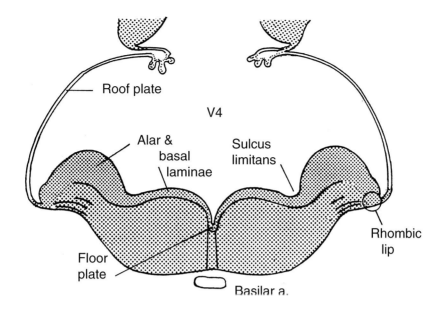

Roof plate

V4

Alar & basal laminae

Sulcus limitans

Floor plate

Rhombic lip

Basilar a.

Fig. 20-18.

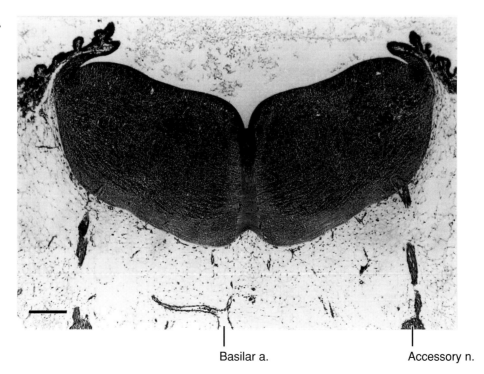

Basilar a.

Accessory n.

TABLE 20-1. Features of the Longitudinal Zones of the Diencephalon: Details for the General Scheme Given in Table 18-1

Zone	Feature	Stage	Fig.
1. Epithalamus	Habenular nucleus	15	19-9
	Epiphysis	16	16-13
	Posterior commissure	17	19-4
2. Dorsal thalamus	Nucleus of posterior commissure	15	
	Lateral geniculate body (dorsal part)	**Fetal period**	
	Sulcus medius	15–16	16-13
			17-11
			18-6
			21-12
3. Ventral thalamus	Lateral geniculate body (ventral part)	21	21-12
	Hypothalamic sulcus	15	15-6
			16-12
			17-11
4. Subthalamus	Subthalamic nucleus	16	21-10
	Globus pallidus externus	19–20	21-13
	Globus pallidus internus*	21	21-12
	Faint, unnamed sulcus	15	15-6
5. Hypothalamus *sensu lato*	Chiasmatic plate	10	10-6
			12-4
			15-8
	Hypothalamic cell cord	14	16-10
	Preoptico-hypothalamotegmental tract	14	19-8
	Interstitial nucleus	14	14-6
	Medial ventricular eminence	14	16-10
	Neurohypophysial diverticulum	15–16	17-12
			21-13
	Mamillary nuclei	15–16	21-9
			22-9

This table provides details for the general scheme given in Table 18-1.
The figure references are to photomicrographs.
* Entopeduncular nucleus.

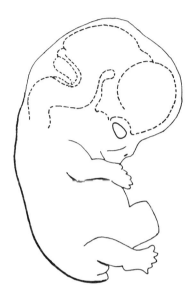

Stage 21: The First Appearance of the Cortical Plate in the Cerebral Hemispheres

---

**Approximately 22–24 mm in Greatest Length
Approximately 50 Postfertilizational Days**

Fig. 21-1. Right lateral view of an embryo of stage 21 with the brain superimposed (CEC 632). From O'Rahilly, Müller, and Bossy (1986).

An important feature is the appearance of the cortical plate within the primordial plexiform layer, adjacent to the lateral ventricular eminence (the future corpus striatum). This makes it possible to distinguish subpial and subplate layers, corresponding respectively to future layer 1 and the white matter of the neopallium. The lateral prosencephalic fasciculus (*Stammbündel* of His) is prominent and unites the telencephalon and the diencephalon. The internal capsule, however, is not yet present in the absence of the appropriate neocortical connections. Clinically important relays of the subthalamus are distinguishable: the subthalamic nucleus proper, the entopeduncular nucleus (future globus pallidus internus), and the globus pallidus externus. The rostral surface of the cerebellar plate has developed a longitudinal elevation that contains the inferior cerebellar peduncle. A distinct feature of the cranial nerves from stage 21 onwards is the presence of multiple glial cells (olfactory and optic nerves) and neurilemmal (Schwann) cells between the fibers. The nasal septum becomes cartilaginous. "Membrane" bones develop: the mandible and the maxilla are always present. Further details: Müller and O'Rahilly (1990b).

239

Fig. 21-2. Right lateral view of the brain (CEC 632) with the membranous labyrinth added. A flat surface marks the site of the future insula. Frontal, occipital, and temporal poles are distinguishable (α, β, γ). The cerebral hemispheres overlap more than half of the surface of the diencephalon. The isthmic groove has deepened. Between 6 and $7\frac{1}{2}$ weeks the head rises in position. This is largely because at stage 21 the growth and expansion of the trunk are such that it could not remain in the position it occupied at stage 18 (although in both stages it rests on the ventral wall of the trunk). A number of features typical of this stage were described by Hochstetter (1919, his embryos Ha3 and Peh4).

Fig. 21-2.

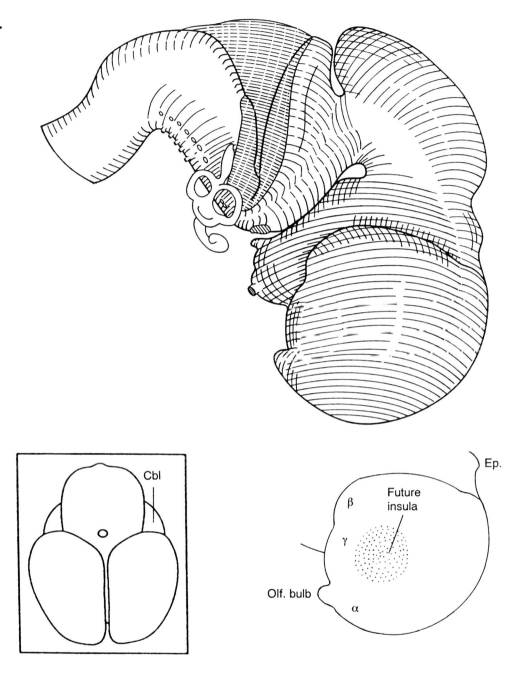

Fig. 21-3. Graphic reconstruction from transverse sections to show a median view of the brain (CEC 632). The asterisk indicates the junction with the spinal cord. Growth of the medial and lateral ventricular eminences transforms the formerly hemispherical lateral ventricle into a C-shaped cavity, which is continuous rostrally with the olfactory ventricle. The first indication of anterior and inferior horns can now be seen in the lateral ventricle (O'Rahilly and Müller, 1990). The pineal recess has formed. Ependymal cells over the posterior commissure form the subcommissural organ. The floor of the rhombencephalon is bent sharply, as described by Hochstetter (1919), and a transverse groove, the sulcus transversus rhombencephali, results. The isthmic recess (short arrow) is a guide to the interpeduncular nucleus. The levels of Figures 21-17 and 21-18 are indicated. Interrupted lines delimit the rhombencephalon, mesencephalon, diencephalon, and telencephalon.

Striatal arteries in this embryo were shown by Padget (1948, Fig. 21).

Precision

In the embryo the caudal border of the mesencephalon passes rostral to the isthmus

---

Fig. 21-3.

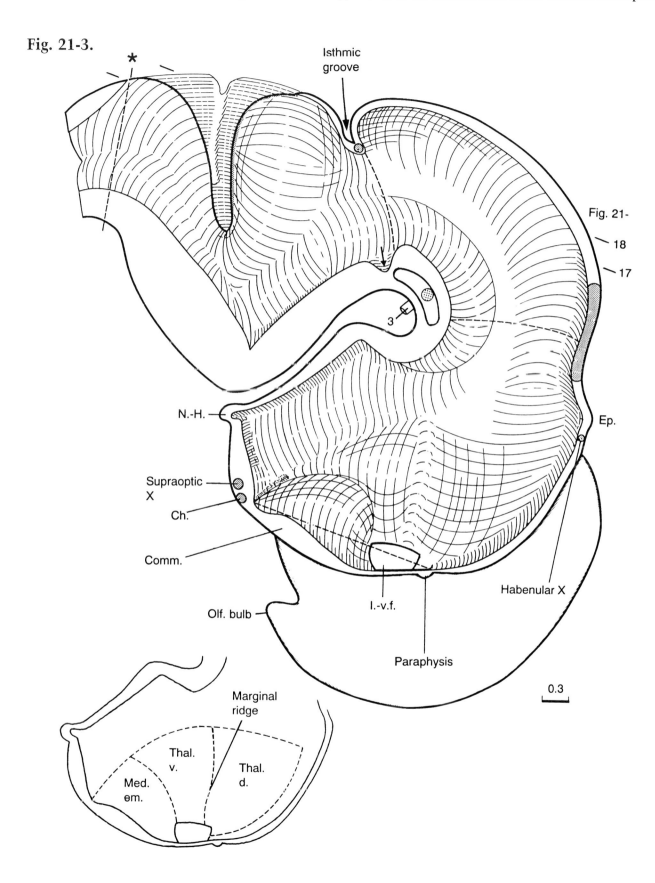

Fig. 21-4. (**A**) The overlap between the left cerebral hemisphere and the left half of the diencephalon (CEC 632). The positions of the subthalamic nuclei (medial and lateral mamillary nuclei, subthalamic nucleus proper, entopeduncular nucleus, and globus pallidus externus) are shown schematically. The ventral part of the lateral geniculate body has developed (Table 20-1). The hippocampus, area dentata, area epithelialis, and the choroid fissure are indicated on the medial wall of the left hemisphere, which is shown as if transparent. The hippocampus reaches almost as far as the temporal pole.

The site of the future lamina affixa, which at this stage overlies the ventral thalamus, is marked by a dagger. The asterisk at the base of the telencephalon is at the site of a cistern. Parts not visible from the surface are shown by interrupted lines. The horizontal interrupted line delimits the diencephalon from the telencephalon.

(**B**) Levels of Figures 21-6 to 21-15, which, because they are from a different embryo (CEC 8533), do not necessarily show a perfect fit.

Fig. 21-4.

A

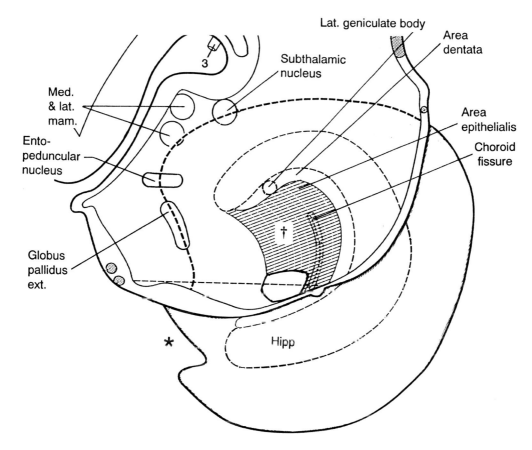

Lat. geniculate body

Subthalamic nucleus

Area dentata

Med. & lat. mam.

Area epithelialis

Ento-peduncular nucleus

Choroid fissure

Globus pallidus ext.

†

*

Hipp

B

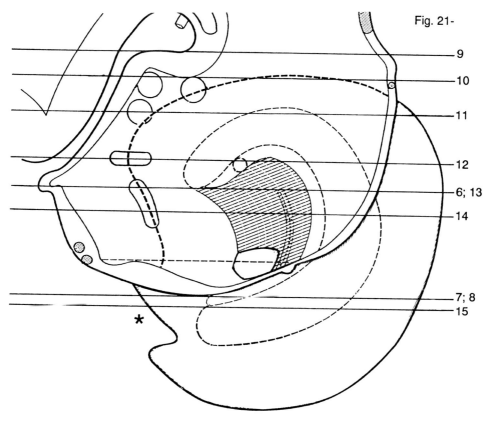

Fig. 21-

9

10

11

12

6; 13

14

7; 8
15

*

Fig. 21-5. An almost median section (CEC 1008). The olfactory and lateral ventricles are continuous. Choroid folds can be seen in the lateral and fourth ventricles. In the diencephalon, the zona limitans intrathalamica is distinguishable between the dark, dorsal area (dorsal thalamus) and the less dark, ventral area (ventral thalamus). The posterior commissure is partly diencephalic and partly mesencephalic (commissure of the superior colliculi). The interpeduncular nucleus is immediately rostral to the tuberculum interpedunculare of the isthmus, which segment includes also the trochlear commissure and the isthmic recess. In the cerebellum, the internal fiber layer is detectable. The sulcus transversus rhombencephali is produced by the sharp bend of the floor of the rhombencephalon. The inferior olivary nucleus is ventral in the rhombencephalon. The base of the chondrocranium shows the dorsum sellae and the hypophysial fossa (containing the hypophysis cerebri), and continues rostrally into the nasal septum. The dens of cervical vertebra 2 is evident.

Fig. 21-5.

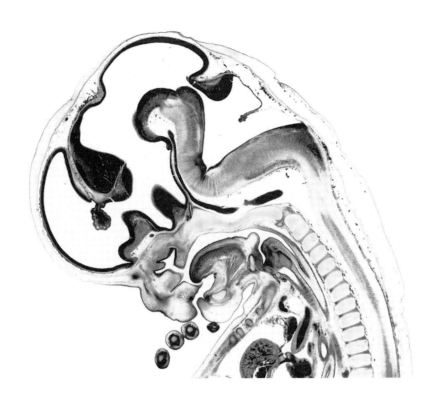

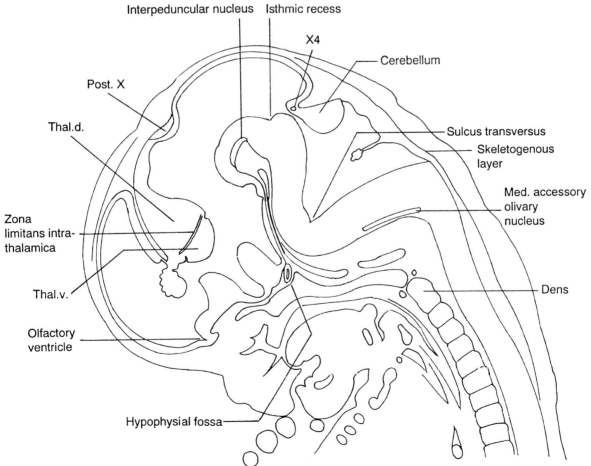

The levels of Figures 21-6 to 21-8 (CEC 8553) are shown in Figure 21-4B. The bars represent 0.1 mm.

Fig. 21-6. A portion of the right cerebral hemisphere adjacent to the diencephalon. The groove between the two (di-telencephalic sulcus) is filled with loose mesenchyme. The choroid plexus now presents stumpy villi limited by three to four rows of epithelial cells. The layer adjacent and ventral to the plexus is the future lamina affixa, which at this stage lies opposite the ventral thalamus. A deep groove, the sulcus terminalis, is situated medial to the medial ventricular eminence. The germinal zone (matrix and subventricular layer) of the ventricular eminences is bordered immediately by the postmitotic layer, without an intervening intermediate zone. The cortical plate, which is typical of stage 21, has begun to form opposite the ventricular eminences. It was seen in embryo CEC 8553 by Molliver et al. (1973). The transition from the hemisphere to the diencephalon is the hemispheric stalk, which contains a thick bundle of fibers, the lateral prosencephalic fasciculus (*Stammbündel* of His). The telencephalic area adjacent to it is the amygdaloid area. The diencephalic nucleus ventral to the lateral prosencephalic fasciculus is the globus pallidus externus. From Müller and O'Rahilly (1990b).

The hemispheric stalk seen in this figure is the original connection between the diencephalon and the telencephalon. It will become greatly enlarged by fibers and tracts, especially by the continuation of the internal capsule.

248

Fig. 21-6.

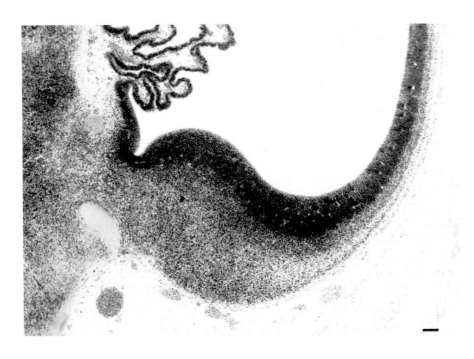

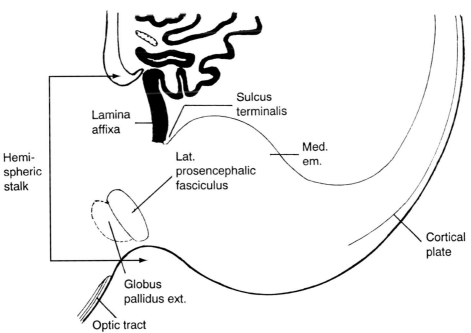

Fig. 21-7. The cortical plate is visible within the cell-poor primordial plexiform layer at the periphery of the ventricular eminences. The plate separates the former primordial plexiform layer into the subpial layer, which is future layer 1, and the subplate (Fig. 6-3). The subplate contains thalamocortical fibers that arrived in the primordial plexiform layer already at the previous stage. Penetration of the cortical plate by mono-amine fibers occurs at the end of trimester 1 (Verney et al., 1993). It is to be noted that the subpial layer and the subplate appear during the embryonic period and not, as has been claimed (Kostović and Rakic, 1990), in the middle third of prenatal life. Transient fibers in the subplate are illustrated in Figure 23-20. The intermediate layer is adjacent to the subventricular layer. Glial production begins from stem cells in the subventricular layer. From Müller and O'Rahilly (1990b).

Fig. 21-8. An overall view of the septal area showing the nucleus of the diagonal band. The prosencephalic septum is closely related to the hippocampal region, which lies dorsomedially. A faint groove separates the lateral and medial ventricular eminences. The cortical plate of the neocortex is contiguous to the pyriform cortex. The lateral olfactory tract is visible. The loose tissue surrounding the base of the telencephalon is a basal cistern.

Neurochemical resemblances have been recorded in the rat between the medial ventricular eminence and the globus pallidus. Also in the rat it has been found that most of the cells of the lateral ventricular eminence become acetylcholinesterase-positive and dopamine-receptive, whereas very few of the cells of the medial eminence do so. Between stages 19 and 23 large interneurons form (Freeman et al., 1995). Most telencephalic neurons arise in the ventricular and subventricular layers. In addition, neocortical GABA-expressing interneurons are believed to be derived (in the mouse) from the lateral ventricular eminence. Indeed, in the human (at 26 mm) GABA-positive cells have been found dorsal and ventral to the developing cortical plate (Zecevic et al., 1995). Striatal progenitors do not proliferate in a strict stem cell mode i.e., a stem cell that would give rise to one postmitotic cell and one mitotic daughter cell, which would then continue to divide in a similar manner.

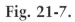

Fig. 21-7.

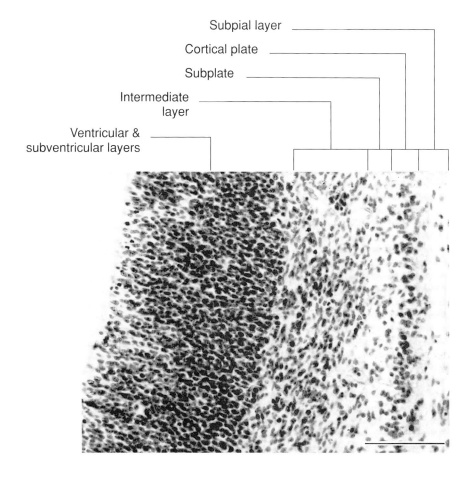

Subpial layer

Cortical plate

Subplate

Intermediate
layer

Ventricular &
subventricular layers

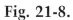

Fig. 21-8.

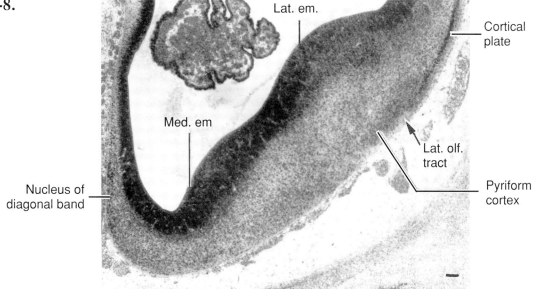

Lat. em.

Cortical
plate

Med. em

Lat. olf.
tract

Nucleus of
diagonal band

Pyriform
cortex

The levels of Figures 21-9 to 21-15 (CEC 8553) are shown in Figure 21-4B. The bars represent 0.2 mm.

Fig. 21-9. The di-mesencephalic transition showing the mamillary area with its budding surface (*"leicht höckerige Oberfläche,"* Hochstetter, 1919; *"mamelones de crecimiento,"* Orts Llorca, 1977). The buds are indicated by arrows. The habenulo-interpeduncular tract runs between the ventricular and intermediate layers, and this part of the section is the caudal area of the diencephalon. Ventrally, its median cellular material seems to be a continuation of the interpeduncular nucleus of the midbrain. Large meshes occur in the subdural space and are generally near the cerebral wall, whereas smaller meshes are found near the skeletogenous layer. From Müller and O'Rahilly (1990b).

Fig. 21-10. Section through the mamillary recess showing the migratory stream from the mamillary area to the subthalamic nucleus. The fibers, which are from the mamillotegmental tract, arise in the lateral, as well as the medial, mamillary nucleus. From Müller and O'Rahilly (1990b).

Fig. 21-11. The mamillothalamic tract runs from the lateral mamillary nucleus to the thalamus. The nucleus appears on each side as a dark, basal area. From Müller and O'Rahilly (1990b).

Fig. 21-9.

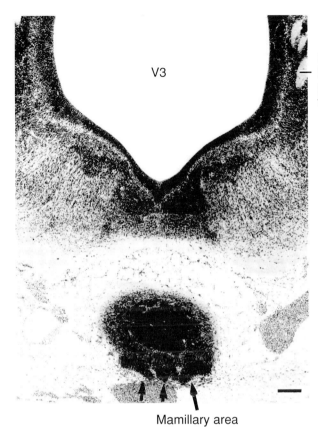

V3

Habenulo-
inter-
peduncular
tract

Mamillary area

Fig. 21-10.

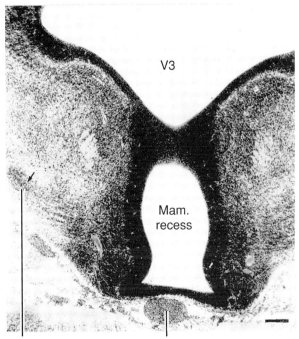

V3

Mam.
recess

Subthalamic
nucleus

Basilar a.

Fig. 21-11.

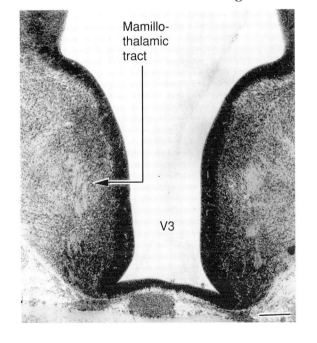

Mamillo-
thalamic
tract

V3

Fig. 21-12. The ventral part of the lateral geniculate body at the level of the sulcus medius, and the entopeduncular nucleus of the subthalamus. The entopeduncular nucleus (globus pallidus internus) is at first at a more caudal level than the globus pallidus externus. From Müller and O'Rahilly (1990b).

Fig. 21-13. Fibers of the optic tract, the globus pallidus externus, and the lateral prosencephalic bundle (*Stammbündel* of His). The cellular bridge between the medial ventricular eminence and the thalamus is important in the formation of the pulvinar during the fetal period (Rakic and Sidman, 1969). The medial ventricular eminence contains the amygdaloid area (Fig. 6-2). The central part of the neurohypophysis is visible between the lateral parts of the adenohypophysis. From Müller and O'Rahilly (1990b).

Fig. 21-12.

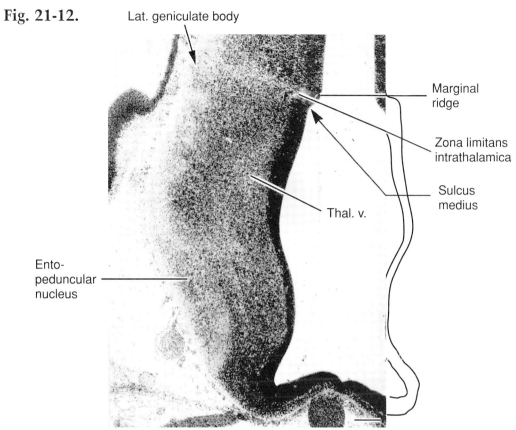

Lat. geniculate body

Marginal ridge

Zona limitans intrathalamica

Sulcus medius

Thal. v.

Ento-peduncular nucleus

Fig. 21-13.

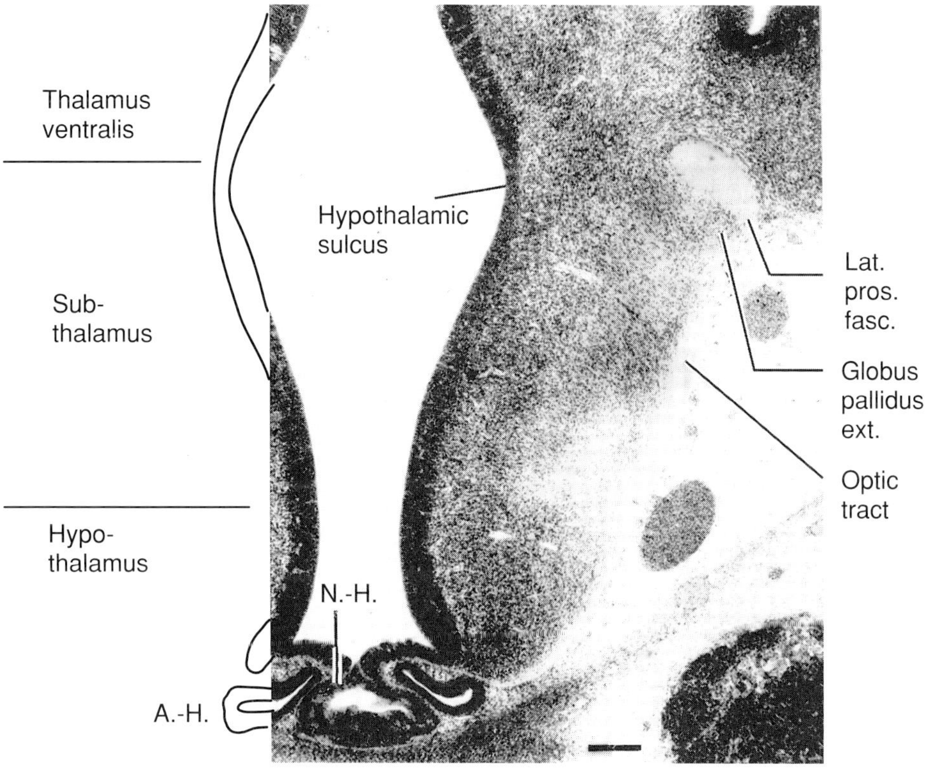

Thalamus ventralis

Hypothalamic sulcus

Sub-thalamus

Lat. pros. fasc.

Globus pallidus ext.

Optic tract

Hypo-thalamus

N.-H.

A.-H.

255

Fig. 21-14. The globus pallidus externus in a more rostral area. The lateral prosencephalic bundle is surrounded by fibers of the fasciculus lenticularis (arrowhead).

Fig. 21-15. The hippocampus and adjacent areas. The root of the choroid plexus continues into the area epithelialis. From there, the following zones can be traced upwards: area dentata, hippocampus and subiculum, and mesocortex. In the hippocampus, marginal and pyramidal cells can already be distinguished (Müller and O'Rahilly, 1990b). The telencephalon is separated from the diencephalon by loose mesenchyme. The stria medullaris thalami and the folded roof of the third ventricle are visible. From Müller and O'Rahilly (1990b).

Fig. 21-16. Schematic representation of the development of the tentorium cerebelli at stage 21. The medial part is shown by hatching, the lateral parts by black arrows. From O'Rahilly and Müller (1986).

Fig. 21-14.

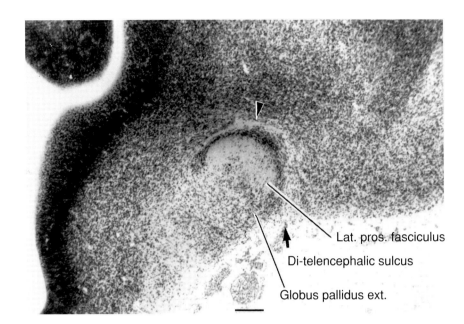

Lat. pros. fasciculus

Di-telencephalic sulcus

Globus pallidus ext.

Fig. 21-15.

Fig. 21-16.

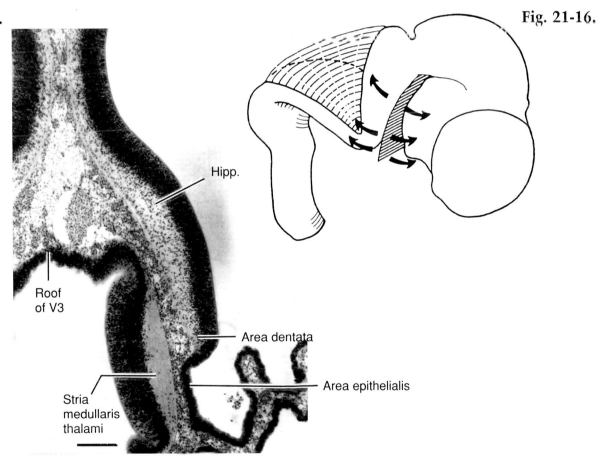

Hipp.

Roof
of V3

Area dentata

Stria
medullaris
thalami

Area epithelialis

257

Fig. 21-17. General view of the cerebellum (CEC 8553) at the level shown in Figure 21-3. Choroid villi are present in the choroid fold and in the wall of the lateral recess of the fourth ventricle. The internal cerebellar swelling, which is lateral to the sulcus limitans, consists mainly of cellular columns of the ventricular layer. A lighter area represents the layer of the future pyriform (Purkinje) cells, followed by the internal fiber layer. The dark area near the lower part of the section, which is the rostral portion of the cerebellar plate, is the primordium of the dentate nucleus (between arrowheads). The external fiber layer is entirely at the periphery. The area between the two arrowheads is a small bulb, which, more ventrally, contains fibers of the inferior cerebellar peduncle. Bar: 0.2 mm.

Fig. 21-18. The internal cerebellar swellings (CEC 8553) at the level shown in Figure 21-3. The vertical columns of the ventricular layer are distinct. Numerous blood vessels penetrate almost as far as the ventricular surface. The rhombic lip has no marginal layer. Bar: 0.2 mm.

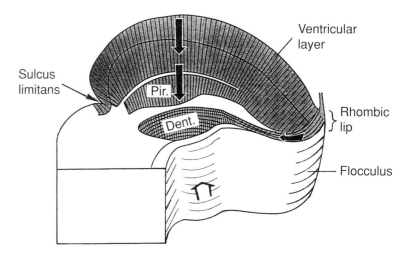

In this schematic interpretation of the section the open arrow indicates the ascending fibers of the inferior cerebellar peduncle, the black arrows the direction of the migrating cells.

Fig. 21-17.

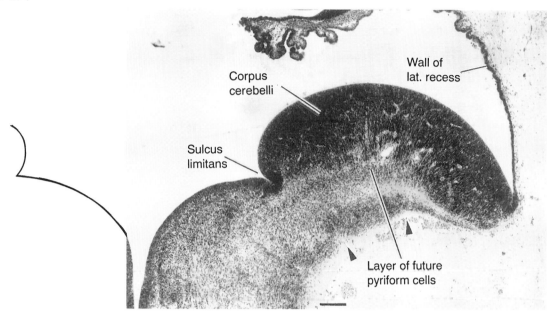

Fig. 21-18.

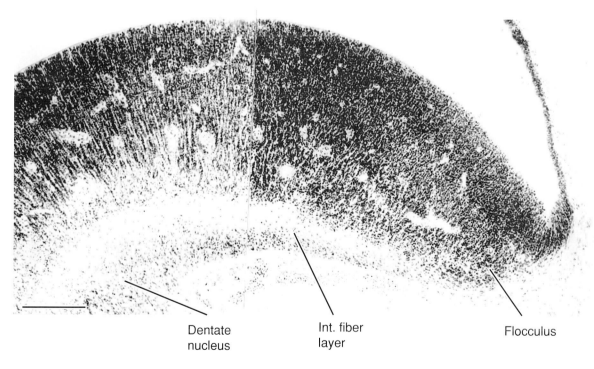

Fig. 21-19. Right lateral views to show the ventricular cavities (indicated in black): (**A**) stage 13, (**B**) stage 15, (**C**) stage 17, and (**D**) stage 21. The ventricles at stage 23 are illustrated in Figure 23-25.

The stippled structures are the otic vesicle, the trigeminal ganglion (in A only), and the optic vesicle, cup, and eye. From O'Rahilly and Müller (1996b).

<u>Important</u>

It should be stressed that, although the third ventricle is mostly diencephalic, its preoptic portion is telencephalic. This rostral part is visible in Figure 21-3 below the interrupted line through the forebrain.

Fig. 21-19.

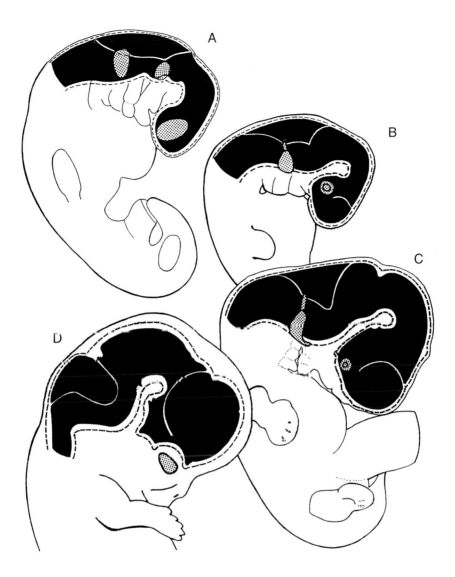

Fig. 21-20. The arterial system at about 6 to 7 postfertilizational weeks. The internal carotid artery is shown in black, and the basilar by horizontal hatching.

(**A**) and (**B**) The arteries at stage 17 (CEC 940 and CEC 1771, respectively). New vessels that can now be identified include the anterior and middle cerebral (AC, MC), and the anterior and posterior choroid arteries. The vertebral artery is formed by anastomoses between the cervical segmental arteries.

(**C**) and (**D**) The arteries at stage 21 (CEC 623) showing the anterior, middle, and posterior cerebral vessels. The anterior communicating artery is present, so that the circulus arteriosus is now complete. The choroid plexuses of the lateral and fourth ventricles are included. These drawings are based on graphic reconstructions made by Padget (1948), whose work should be studied for further details. The venous system at stages 18, 19, 20, and 21 has been illustrated by Padget (1957, Figs. 6, 9, 11, and 10). The arterial system at the end of the embryonic period is shown in Figures 23-29 and 23-30.

Abbreviations: AC, anterior cerebral; AICA, anterior inferior cerebellar artery; DA, ductus arteriosus; MC, middle cerebral; PC, posterior cerebral; P.co., posterior communicating; PICA, posterior inferior cerebellar artery; PT, pulmonary trunk.

Fig. 21-20.

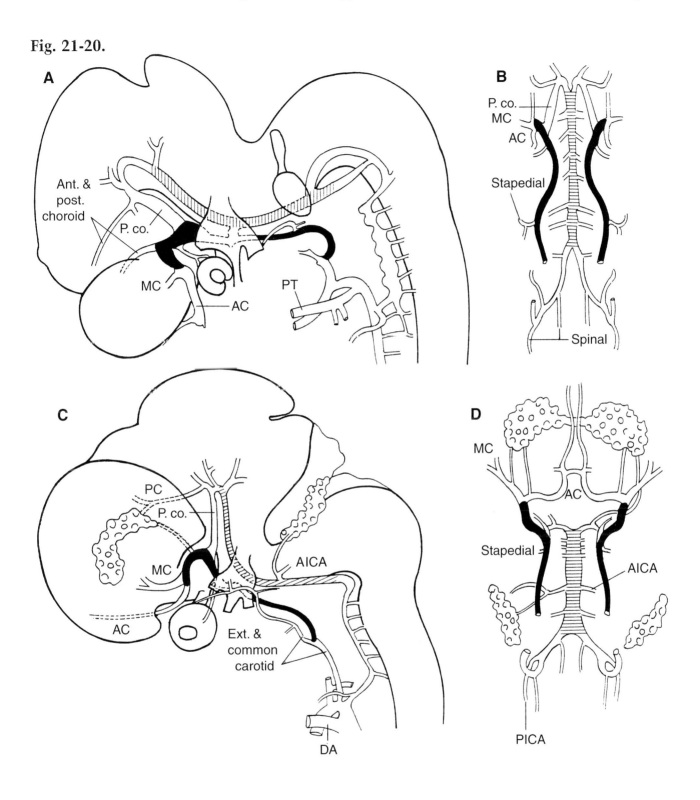

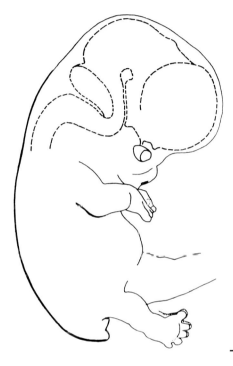

Stage 22: The Internal Capsule and the Olfactory Tract

Approximately 23–28 mm in Greatest Length
Approximately 52 Postfertilizational Days

Fig. 22-1. Right lateral view of an embryo (CEC 8394) of stage 22 with the brain (CEC 1458) superimposed. From O'Rahilly, Müller, and Bossy (1986).

The internal capsule and its connections to the neopallium are now present. Outlets lead (1) to the epithalamus, (2) to the dorsal thalamus, and (3) to the mesencephalon. The claustrum develops, and a clear developmental relationship exists between it and the intermediate layer of the olfactory bulb. The globus pallidus externus moves towards a telencephalic position. Further details: Müller and O'Rahilly (1990b).

265

Fig. 22-2. Right lateral view of the brain (CEC 840). The cerebral hemispheres cover about three-quarters of the diencephalon. The three poles (α, β, γ) are distinguishable. The mesencephalon is "ballooning out" (Bartelmez and Dekaban, 1962), sits on top of the brain, and is higher than the cerebellar plates. Its delineation, therefore, is easier than in earlier stages. The inferior colliculus forms a slight bulge on top of the *Blindsack*. The isthmus is markedly narrow. The posterolateral fissure, which delineates the future flocculus, has become a sharp boundary. The cerebellar plates are no longer as wide as the cerebral hemispheres (see inset). A reconstruction of the cranial nerves (CEC 1458) is available (Müller and O'Rahilly, 1991, Fig. 4).

Fig. 22-2.

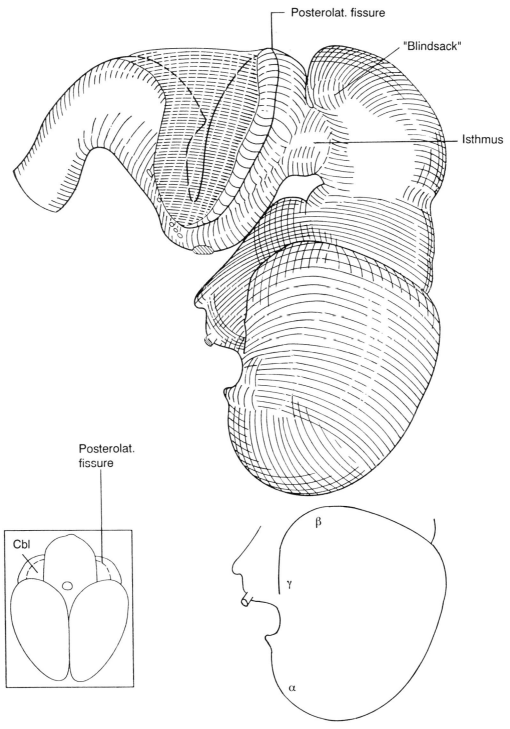

Fig. 22-3. Graphic reconstruction prepared from transverse sections to show a median view of the brain (D-10269 combined with features of CEC 1458). The asterisk indicates the junction with the spinal cord. The internal relief is shown, and the structures of the medial wall of the left hemisphere are projected as interrupted lines: the caudal extent of the cerebral hemispheres, the area dentata, and the hippocampus. The hippocampus extends between the occipital pole and the prosencephalic septum. The marginal ridge separates the diencephalon into halves: the dorsal thalamus on one side, and the ventral thalamus, subthalamus, and hypothalamus on the other. The pineal recess (arrow at right) is still undivided. The isthmic groove (upper arrow) and the isthmic recess (lower arrow) are also marked. The commissural plate has become thicker. No fusion takes place during the embryonic period proper between the cerebral hemispheres, as was clearly understood and stated by Hochstetter (1919).* The approximate levels of Figures 22-7 to 22-12 are indicated, although the fit does not correspond completely, because these are from different embryos. (For example, in Figure 22-7 the interpeduncular fossa is slightly more dorsal than in Figure 22-3.) A three-dimensional reconstruction, prepared ultrasonically, of the ventricles *in vivo* in an embryo of 24 mm is illustrated by Blaas et al. (1995).

---

* "Nicht der kleinste Umstand aber deutet darauf hin, dass die zu beobachtende Dickenzunahme etwa auf eine Verwachsung der unmittelbar an die Kommissurenplatte anschliessenden Abschnitte der medialen Hemisphärenwände zurückzuführen wäre" (p. 109). See also definition of Massa commissuralis in Chapter 6, this volume.

Fig. 22-3.

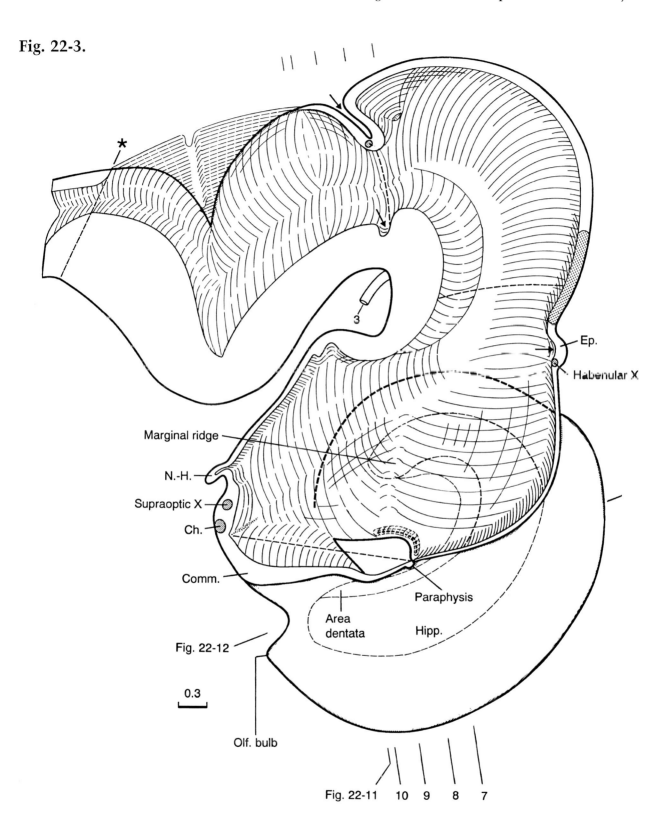

* \
3

Ep.

Habenular X

Marginal ridge

N.-H.

Supraoptic X

Ch.

Comm.

Paraphysis

Fig. 22-12

Area
dentata

Hipp.

0.3

Olf. bulb

Fig. 22-11   10   9   8   7

Fig. 22-4. Median view to show elements that are important in understanding the internal capsule. The lateral ventricular eminence, which gives rise to the future corpus striatum, is projected onto the medial surface to show its extent. The fibers of the lateral prosencephalic fasciculus (*Stammbündel* of His) arise in the neopallial wall and descend lateral to the lateral ventricular eminence. The fibers, having traversed the hemispheric stalk, ascend in the diencephalic wall and spread into, among other structures, the dorsal thalamus. All the structures indicated are shown as if the prosencephalon were transparent.

It has been found (in the hamster) that thalamocortical fibers (stage 21) are present before corticothalamic fibers become visible in the internal capsule.

Important

Contrary to the opinion of certain authors in the past (including His), what appears to be a fusion between the cerebral hemisphere and the diencephalon is a thickening of the thalamic wall at the di-telencephalic sulcus as the internal capsular fibers begin to pass through it. This was appreciated by Hochstetter (1929) and Sharp (1959), as well as by Bartelmez (cited by Padget, 1957).

Fig. 22-4.

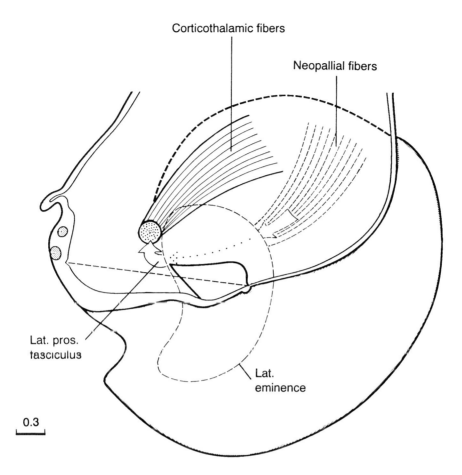

Corticothalamic fibers

Neopallial fibers

Lat. pros.
fasciculus

Lat.
eminence

0.3

Fig. 22-5. Left lateral view of a reconstruction of the brain and chondrocranium (CEC 1458). The asterisk indicates the junction with the spinal cord. The basal portions of the skull are present in cartilage. The basolateral and lateral walls are still far from complete, but the following are discernible: the greater and lesser wings of the sphenoid; the otic capsule; and the parietal plate, which is not yet fused with the plate of the other side. Hence the foramen magnum has not yet developed. The chondrocranium of stage 22 is compared with that of stage 23 in Figure 23-8. From Müller and O'Rahilly (1991).

Fig. 22-5.

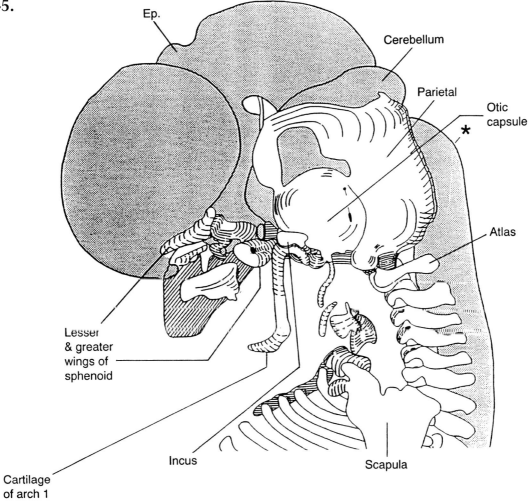

Ep.

Cerebellum

Parietal

Otic capsule

*

Atlas

Lesser & greater wings of sphenoid

Incus

Scapula

Cartilage of arch 1

Fig. 22-6. A schematic representation of the development of the internal capsule (based on reconstructions of G-24). Modified from Müller and O'Rahilly (1990b).

(**A**) Dorsal view of the opened right hemisphere showing the internal capsule in relation to the lateral ventricular eminence. Neopallial fibers (between the black arrowheads), which are an essential component of the definitive internal capsule, are shown on their way from the neopallium, lateral to the ventricular eminence and running to the lateral prosencephalic fasciculus (cf. Fig. 22-11). The first fibers can be traced to an area comparable to the later postcentral gyrus. The lateral ventricular eminence has grown more rapidly than the medial, which is adjacent to the hemispheric stalk. A faint groove called the intereminential sulcus by the present writers is distinguishable between the eminences.

The neurons for the neostriatum arise during stages 21–23, as has been shown in rhesus. It has been found that the histochemical development of the nucleus accumbens resembles that of the lateral ventricular eminence.

(**B**) A right lateral view showing the internal capsule in more detail. The neopallial fibers (black arrowheads) between the primordia of the future caudate nucleus medially, and the putamen laterally, accumulate in the thick lateral prosencephalic fasciculus (*Stammbündel* of His) before entering the diencephalon. Finally they continue in three main groups: epithalamic, thalamic, and mesencephalic (white arrows). The main bundle is arched over by the stria terminalis, which is composed chiefly of fibers that can be traced to the medial part of the amygdaloid nuclei.

(**C**) Also a right lateral view: the cortical plate at stage 22 (stippled area) extends over half the surface of the neopallium, and its increase from stage 22 to stage 23 is shown.

Fig. 22-6.

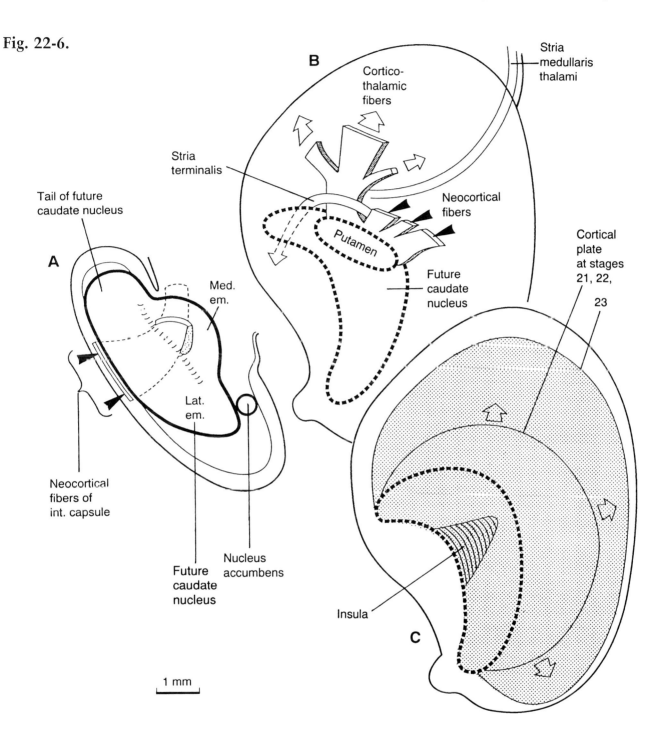

Figures 22-7 to 22-11. The levels of these sections (CEC 8394) are indicated in Figure 22-3. The left side is cut at a deeper level than the right. The sections of Figures 22-7 to 22-9 and of Figure 22-11 were selected by Bartelmez and Dekaban (1962), who completed their study with stage 22. The bars represent 1 mm.

Fig. 22-7. The lateral ventricular eminence, hippocampus, and choroid plexus are visible. The folded roof of the diencephalon is adjacent to the stria medullaris thalami on each side. The dorsal thalami appear dark. The mesencephalic ventricle (future aqueduct) and its prolongation into the right inferior colliculus are evident. The fiber masses in the tegmentum are increasing. The medial longitudinal fasciculus is visible on each side. Dorsal to the main mesencephalic ventricle, the white lines are fibers leading to the trochlear decussation.

Fig. 22-8. The cortical plate is evident on each side and is mostly opposite the ventricular eminences at the site of the future insula. At the beginning of its appearance a part of the cortical plate contains early-generated subplate cells (McConnell et al., 1989), which leave the cortical plate and reside in the subcortical plate. They are responsible for the descending axons that run in the intermediate zone and reach the internal capsule. A faint groove can be seen between the medial and lateral eminences. The sulcus terminalis is medial, towards the diencephalon. The inferior horn of the left lateral ventricle is evident. The diencephalic area dorsal to the hypothalamic sulcus is mainly ventral thalamus. In the isthmus, the tegmentum is filled with fibers, including the medial longitudinal fasciculus. The cerebellar plate is visible to the left of the isthmus.

Fig. 22-7.

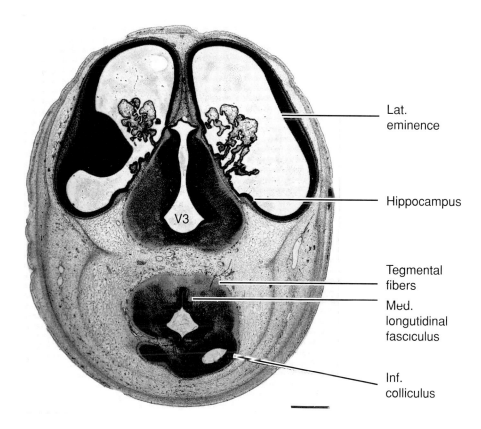

Lat. eminence

Hippocampus

Tegmental fibers

Med. longutidinal fasciculus

Inf. colliculus

V3

Fig. 22-8.

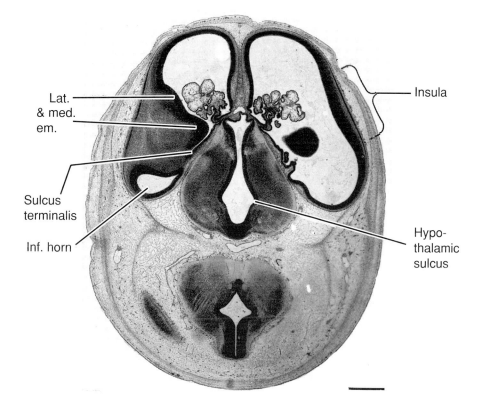

Lat. & med. em.

Sulcus terminalis

Inf. horn

Insula

Hypo- thalamic sulcus

Fig. 22-9. This section, at the level of the interventricular foramina, shows the lateral prosencephalic fasciculus (*Stammbündel* of His) on the left side. The sulcus terminalis is the internal boundary between telencephalon and diencephalon. The mamillary region and the mamillothalamic tract are visible. The internal cerebellar swellings almost fill the fourth ventricle. The fibers penetrating it (on the left side) belong mainly to the inferior cerebellar peduncle. The lateral portions of the tentorium cerebelli are evident here as well as in the other sections.

Fig. 22-10. At the right, fibers can be seen arising in the neopallium and running towards the *Stammbündel*, which is visible at the di-telencephalic borderline (hemispheric stalk). The stalk lies between the sulcus terminalis on the ventricular and the di-telencephalic sulcus on the external surface. The mamillary region still shows. At the rostral surface of the left cerebellar plate, the lighter triangular area is the inferior cerebellar peduncle. To its left is the flocculus, and to its right is the area of the dentate nucleus.

Fig. 22-9.

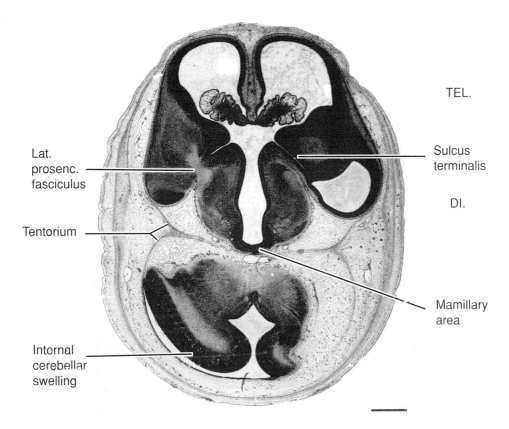

Lat. prosenc. fasciculus

TEL.

Sulcus terminalis

DI.

Tentorium

Mamillary area

Intornal cerebellar swelling

Fig. 22-10.

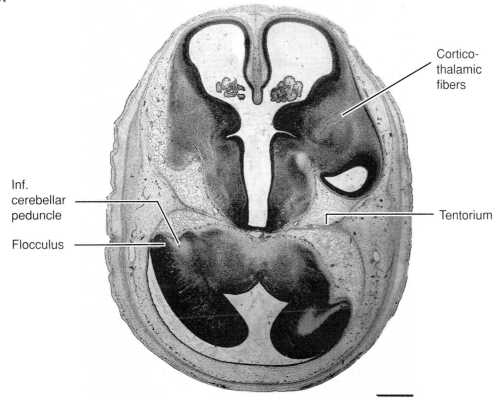

Cortico-thalamic fibers

Inf. cerebellar peduncle

Flocculus

Tentorium

Fig. 22-11. The entire extent of the internal capsule is visible in the right hemisphere. Some villi are present in the thin wall of the lateral recess of the fourth ventricle. Although skeletal elements are not encountered as far dorsally as this level, the skeletogenous layer is clearly delimited (cf. Fig. 22-14B).

Fig. 22-12. The primordium of the claustrum develops as a condensed stream of neurons that extends from the area caudal to the olfactory bulb and along the lateral ventricular eminence to the future insular region. The level of the section is shown in Figure 22-3. Later in trimester 1, cells of the subventricular layer of the olfactory bulb will form the subpial granular layer. Bar: 0.2 mm.

Fig. 22-11.

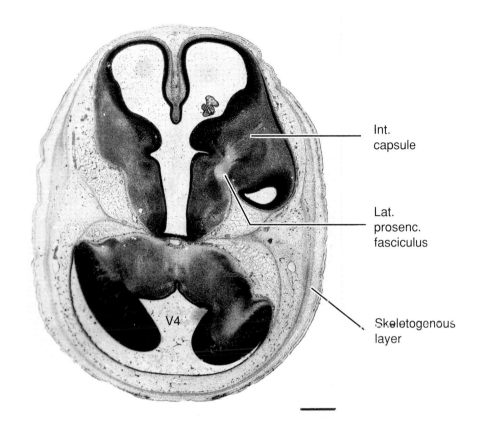

Int. capsule

Lat. prosenc. fasciculus

Skeletogenous layer

V4

Fig. 22-12.

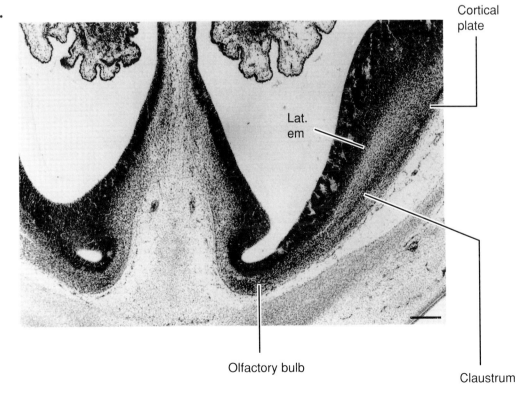

Cortical plate

Lat. em

Olfactory bulb

Claustrum

281

Fig. 22-13. The choroid folds of the fourth ventricle as seen in a coronal section (D-9886) through the rhombencephalon. The first inset drawing indicates the field shown in A. The second illustrates the migration pathways in the rhombencephalon: (1) from the rhombic lip along the external surface of the brain stem, and (2) from the entire ventricular layer into the alar and basal laminae.

(**A**) The ependyma of the lateral recess presents small villi, whereas the choroid folds more medially show large villi. The rhombic lip is well developed but differs in shape depending on the stage and the precise region (e.g., Fig. 21-18). In addition to the median sulcus, the sulcus limitans is distinguishable on each side. The tractus solitarius (asterisk) is visible inside the alar lamina. Dark areas on both sides of the median raphe are the rostral parts of the inferior olivary nuclei. ×36.

(**B**) A view at higher power. Blood vessels have penetrated the choroid folds. The tall neurons of the hypoglossal nucleus are discernible medially, adjacent to the matrix of the basal lamina (dagger). ×87.

The choroid pleuxus of the fourth ventricle, from its first appearance at stage 19, is more advanced than that of the telencephalon. Apertures are not present yet. The choroid plexus will undergo enlargement and differentiation, including the production of more villi and the appearance of two types of ependymal cells, dark and light. Further details: O'Rahilly and Müller (1990).

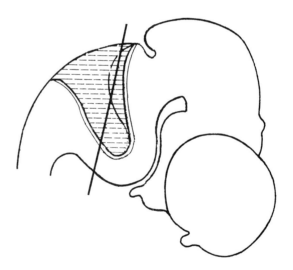

Fig. 22-13.

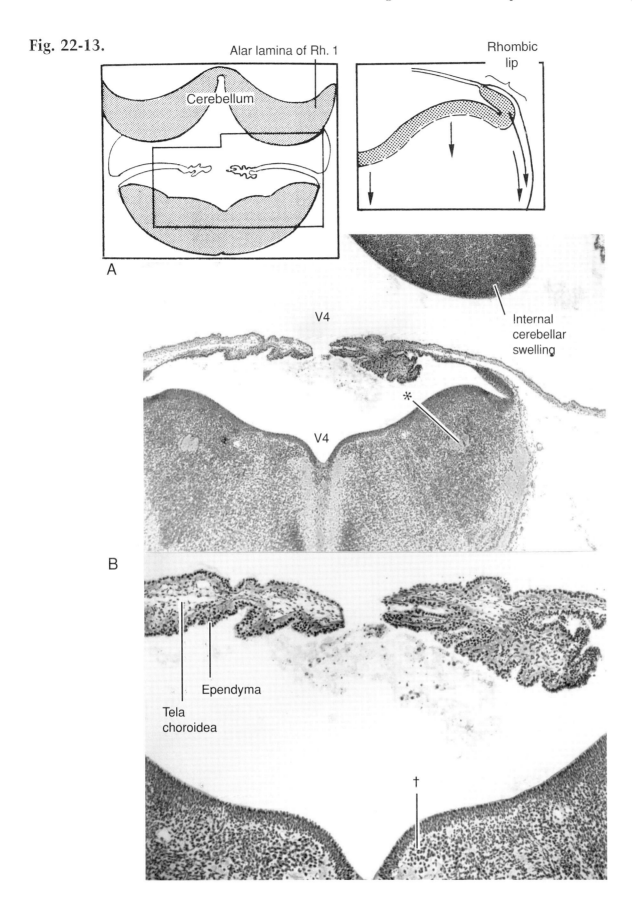

Fig. 22-14. Schematic representation of the development of the cranial meninges.

(**A**) At approximately $3\frac{1}{2}$ postfertilizational weeks, mesenchyme from various sources surrounds the brain, and blood vessels are present. The sources probably include prechordal plate, unsegmented paraxial mesenchyme, segmented paraxial (somitic) mesenchyme, ectomesenchyme (neural crest), and neurilemmal cells (neural crest). The pia mater develops between the blood vessels and the cerebral wall. A dense skeletogenous layer forms at the periphery and veins are situated on its internal aspect. As the meningeal vessels are transformed into arteries and veins, they become progressively isolated from the CSF compartment (Marín-Padilla, 1988b).

(**B**) Approximately 7 postfertilizational weeks, the dural limiting layer appears between the pia and the skeletogenous layer. Large meshes form in the future subarachnoid space, smaller meshes between the dural limiting and skeletogenous layers (in the pachymeninx). Cartilage and intramembranous bone are forming within the skeletogenous layer. The veins (dural sinuses) on the internal aspect of the skeletogenous layer are now intradural in position. Modified from O'Rahilly and Müller (1986).

The leptomeningeal cells establish perivascular spaces around the arachnoidal and pial vessels, and these drain into the perivascular lymphatic system of the extracranial vasculature (Marín-Padilla, 1988b).

(**C**) Scheme of the meninges in the adult. So-called subdural hemorrhage is within the dural border layer and hence is intradural. Based largely on Schachenmayr and Friede (1978) and Alcolado et al. (1988).

The development of the cranial meninges was investigated by Hochstetter (1939) among others, and the complicated origin of these membranes from several sources (including the prechordal plate, parachordal mesoderm, and neural crest) was studied by O'Rahilly and Müller (1986). The loose mesenchyme around most of the brain at stage 13 (Fig. 13-5) is termed the primary meninx. At stage 17 the dural limiting layer begins to form basally (Fig. 17-6) and the skeletogenous layer of the head soon becomes visible (Fig. 22-14). At stage 23 the pachymeninx and the leptomeninx are distinguishable in the head (Fig. 23-9).

The spinal meninges have been investigated particularly by Hochstetter (1934) and Sensenig (1951). The future pia mater, derived from neural crest cells, can be detected at stage 11 and, at stage 15, the primary meninx is represented by a loose zone between the vertebral primordia and the neural tube. At stage 18 the mesenchyme adjacent to the vertebrae becomes condensed as the dural lamella. At stage 23 the dura lines the vertebral canal completely and the future subarachnoid space is becoming cell-free. The arachnoid, however, does not appear until either trimester 3 or postnatally, although a much earlier artifact has frequently been mistaken for it.

Fig. 22-14.

A

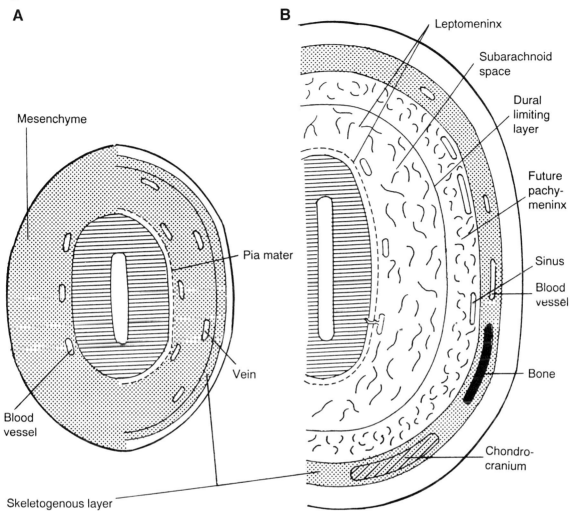

Mesenchyme

Pia mater

Vein

Blood vessel

Skeletogenous layer

B

Leptomeninx

Subarachnoid space

Dural limiting layer

Future pachy-meninx

Sinus

Blood vessel

Bone

Chondro-cranium

C

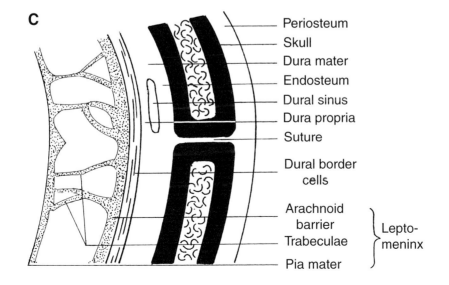

Periosteum

Skull

Dura mater

Endosteum

Dural sinus

Dura propria

Suture

Dural border cells

Arachnoid barrier

Trabeculae

Pia mater

Lepto-meninx

Comments on Neuroteratology (Stage 22)

Exencephaly. The second phase in the development of anencephaly is the exposure of a highly developing and well-differentiated brain during the embryonic period proper. A number of examples are available in the literature (Table 3 of Müller and O'Rahilly, 1991). The condition includes either cranioschisis or craniorhachischisis. An examination of anencephaly at stage 22 has shown that the brain attains a high degree of differentiation before disintegration takes place during the fetal period (Müller and O'Rahilly, 1991). The skeletal covering, however, can become deviated very early, so that the typical features of an anencephalic skull can be present before the characteristics of an anencephalic brain. Moreover, even as early as stage 22, variations in anencephaly are noteworthy.

In their useful book on anencephaly, Lemire, Beckwith, and Warkany (1978) illustrate 56 instances of embryos/fetuses that range from 17 mm (22 mm when fresh) to 345 mm (360 mm when fresh) in C-R length.

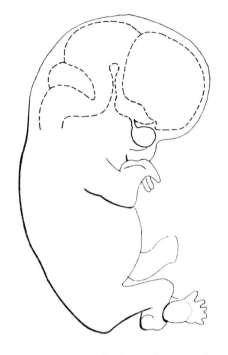

Stage 23: The Brain at the End of the Embryonic Period

Approximately 27–31 mm in Greatest Length
Approximately 56 Postfertilizational Days

Fig. 23-1. Right lateral view of an embryo of stage 23 (CEC 9226) with the brain superimposed. From O'Rahilly, Müller, and Bossy (1986).

Stage 23, 8 postfertilizational weeks, is stressed here because this is the close of the embryonic period proper. The cortical plate covers almost the whole neopallial surface. The hippocampus has reached the temporal pole; its cells exhibit the largest intercellular distances in the entire brain. The insula appears as an indented area. In the corpus striatum the primordia of the caudate nucleus and the putamen are recognizable, and the globus pallidus externus has moved into a telencephalic position. The anterior commissure begins to develop in the commissural plate, which has gained in thickness. It needs to be stressed that the telencephalon and the diencephalon are not fused. The optic tract reaches the ventral portion of the lateral geniculate body. The dorsal thalamus occupies approximately half of the medial diencephalic surface. In addition to the ventricular layer, which is found in all parts of the brain, the rhombic lip has a germinative role. It produces the external germinal layer of the cerebellum, which has begun to spread over the rostral surface of the flocculus. The rhombic lip also

287

gives off olivo-arcuate and pontine migratory sheets. The cerebellar commissures have appeared. Two cerebellar peduncles, the inferior and the superior, are distinguishable. The presence of the pyramidal decussation is noted for the first time during the embryonic period. A reconstruction of the arteries at stage 23 is presented for the first time. The brain at stage 23 is far more advanced morphologically than is generally appreciated, to such an extent that functional considerations are imperative. The arrangement of the rhombencephalic nuclei and tracts at 8 weeks is very similar to that present in the newborn. It is likely that the rapid growth of the rhombencephalon during the embryonic period proper is associated with correspondingly early functional activity. Further details: Müller and O'Rahilly (1980, 1990a,b), O'Rahilly and Müller (1990).

Important

The term basal nuclei is best reserved for the basal structures affected pathologically in so-called extrapyramidal motor diseases, i.e., the corpus striatum, the subthalamic nucleus, and the substantia nigra (Fig. 6-2). The inclusion of the claustrum and the amygdaloid body, however, has little to recommend it.

Fig. 23-2. Lateral view (reversed) of the brain (CEC 5154), drawn by Mary M. Cope from a reconstruction and published by Gilbert (1957). This stage was not included by Bartelmez and Dekaban (1962). The insula, previously recognizable by its flat surface (stages 18–20), is now clearly indented. Almost the entire diencephalon is covered by the cerebral hemispheres, so that the epiphysis cerebri is no longer visible in this embryo, although it is in some others of the same stage (Fig. 23-4). Contrary to the opinion of certain authors in the past, the telencephalon and the diencephalon are not fused: they are separated from each other by a thin sheet of mesenchyme.

The interrupted circle around the key drawing serves to emphasize that the brain is more compact than in the previous stage. This is related in part to the progression of such C-shaped features as the hippocampus, the corpus striatum, and the entire cerebral hemispheres.

The inset shows the topographical changes of the hemispheric poles from stage 18 (continuous line) to stage 23 (dotted line). From O'Rahilly, Müller, and Bossy (1986).

Fig. 23-2.

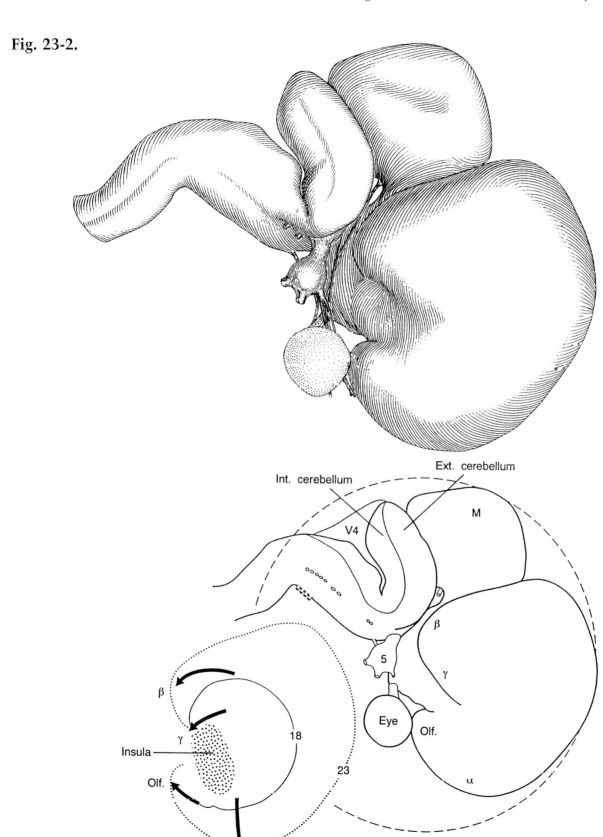

Fig. 23-3. The cranial nerves.

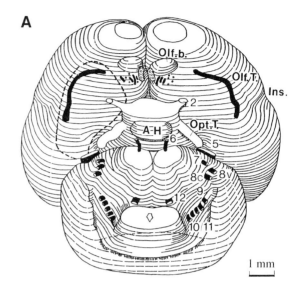

(**A**) A basal view of the brain at stage 23 (*Perspektomat* reconstruction of CEC 9226) showing most of the cranial nerves. The mesencephalon and nerves 3 and 4 are hidden. The combined cerebral hemispheres are now wider than the cerebellum. From Müller and O'Rahilly (1990b).

(**B**) Reconstruction of the cranial nerves (CEC 9226) in relationship to some of the "membrane" bones and to the surface of the head. The arrangement of the nerves is now very complex and resembles the adult pattern. The laryngeal nerves are a good example of this (Müller et al., 1981, 1985). Interestingly, small branches that are easily overlooked in the adult can readily be followed in embryos and fetuses. The recurrent branch of the trochlear nerve is a case in point. The skeletal surroundings of the nerves, however, are still in an unfinished state. The facial nerve, for example, is surrounded only by mesenchyme instead of bone, and neither the cribriform plate nor the foramen ovale has formed. All the cranial autonomic ganglia are present. The main divisions of the trigeminal nerve (5) are marked by superscripts 1, 2, and 3. The sheaths of cranial nerves 3, 4, and 5 are partly meningeal and partly peripheral in type (Kehrli et al., 1995).

290

Fig. 23-3.

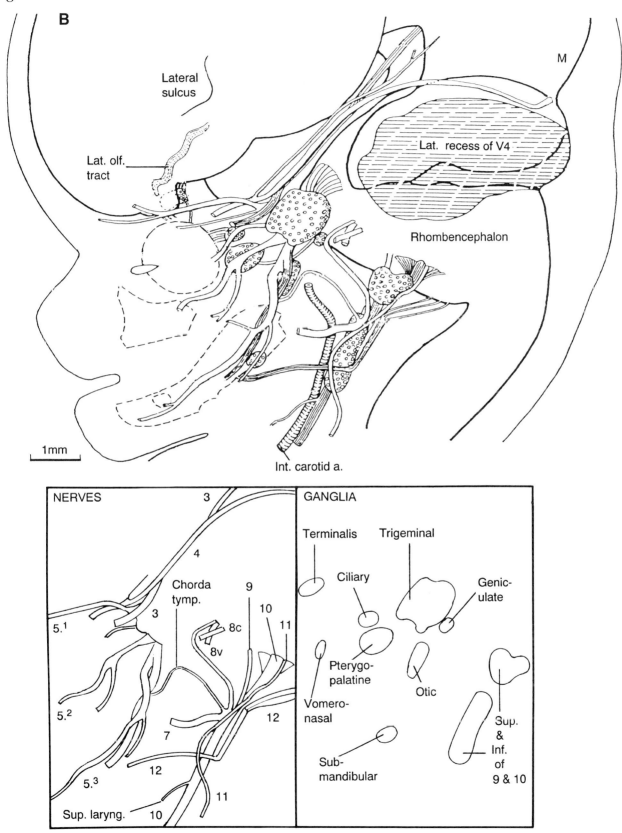

B

Lateral
sulcus

Lat. olf.
tract

Lat. recess of V4

M

Rhombencephalon

1mm

Int. carotid a.

NERVES	GANGLIA
3	Terminalis Trigeminal
4	Ciliary Geniculate
Chorda tymp.	
9	
5.¹	10
3	11
8c	Pterygo-palatine
8v	Vomeronasal Otic
5.²	
7	12
12	Sub-mandibular Sup. & Inf. of 9 & 10
5.³	
Sup. laryng. 10	
11	

291

Fig. 23-4. Graphic reconstruction prepared from transverse sections to show a median view of the brain (CEC 9226) in which the internal relief is based on an unpublished *Perspektomat* reconstruction. The asterisk indicates the junction with the spinal cord. The outline of the left hemisphere is continued as an interrupted line. Only small portions of the diencephalic surface remain uncovered by the hemispheres. The ditelencephalic sulcus is filled with mesenchyme (Figs. 23-17 and 23-22) and the only bridge is that present since the beginning, which is now termed the hemispheric stalk. The stalk contains fibers between the thalamus and the hemisphere, and these travel in the lateral prosencephalic fasciculus, as seen already in the previous stage (Fig. 22-6). Corticothalamic fibers arise in proximity to the future central sulcus, probably in the area that corresponds to the future precentral and/or postcentral gyrus. The commissural plate is very thick and, in some embryos, is approached by fibers of the anterior commissure. Lateral strands leading to the site of the commissure can be observed before crossing fibers are present. The choroid fissure is now longer. The fissure and the hippocampus are shown as if the prosencephalon were transparent. The height of the diencephalon from the chiasmatic plate to the epiphysis is appreciable. The suprapineal recess has developed. The marginal ridge, which separates the dorsal from the ventral thalamus, ends at the level of the interventricular foramen. In this embryo the fibers of the posterior commissure are separated from those of the commissure of the superior colliculi, which latter has two portions. If not earlier, then at least at stage 23 it would seem to be legitimate to use the terms basal nuclei and corpus striatum, and their various components (Fig. 6-2).

The internal ridge in the mesencephalon does not seem to indicate the border between neuromeres M1 and M2. The isthmic recess has become a shallow groove. Dopaminergic neurons are no longer produced in the ventrocaudal proliferative area of the mesencephalon, as they were from $6\frac{1}{2}$ to $7\frac{1}{2}$ weeks (Freeman et al., 1991).

A commissure of considerable size situated adjacent to the isthmic recess seems to be the decussation of the superior cerebellar peduncles (Cooper, 1946a). The cerebellum is not visible in its whole extent because portions of it extend ventrally and laterally, and are hidden by the rhombencephalic tegmentum. The cerebellar commissures contain, from rostral to caudal: (1) decussating fibers of the mesencephalic trigeminal root, (2) decussating vestibulocerebellar fibers, and (3) fibers from the area that includes the dentate nucleus. These ontogenetic data have been partly described by other authors, although only commissure No. 3 seems to correspond with the adult condition. The decussation of the trochlear nerves is rostral to the cerebellar commissures.

At the cerebrospinal junction two bundles are found: the fasciculus cuneatus (larger) and the fasciculus gracilis (smaller). They form the decussation of the medial lemnisci. More caudally, the pyramidal decussation is shown. The pyramidal tract and its decussation become definitive bundles only at this stage.

The levels of Figures 23-12, 23-14 to 23-17, and 23-22 are indicated.

Fig. 23-4.

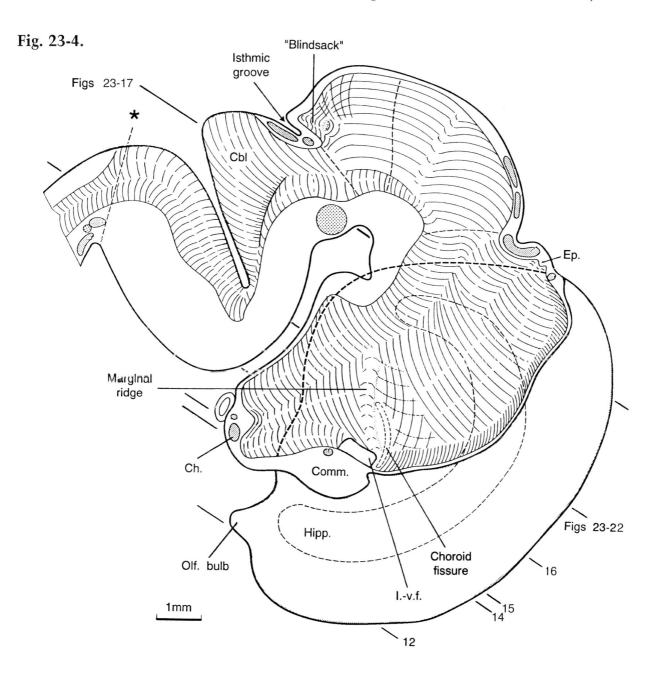

Fig. 23-5. The medial aspect of the left cerebral hemisphere and the left half of the diencephalon (D-122) are shown, including the lateral ventricular eminence and striatothalamic fibers. The thick part of the commissural plate (cf. Fig. 23-4) has also been called *massa commissuralis*. It is penetrated later in trimester 1 by fibers of the fornix. The central stem of the chondrocranium is shown by horizontal hatching. The levels of Figures 23-18 to 23-20, 23-23, and 23-24 arc indicated.

A basal view of the brain at stage 23 (CEC 9226) is shown in Figure 23-3A.

Fig. 23-5.

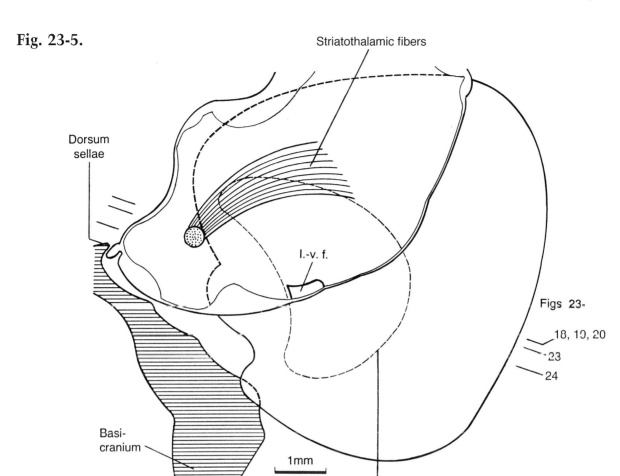

Striatothalamic fibers

Dorsum
sellae

l.-v. f.

Figs 23-

18, 19, 20

23

24

Basi-
cranium

1mm

Lat. eminence

Fig. 23-6. A sagittal (almost median) section (CEC 5422). The (left) cerebral hemisphere is seen to expand basally into the caudally directed olfactory bulb. The choroid plexus and the medial ventricular eminence are evident. The gray area caudal to the eminence is the striatothalamic radiation (lateral prosencephalic fasciculus). The hypophysis can be seen lying in the hypophysial fossa. Caudally in the mesencephalon, the (left) inferior colliculus contains a ventricular outpocketing. The skeletogenous layer of the head (Fig. 22-14B) and the subarachnoid space are recognizable. The amount of mesenchyme external to the skeletogenous layer is increasing. A reconstruction of the vertebral column of this embryo has been published (O'Rahilly, Müller, and Meyer, 1980, Fig. 3; O'Rahilly, Müller, and Meyer, 1983, Fig. 1).

Some 33 cartilaginous vertebrae are arranged in a flexed column approximately 20–23 mm in length. They do not yet show spinous processes, however, and hence a normal spina bifida occulta may be said to be present throughout the length of the column (O'Rahilly, Müller, and Meyer, 1980).

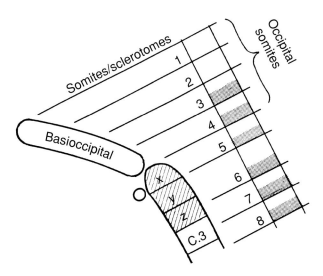

A key for the interpretation of the occipitocervical region seen in Figure 23-6. Four occipital somites develop in the human and give rise to the basi-occipital portion of the skull; X, Y, and Z refer to the three components of the central pillar of the second cervical vertebra (the axis). Further details: O'Rahilly, Müller, and Meyer (1983); Müller and O'Rahilly (1994).

Fig. 23-6.

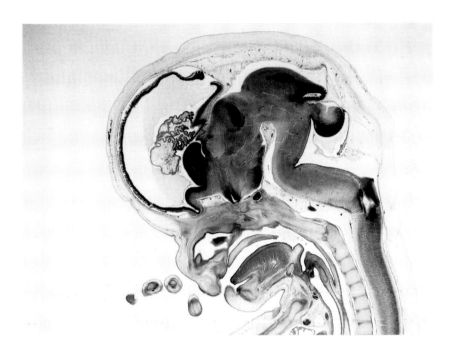

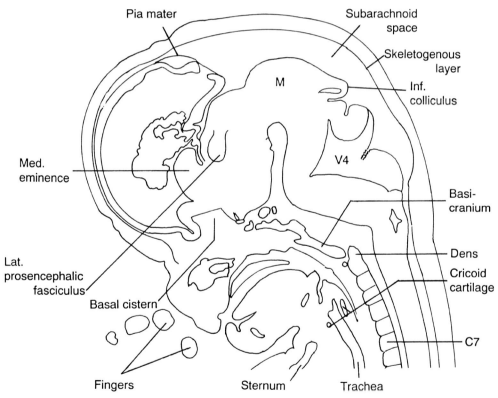

Fig. 23-7. Left lateral view of the brain and skull (CEC 9226). At this stage, as during the previous 5 weeks, the brain dominates the morphological appearance of the head. The chondrocranium is mainly a basal support for certain parts: the surface of the spheno-ethmoidal cartilage for the anterior part of the olfactory bulb; the sphenoid for the hypothalamus and the hypophysis. The mesencephalon and the cerebellum, however, lack such a basal cartilaginous support. The pons is buttressed mediobasally by the basisphenoid and laterobasally by the cochlear portion of the otic capsule. The portions of the eye and brain covered by skeletal elements are shown by interrupted lines.

The protective covering of the superolateral surface of the cerebral hemispheres is beginning to be strengthened by the frontal bones. The lateral portions of the cerebellum and of the pons and medulla oblongata are encased by the parietal laminae and by the tectum posterius and pilae occipitales. The foramen magnum is very extensive, portions of the medulla oblongata being surrounded by mesenchyme only. The cartilages of the pharyngeal arches, including the first (Meckel's), are well developed: those for the auditory ossicles, styloid process, and hyoid and laryngeal cartilages (Müller, O'Rahilly, and Tucker, 1981). The neural arches of the vertebrae have not fused across the median plane. The normal spina bifida totalis characteristic of stage 23 has been studied in detail (O'Rahilly, Müller, and Meyer, 1980, 1983, 1990a,b). From Müller and O'Rahilly (1980).

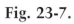

Fig. 23-7.

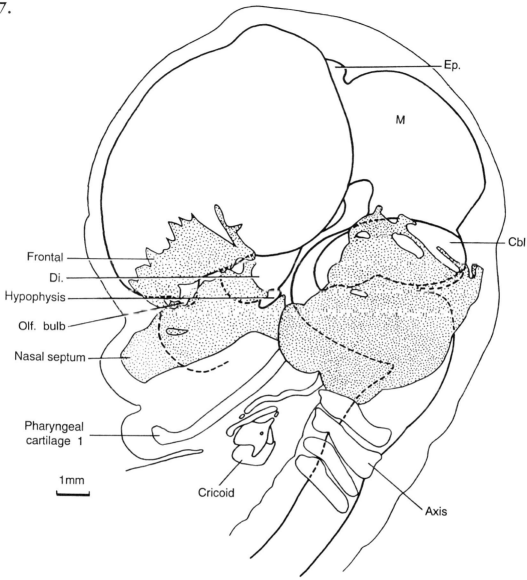

Fig. 23-8. Dorsal (superior) schematic views of the chondrocranium at stage 22 (CEC 1458) and stage 23 (CEC 9226), drawn to the same scale.

(**A**) The main components of the skull are listed on the left, the chief foramina and future canals on the right. At the junction of the basisphenoid, basioccipital, greater wing of the sphenoid, and petrous temporal, the carotid foramen is visible (in black).

(**B**) The internal acoustic foramen (future meatus) is again evident in the petrous temporal, the jugular foramen is situated posteriorly, and the hypoglossal foramen lies close to the foramen magnum. The thick black, vertical line in both A and B is the notochord in transit from the dens to the cranial base. Comparison shows that very considerable progress has occured within 2 or 3 days. The main changes are the acquisition of the nasal capsule, the widening of the greater wings of the sphenoid (which support the cerebral hemispheres), and the formation of the parietal laminae (which include the foramen magnum). The occipital part of the brain sits in a skeletal bowl, from which, however, it is protected by fluid-filled mesenchyme (as in the area between the rhombencephalon and the basicranium in Fig. 23-6). The inventory of the "membrane" bones is almost complete in some embryos of stage 23. Further details: Müller and O'Rahilly (1980). From Müller and O'Rahilly (1991).

Fig. 23-8.

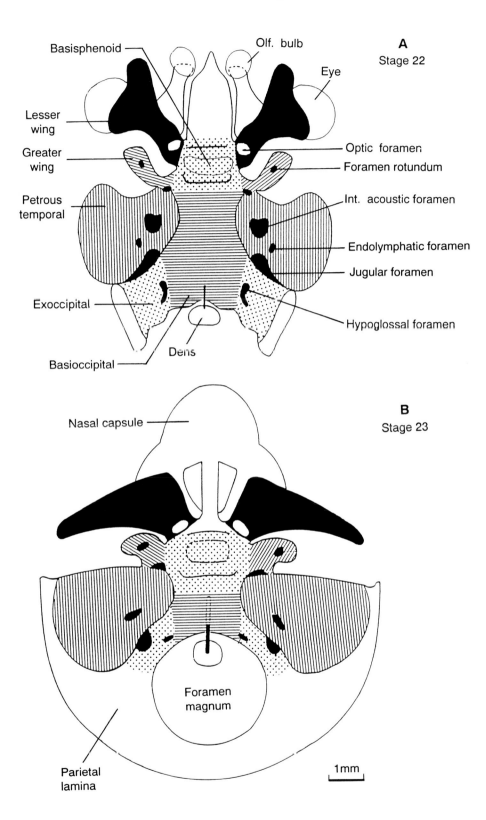

A
Stage 22

Basisphenoid

Olf. bulb

Eye

Lesser wing

Greater wing

Optic foramen

Foramen rotundum

Petrous temporal

Int. acoustic foramen

Endolymphatic foramen

Jugular foramen

Exoccipital

Hypoglossal foramen

Dens

Basioccipital

B
Stage 23

Nasal capsule

Foramen magnum

Parietal lamina

1mm

301

Fig. 23-9. The dura mater (CEC 7425, silver-impregnated). The falx cerebri is clearly formed from the skeletogenous layer, beginning at the level of the future crista galli. Most of the tissue between the cerebral hemispheres is still leptomeningeal, whereas the dural limiting layer is fibrous. The primordium of the superior sagittal sinus is visible at the edge of the developing falx. The beginnings of the transverse and occipital sinuses are also present and are intradural. Bars: 0.2 mm. From O'Rahilly and Müller (1986).

Fig. 23-10. A coronal section (CEC 7425) showing a subarachnoid cistern situated between the olfactory bulb and the optic nerve. Most of the cisterns found in the adult are now present. Bar: 0.2 mm. From O'Rahilly and Müller (1986).

Fig. 23-9.

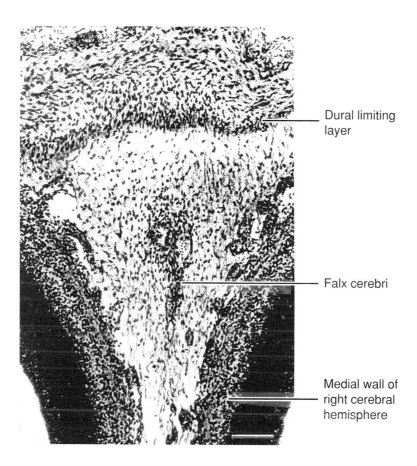

Dural limiting layer

Falx cerebri

Medial wall of right cerebral hemisphere

Fig. 23-10.

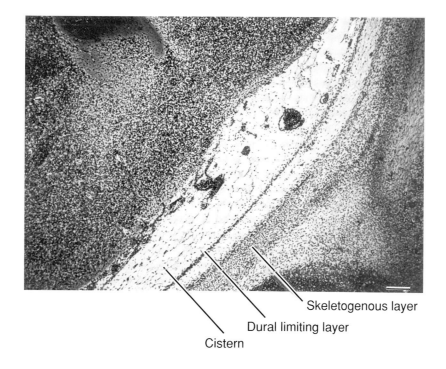

Skeletogenous layer

Dural limiting layer

Cistern

Fig. 23-11. Right lateral reconstruction to show (stippled) the tentorium cerebelli (CEC 9226). The medial part of the tentorium still extends from the sellar region to the mamillary area, but it is becoming thinner. It separates incompletely two future subarachnoid areas: (1) that of the telencephalon and diencephalon, and (2) that of the rhombencephalon, including the cerebellum. In this reconstruction only the lateral parts are represented: the rostrolateral and the caudolateral, joined at the future tentorial notch, which is continuous with the medial part. The development of the tentorium during the fetal period is complicated, but has been well schematized by Markowski (1922). From O'Rahilly and Müller (1986).

Figures 23-12 and 23-14 to 23-17 are transverse sections (No 9226) that give an overall view of the cerebral hemispheres. The levels are indicated in Figure 23-4. The bars represent 1 mm. From Müller and O'Rahilly (1990b).

Fig. 23-12. A section through the eyes, nasal cavity, and pharynx. The cortical plate extends even to the rostralmost levels. The primordium of the falx cerebri appears as a septum between the two olfactory bulbs. It extends from the skeletogenous layer towards and into the longitudinal fissure. The closeness of the two cerebral hemispheres can be appreciated here and also in Figures 23-14 and 23-15.

Fig. 23-11.

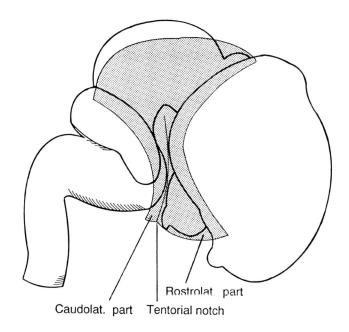

Caudolat. part   Tentorial notch   Rostrolat. part

Fig. 23-12.

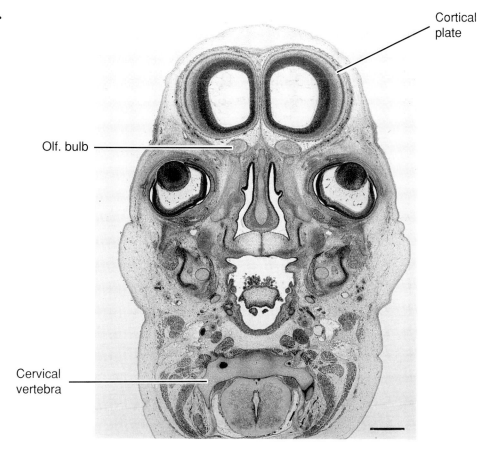

Cortical plate

Olf. bulb

Cervical vertebra

305

Figure 23-13. The eye at the end of the embryonic period.

(**A**) General view (CEC 9226). At about 12 weeks the rim of the optic cup will differentiate into the ciliary region and the iris will begin to develop. The front part of the optic cup will then become the ciliary and iridial parts of the retina, to which other layers will be added externally. Further details: O'Rahilly (1966, 1975, 1983).

The slight separation between the pigment layer (No. 1) and the remaining layers (Nos. 2–10) of the retina seen here in a few places is the site of the former optic ventricle (Fig. 14-7) and shows where so-called detachment of (in reality a separation within) the retina would occur.

(**B**) Section through the retina of the same embryo. Of the 10 layers that are characteristic later, layers 1, 3, 9, and 10 are present here. ×400.

Of the direct derivatives of the neuroepithelium of the optic cup (Figs. 14-7 and 15-7), the external "neuroblastic" layer will give rise to layers 4, 5, and 6 (external nuclear, external plexiform, and internal nuclear) and the transient fiber zone to layer 7 (internal plexiform); both "neuroblastic" layers will contribute to layer 8 (ganglion cells). All 10 layers will be present by 120 mm GL. ×52. Further details: Rhodes (1979).

The eye arises from (1) neural ectoderm (the retinal disc), (2) somatic ectoderm (the lens disc and anterior epithelium of the cornea), (3) neural crest (probably the stroma and posterior epithelium of the cornea, the sclera and choroid, and the ciliary muscle), and (4) mesoderm (the sclera and uvea). In contrast, the internal ear arises from somatic ectoderm, and the vestibular and cochlear ganglia mostly from neural crest. The otic and epipharyngeal discs associated with ganglia of the cranial nerves were regarded by Streeter as islands of neural ectoderm (Table 7-1).

Fig. 23-13.

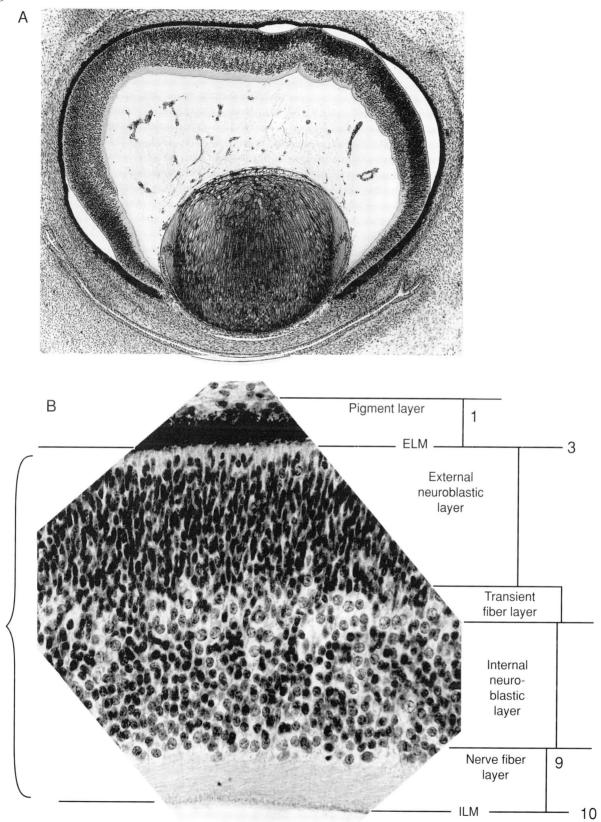

Fig. 23-14. A section along the base of the skull. The internal ear is shown on each side. A small, basal part of the diencephalon can be seen at the level of the tuberculum sellae. The optic chiasma and the third ventricle are visible. The mesenchyme surrounding the diencephalon and telencephalon basally is the meshwork of a basal cistern. The cerebral hemispheres contain the septal area with the nucleus accumbens, the hippocampus, and the lateral ventricular eminence, which last is the primordium of the caudate nucleus. Ontogenetically, the nucleus accumbens is more closely related to the corpus striatum than to the septal nuclei. In addition, its origin is possibly related to the medial ventricular eminence (Sidman and Rakic, 1982).

Fig. 23-15. A section through the hypophysial fossa, the adenohypophysis, and the optic chiasma. A small, basal part of the diencephalon and third ventricle is included. The prosencephalic septum is prominent. The sulcus terminalis limits it laterally, towards the beginning of the medial ventricular eminence. At this level the lateral eminence is mainly caudate nucleus.

Fig. 23-14.

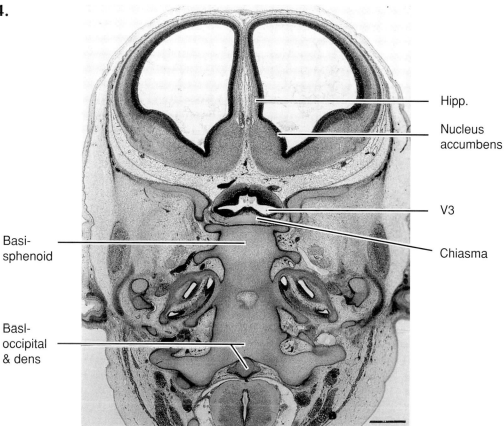

- Hipp.
- Nucleus accumbens
- V3
- Chiasma
- Basi-sphenoid
- Basi-occipital & dens

Fig. 23-15.

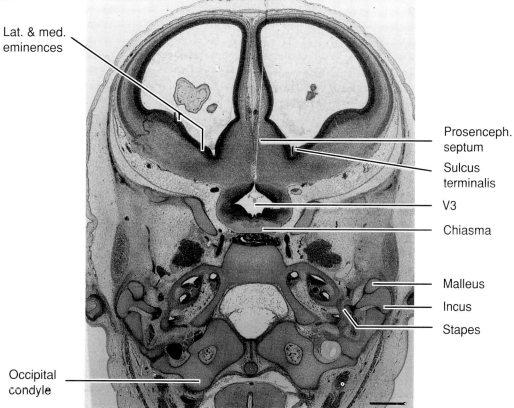

- Lat. & med. eminences
- Prosenceph. septum
- Sulcus terminalis
- V3
- Chiasma
- Malleus
- Incus
- Stapes
- Occipital condyle

Fig. 23-16. A section through the insular region and the left interventricular foramen. The cortical plate, which first appeared at stage 21 in the insular region, is thickest there, partly because of the increase of the intercellular spaces. The internal capsule, putamen, and globus pallidus externus are visible. The gray band lateral to the putamen is the claustrum. The choroid plexus at this time has become lobular, the epithelium is low prismatic, and the gelatinous stroma resembles that in the umbilical cord (Ariëns Kappers, 1966). The insula becomes buried during the fetal period and will possess extensive connections, as well as numerous functions (Augustine, 1996).

In the key drawing, arrows indicate the course of the internal capsule. Its fibers, mostly thalamocortical, become dispersed in the intermediate layer and the subplate of the neopallium. Some fibers may be corticothalamic, although it is doubtful that they reach the thalamus already.

The developing corpus striatum is composed of several neurochemically defined populations, and neuropeptide genes are expressed during trimester 2 (Brana et al., 1995). Moreover, the subependymal germinal layer is voluminous at this time, whereas the matrix disappears near birth. Neuropeptide gene expression is already under dopamine control through innervation from the substantia nigra (Freeman et al., 1995). The density of dopaminergic innervation is greatest caudal to the genu of the corpus callosum (Verney, 1993). Most if not all striatal neurons bear dopamine receptors (Brana et al., 1996). In addition to the nigrostriatal influence, corticostriatal inputs are believed to be important.

Fig. 23-16.

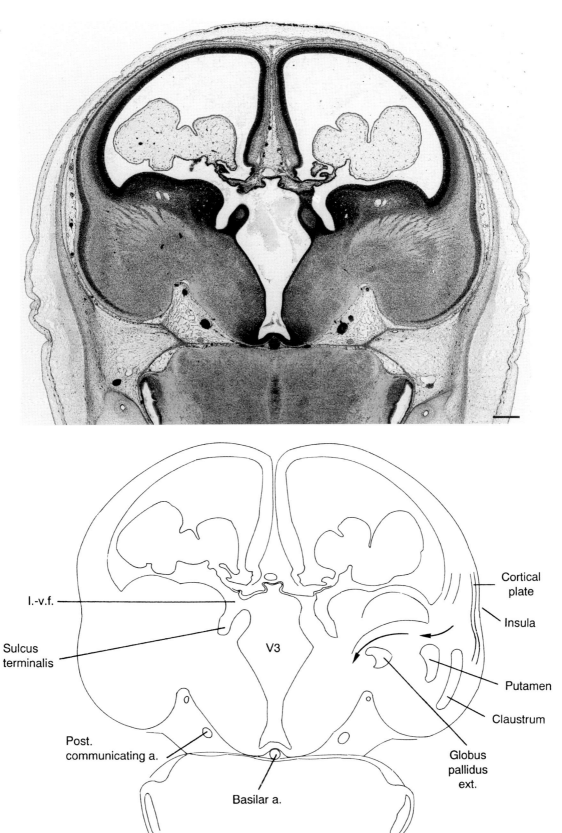

Fig. 23-16, continued. Further details of the important photomicrograph on the preceding pages are emphasized here.

The sulcus terminalis is the site of the future thalamostriate vein and is parallel to the stria terminalis, which is recognizable already at stage 22 (Fig. 22-6B). The order of structures, from medial to lateral, is (1) hippocampus (still prominent rostrally), (2) choroid fissure and plexus, (3) thalamus and lamina affixa, (4) sulcus terminalis, and (5) caudate nucleus. Arrows indicate the internal capsule.

Later in prenatal life the corpus callosum and the fornix become interposed between the rostral remains of the hippocampus and the choroid fissure. Then the order of structures is similar to that in the adult, as shown in the lower drawing: (1) indusium griseum and longitudinal striae (rostral remains of the hippocampus), (1a) corpus callosum and fornix, (2) choroid fissure and plexus, (3) thalamus and lamina affixa, (4) thalamostriate vein and stria terminalis (in the sulcus terminalis), and (5) caudate nucleus.

The internal capsule (arrows) passes first between two telencephalic structures (finer stippling), the caudate nucleus and the putamen, and then between two diencephalic structures (coarser stippling), the thalamus and the globus pallidus.

Fig. 23-16.

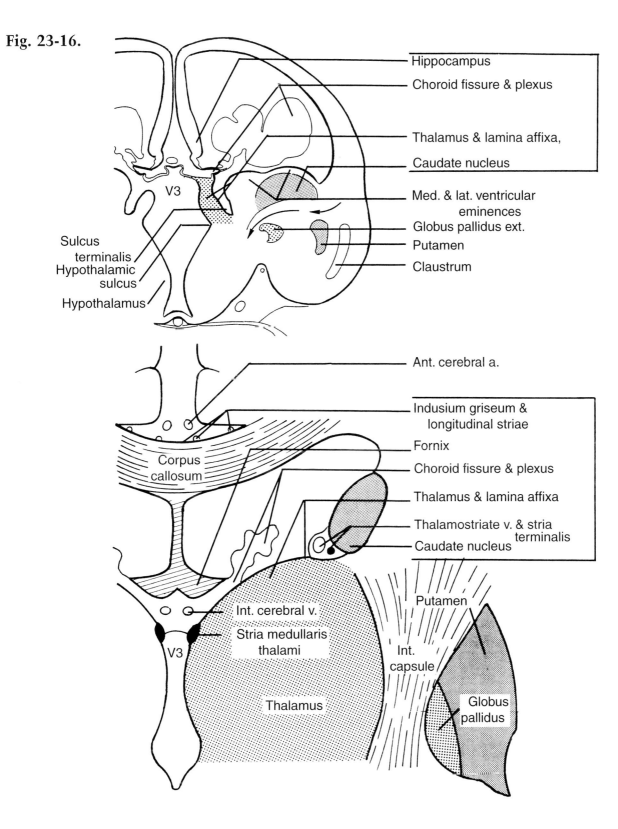

Hippocampus

Choroid fissure & plexus

Thalamus & lamina affixa,

Caudate nucleus

Med. & lat. ventricular
    eminences
Globus pallidus ext.
Putamen
Claustrum

V3

Sulcus
    terminalis
Hypothalamic
    sulcus
Hypothalamus

Ant. cerebral a.

Indusium griseum &
    longitudinal striae
Fornix
Choroid fissure & plexus
Thalamus & lamina affixa
Thalamostriate v. & stria
    terminalis
Caudate nucleus

Corpus
callosum

Putamen

Int. cerebral v.
Stria medullaris
    thalami
V3

Int.
capsule

Thalamus

Globus
pallidus

Fig. 23-17. A section through the interpenduncular fossa, which appears in the middle of the photomicrograph. The dorsal thalamus, which has enlarged considerably, is evident at this level and is characterized by a dark (subventricular) layer and a clearer superficial (intermediate) layer. The matrix is still in its migrational period (Richter, 1965). Its ventricular zone is still thicker than that of the ventral thalamus. A mesenchymal sheet, the primary meninx, is noteworthy between the diencephalon and the cerebral hemispheres.

The cerebellum has developed an external germinal layer, the extent of which has been reconstructed (Müller and O'Rahilly, 1990b, Fig. 2B; Müller and O'Rahilly, 1990c, Fig. 1A). The fibers in the cerebellum are mostly from the inferior cerebellar peduncle, rostral to which the dentate nucleus can be distinguished. (See also the scheme in Fig. 21-18.) A small rectangular section through the interpeduncular fossa, containing numerous small blood vessels, is visible below the third ventricle.

Fig. 23-17.

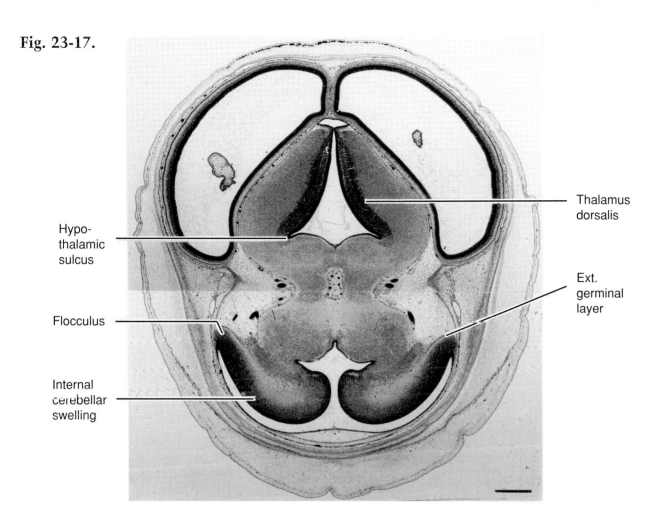

Thalamus
dorsalis

Hypo-
thalamic
sulcus

Ext.
germinal
layer

Flocculus

Internal
cerebellar
swelling

Figures 23-18 to 23-20 show sections through the frontal part of the neopallium of a silver-impregnated embryo (D-122). The levels are indicated in Figure 23-5. The bars represent 0.05 mm. From Müller and O'Rahilly (1990b).

Fig. 23-18. A section through an area in which a cortical plate has not yet developed. The primordial plexiform layer contains bipolar horizontal and other neurons. Radial fibers can be seen between the vertically arranged cells of the ventricular layer. The cell columns ("proliferative units" of Rakic) are defined by glial septa. The postmitotic cells migrate towards the periphery, and the bipolar radial glial cells are believed to guide them.

Fig. 23-19. An overall view of an area that shows the cortical plate, which is situated within the former cell-sparse primordial plexiform layer (Fig. 6-3). The plate now consists of five or more cellular rows that have migrated radially from the ventricular layer. The elements of the cortical unit and those of the proliferative unit form an ontogenetic column (Rakic). The following are present from the ventricular towards the pial surface: ventricular layer, intermediate layer, subplate, cortical plate, and subpial layer. Tangentially arranged nerve fibers are seen in the subpial layer, which is future cortical layer 1, and also between the cortical plate and the intermediate layer (shown also in Fig. 23-20). The latter fibers are specific thalamic afferents, which are transiently in the subplate before they invade the cortical plate. The early monoamine projection to the subplate that has been shown at about this time is believed to be permanent, although direct data in the human are lacking. Fibers from catecholamine neurons enter the intermediate layer (Zecevic and Verney, 1995). Nigrostriatal fibers arrive in the hemispheres at 8 weeks (Freeman et al., 1991). Other afferents are from the brain stem and the basal part of the prosencephalon.

The labels for the different zones shown here are based on the fact that the layer internal to the cortical plate is rich in tangential fibers, but poor in cells, which is characteristic of the subplate. The space between the pia mater and the subpial layer is artifactual.

Fig. 23-20. The peripheral part of Figure 23-19 [enlarged area, indicated by rectangle]. Numerous silver-impregnated, tangentially arranged neurites are evident within the subplate. On its first appearance, a part of the cortical plate contains early-generated subplate cells. Later, those cells leave the cortical layer and come to reside in the subcortical layer. They may give off the descending axons that run in the intermediate zone and reach the internal capsule. Although formerly it was thought that only layers 2 to 5 develop from the cortical plate, it is now generally believed that layer 6 is also derived from the plate (Mrzijak et al., 1988).

The first synapses in the brain appear in the two parts of the former primordial plexiform layer in human embryos and fetuses. Already at stage 19, that layer contains horizontal cells corresponding to Cajal-Retzius cells (Larroche and Houcine, 1982), which form the earliest synapses in the neopallium of the human brain (Choi, 1988), probably at stage 17.

316

Fig. 23-18. Ventric. & subventric.

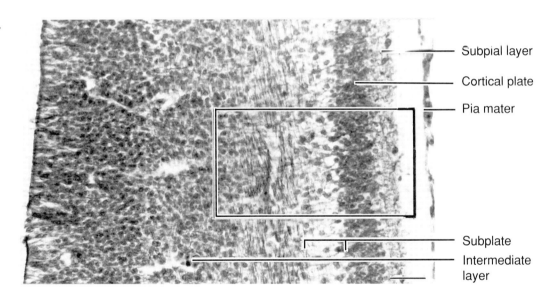

Primordial plexiform layer

Fig. 23-19.

Subpial layer

Cortical plate

Pia mater

Subplate

Intermediate layer

Fig. 23-20.

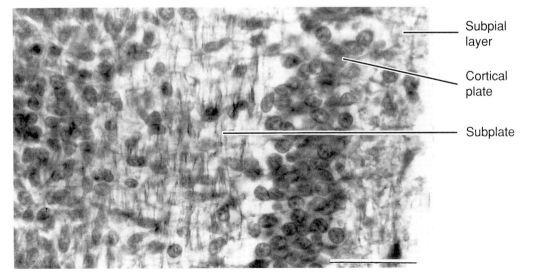

Subpial layer

Cortical plate

Subplate

Fig. 23-21. Formation of the cerebral cortex.

(**A**) The ventricular zone or layer.

(**B**) A marginal zone is added. It is also known as the primordial plexiform layer, because it contains long nerve fibers that arrive early (stages 13–15) from the brain stem. Furthermore, it contains horizontal Cajal–Retzius cells, which are the earliest neurons to be derived from the ventricular layer.

(**C**) An intermediate layer is added between the ventricular and marginal zones. It consists of cells that have migrated peripherally from the ventricular layer.

(**D**) At stage 21 the cortical plate begins to form within the primordial plexiform layer.

(**D′**) medial view of the left half of the brain at 8 weeks.

(**E**) The definitive cerebral cortex of the adult consists typically of six layers. Layers 2–6 are derived from the cortical plate. A giant pyramidal cell is shown in layer 5, and its apical dendrite (a.d.) and axon (a) are indicated.

From O'Rahilly and Müller (1996a).

Fig. 23-21.

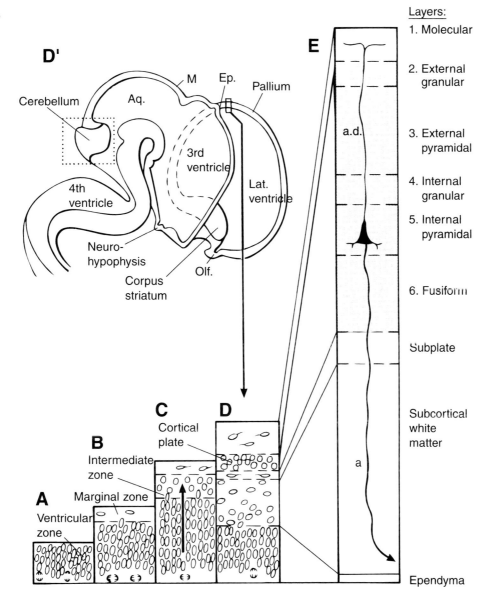

Fig. 23-22. The hippocampus and adjoining areas (CEC 9226) at the level indicated in Figure 23-4. Adjacent to 1, the multilayered epithelial lamina, is 2, the area dentata. Here the cell columns of the ventricular layer have become looser, and an intermediate layer is not present. The hippocampus *sensu stricto*, 3, which reaches the temporal pole at this stage, is characterized in general, as compared with the neocortex, by wide marginal and intermediate layers and a narrow ventricular layer. The cell columns of the ventricular layer are loose, and adjacent to them are cells, the axes of which resemble those of the ventricular layer; they represent probably future pyramidal cells (7). The tangenitally arranged cells in the marginal layer are subpial or marginal cells (6), which were also observed in this early phase of hippocampal development by Humphrey (1965) and Kahle (1969). The distances between individual cells in the intermediate layer of the hippocampus *sensu stricto* are greater than in any other part of the telencephalon. In the absence of special techniques (e.g., radioactive marking) it is scarcely possible to decide whether marginal cells of the present scheme correspond to a first wave of early-generated pyramidal cells or simply represent migrating cells from the area dentata. The mesocortex, 4, is between the hippocampus *sensu stricto* and the neopallium, and possesses the narrowest intermediate layer. The hippocampus *sensu lato* comprises the areas marked 2, 3, and 4.

Mesenchyme is noteworthy between the telencephalic surfaces at the right and the diencephalon at the left. Bar: 0.1 mm. From Müller and O'Rahilly (1990b).

Fig. 23-22.

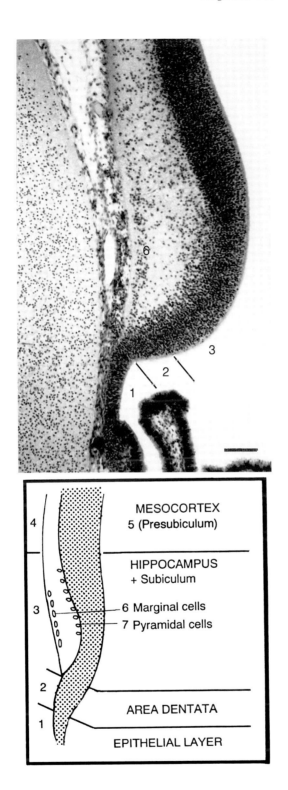

MESOCORTEX
5 (Presubiculum)

HIPPOCAMPUS
+ Subiculum

6 Marginal cells
7 Pyramidal cells

AREA DENTATA

EPITHELIAL LAYER

Figures 23-23 and 23-24 are silver-impregnated sections (D-122), the levels of which are indicated in Figure 23-5. The bars represent 0.2 mm. From Müller and O'Rahilly (1990b).

Fig. 23-23. The medial and lateral ventricular eminences. The sulcus terminalis is evident medially (upper arrow). The subventricular layer of the lateral eminence, from which the caudate nucleus arises, continues into the putamen. The fibers of the external capsule, which are few at this stage, form a sagittal sheet that follows approximately the direction of the olfactory tract, but runs more centrally. The fibers stem mostly from the pyriform area. The fibers of the internal capsule are visible between the putamen laterally and the primordium of the caudate nucleus medially. The globus pallidus externus at this relatively caudal level lies in the hemispheric stalk, whereas more rostrally it is far more telencephalic in position. The internal capsule at this stage contains thalamostriatal, thalamocortical, corticothalamic, and nigrostriatal fibers, probably in that order. (The nigrostriatal bundle can first be discerned at 8 weeks: Freeman et al., 1991.) On their way to and from the diencephalon, the fibers of the internal capsule pass through the hemispheric stalk (His, 1904; Hochstetter, 1919), which is found between two boundaries marked here by arrows: the sulcus terminalis on the ventricular surface (upper arrow), and the di-telencephalic sulcus at the external surface (lower arrow).

Fig. 23-24. A more ventral section at the level of the interventricular foramen (Fig. 23-5). Neopallial fibers, as well as fibers to and from the region of the lateral ventricular eminence, are visible. Those fibers are part of the internal capsule and are mostly thalamocortical. They arise in the nearby dorsal thalamus and cross the di-telencephalic boundary, which is indicated by the sulcus terminalis and the stria terminalis (cf. Fig. 24-7).

322

Fig. 23-23.

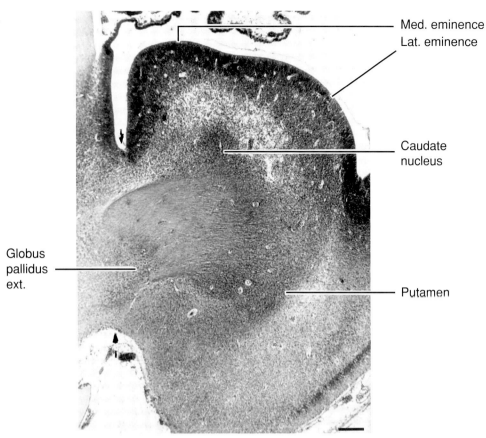

Med. eminence
Lat. eminence

Caudate
nucleus

Globus
pallidus
ext.

Putamen

Fig. 23-24.

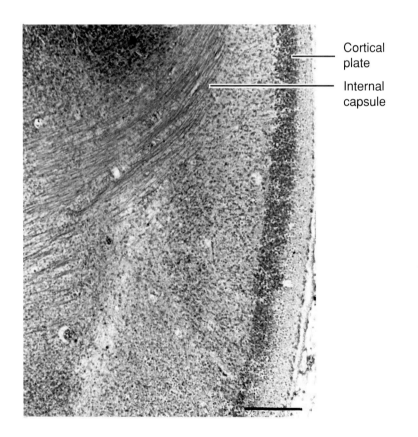

Cortical
plate

Internal
capsule

323

Fig. 23-25. The ventricular system (CEC 9226).

(**A**) A left lateral view showing the now small interventricular foramen, and the overlap between the lateral and third ventricles. Anterior and inferior horns (part of the C formation) are well defined, but the posterior horn has not yet appeared. The future aqueduct is becoming delineated by two narrow regions, one of which is at the isthmus rhombencephali. The area membranacea rostralis is marked by an asterisk. The area membranacea caudalis is indicated by a dagger. Compared with the corresponding areas in stages 17 and 18, the epithelium of the areae membranaceae caudalis et rostralis is cuboidal rather than flat. No apertures are yet present in the roof of the fourth ventricle. The zones with choroid villi in the lateral and fourth ventricles are hatched. From O'Rahilly and Müller (1990).

(**B**) A dorsal view of the ventricular system (CEC 9226). Two pairs of semicircles can be seen: the left and right lateral ventricles rostrally, and the lateral recesses and the main part of the fourth ventricle caudally. The third ventricle is foreshortened in this perspective, whereas the future aqueduct and its bilateral *Blindsack* are seen in their full extent. The area choroidea of the roof of the telencephalon medium consists of two cellular rows and is the thinnest portion of the lamina terminalis. The choroid plexus of one lateral ventricle is shown.

An area membranacea rostralis and an area membranacea caudalis appear at stage 18. The caudal area (marked here by a dagger) has also been termed the saccular ventricular diverticulum (Wilson, 1937) and the central bulge (Brocklehurst, 1969). It is possible that the area permits the passage of cerebrospinal fluid (as suggested in the mouse), in which case a functional rather than a structural median aperture could be said to be present at this time. It has been claimed that the median and lateral apertures (of Magendie and Luschka) are present at 20 and 220 mm, respectively (Brocklehurst, 1969), but further study of this region is required.

It is likely, as has been suggested, that the cerebrospinal fluid is nutritive while vascularization is progressing, while the wall of the brain is increasing in thickness, and while the lateral ventricles are decreasing proportionately. This is supported by the relatively late appearance of capillaries that penetrate the wall of the brain, namely at stages 12 (hindbrain), 13 (midbrain), and 16 (cerebral hemispheres).

From O'Rahilly and Müller (1990, Table 1), who have provided measurements of the ventricular system at this stage. A three-dimensional reconstruction, prepared ultrasonically, of the ventricles *in vivo* in an embryo of 29 mm (Blaas et al., 1998) confirms the accuracy of the more detailed graphic reconstruction shown here.

Fig. 23-25.

A

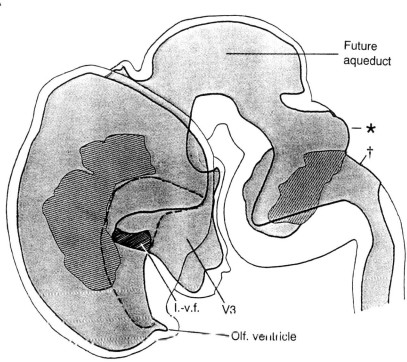

Future aqueduct

∗

†

l.-v.f.　V3

Olf. ventricle

B

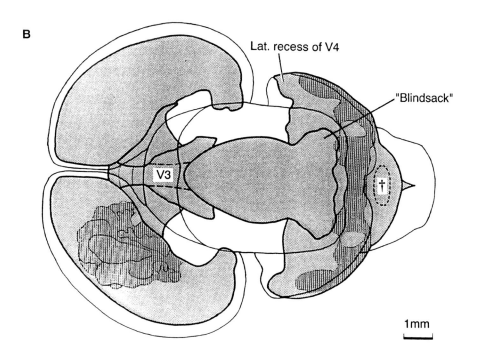

Lat. recess of V4

"Blindsack"

V3

†

1mm

Fig. 23-26. The cerebellum at the end of the embryonic period (D-122).

(**A**) A reconstruction of the brain stem and cerebellum (27 mm) as seen from behind, according to Hochstetter (1929). The roof of the fourth ventricle has been removed along the taenia.

(**B**) Right lateral view of the brain to show the plane of section for C and D.

(**C**) A section near the surface of the mesencephalon and isthmus. The latter shows the decussation of the trochlear nerves, the medial part of the cerebellar plate, and the future superior medullary velum. Hochstetter (1929) stressed the importance of the connection between the left and right halves of the developing cerebellum, somewhat negating the idea of paired cerebellar primordia.

(**D**) A more ventral section, in which caudal is shown uppermost. The external cerebellar swelling (at the right) presents the rhombic lip and the flocculus, the latter now being covered by a thin sheath of external germinal layer, which is given off from the rhombic lip. An adjacent new and smaller swelling (unnamed by both Hochstetter and Larsell) contains the primordium of the dentate nucleus and (in more ventral sections) the inferior cerebellar peduncle. Numerous blood vessels penetrate as far as the ventricular layer. Further details: Müller and O'Rahilly (1990).

Important

The cerebellum develops from the alar plate of both the isthmic and the first rhombencephalic neuromeres. The rhombic lip, which is a part of the alar plate, is not the sole origin of the cerebellum

---

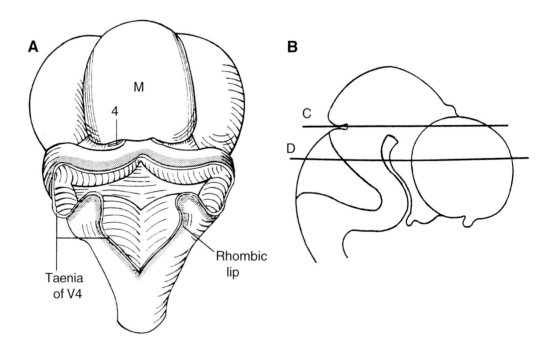

Fig. 23-26.

C

Vascular
plexus

X4

Internal
cerebellar
swelling

V4

D

Sulcus
limitans

Ventricular
layer

Internal
cerebellar
swelling

Alar
lamina

V4

P-L
fissure

Ext.
germinal
layer

Flocculus

Rasal
lamina

Rhombic lip

Fig. 23-27. Dorsal view of a reconstruction of the rhombencephalon (D-122, silver-impregnated), showing nuclei and tracts. The caudal direction is towards the top of the page. The right embryonic half is on the left of the drawing. The cerebellum has not been included. The white line on the right-hand side of the drawing represents the cut edge of the roof of the fourth ventricle. Black triangles indicate the levels of the reconstructed cross-sections in Figure 23-28. The afferent nuclei are marked by small circles, the somatic efferent nuclei by bold stippling, and visceral efferent nuclei are hatched. The nucleus funiculi teretis (*Kappenkern* of the genu of the facial nerve) is included. The two (ascending and descending) intramural parts of the facial nerve are indicated by the numeral 7.

The inset shows the four vestibular nuclei.

The rhombic lip, an important proliferative area in the alar plate, is the source of two superficially situated migratory areas: the so-called olivo-arcuate caudally, and the pontine rostrally. Two of the three migratory areas found at stage 23 have been reconstructed (Müller and O'Rahilly, 1990c, Fig. 1). The term "olivo-arcuate migration" (Essick, 1912), however, is unsatisfactory, because it has been shown (in the monkey) that the olivary nuclei arise mainly from the ventricular layer.

The rhombencephalon at this stage is already very complicated and comparable in many respects to that of the newborn (Fig. 26-6). Its rapid development suggests an early onset of functional activity. From Müller and O'Rahilly (1990c), who give further details.

Fig. 23-27.

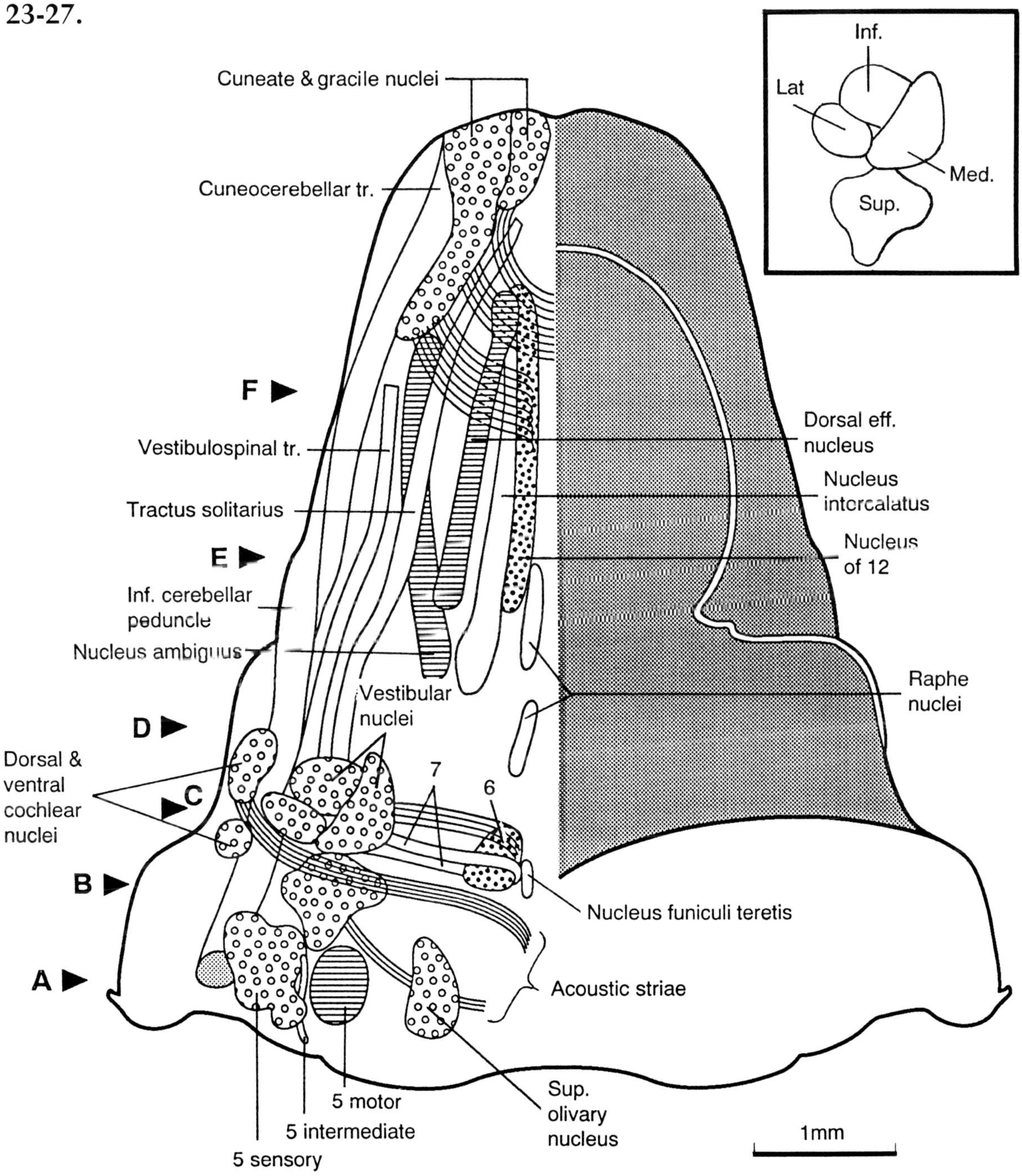

Cuneate & gracile nuclei

Inf.

Lat

Med.

Sup.

Cuneocerebellar tr.

F ▶

Dorsal eff.
nucleus

Nucleus
intercalatus

Vestibulospinal tr.

Nucleus
of 12

Tractus solitarius

E ▶

Inf. cerebellar
peduncle

Nucleus ambiguus

Vestibular
nuclei

Raphe
nuclei

D ▶

Dorsal &
ventral
cochlear
nuclei

C ▶

7

6

B ▶

Nucleus funiculi teretis

A ▶

Acoustic striae

5 motor

5 intermediate

Sup.
olivary
nucleus

5 sensory

1mm

329

Fig. 23-28. Reconstructed coronal sections of the rhombencephalon (D-122). The levels of the sections (A)–(F) in rostrocaudal succession are indicated in Figure 23-27 by black triangles.

(**A**) Section showing the nuclei of the trigeminal nerve and the transition to the cerebellum via the inferior cerebellar peduncle. The position of the trigeminal nuclei here is conditioned by the slight obliquity of this slice. The inset in the lower right-hand corner of the page shows fiber bundles of the motor part, of the intermediate, and of the sensory portion of the trigeminal nerve.

(**B**) Area of the abducent and facial nerves, showing the superior olivary nucleus, and the superior vestibular nucleus and its fibers to the medial longitudinal fasciculus.

(**C**) Entry of the cochlear nerve. Ventral and dorsal cochlear nuclei are lateral to the inferior cerebellar peduncle. The fibers from the dorsal cochlear nucleus that run medially constitute the intermediate acoustic striae. A dagger indicates the tectobulbar and tectospinal tracts.

(**D**) Entry of the sensory glossopharyngeal fibers that run directly to the tractus solitarius. Olivocerebellar fibers can be seen passing towards the inferior cerebellar peduncle.

(**E**) and (**F**) Inferior olivary, vagal, accessory, and hypoglossal nuclei. A small bundle of corticospinal (pyramidal) fibers is present in all the sections. From Müller and O'Rahilly (1990c).

Fig. 23-28.

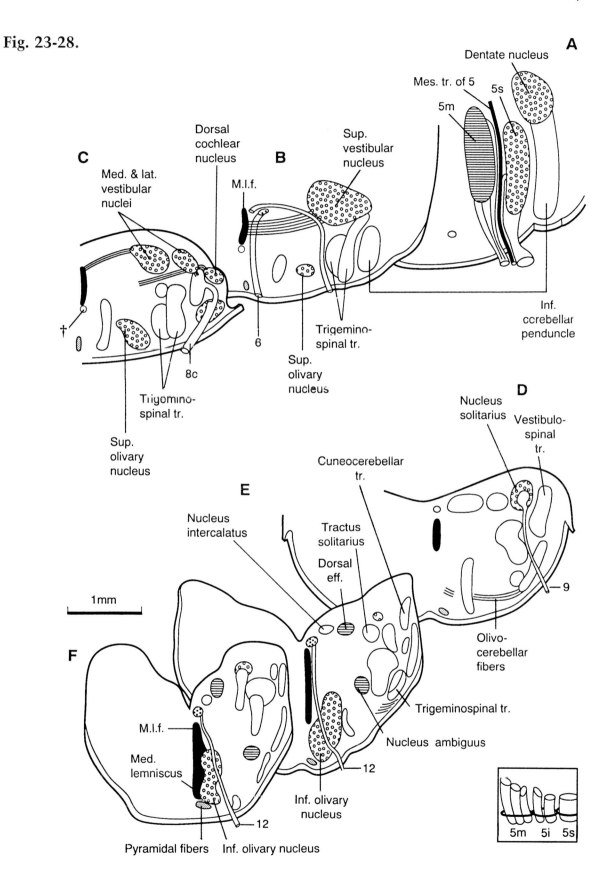

A

Dentate nucleus

Mes. tr. of 5

5s

5m

Dorsal cochlear nucleus

M.l.f.

B

Sup. vestibular nucleus

C

Med. & lat. vestibular nuclei

Inf. cerebellar peduncle

Trigemino-spinal tr.

6

Sup. olivary nucleus

Trigemino-spinal tr.

8c

Sup. olivary nucleus

†

D

Nucleus solitarius

Vestibulo-spinal tr.

Cuneocerebellar tr.

E

Nucleus intercalatus

Tractus solitarius

Dorsal eff.

1mm

F

9

Olivo-cerebellar fibers

Trigeminospinal tr.

Nucleus ambiguus

M.l.f.

Med. lemniscus

12

Inf. olivary nucleus

12

Pyramidal fibers   Inf. olivary nucleus

5m   5i   5s

331

Fig. 23-29. Reconstruction of the arteries in a dorsal view (D-122), with a key drawing on the left. The right and left sides were reconstructed separately, and the two sides are slightly different. Most cranial nerves, the optic chiasma, and part of the optic tracts are shown. The main components of the circulus arteriosus have been present since stage 16 (Fig. 16-6), and the circle has been complete since stage 19 (Fig. 19-17). The arteries to the choroid plexus of the lateral ventricles come from one of the deep branches of the anterior cerebral artery (anterior choroid a.) and from the posterior cerebral artery (posterior choroid a.). Two anterior communicating arteries are present, a frequent finding later in life. Apart from differences in the proportions, the arterial pattern resembles closely that of the adult.

Fig. 23-29.

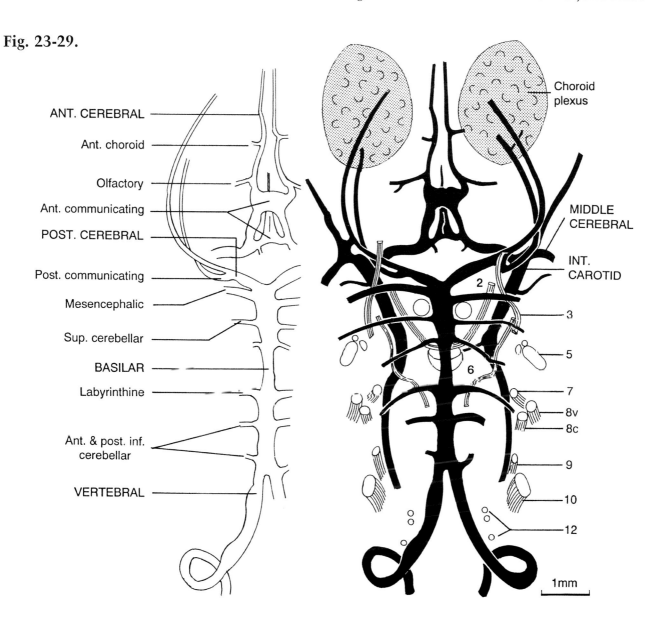

ANT. CEREBRAL

Ant. choroid

Olfactory

Ant. communicating

POST. CEREBRAL

Post. communicating

Mesencephalic

Sup. cerebellar

BASILAR

Labyrinthine

Ant. & post. inf. cerebellar

VERTEBRAL

Choroid plexus

MIDDLE CEREBRAL

INT. CAROTID

2

3

5

6

7

8v

8c

9

10

12

1mm

Fig. 23-30. Reconstruction of the arteries in a right lateral view with a key drawing below. The overlapping that occurs in a dorsal representation is omitted. The posterior communicating artery is clearer than in Figure 23-29. Noteworthy are the serpentine course of the internal carotid and the many striatal branches that penetrate the anterior perforated substance. The ramifications of the middle cerebral are not shown. The anterior cerebral gives off a branch to the olfactory bulb and significant branches to the medial surface of the cerebral hemisphere. An example of the differing proportions in the embryo is seen in the posterior communicating artery, which joins the internal carotid long before the latter divides into the anterior and middle cerebral arteries.

The internal carotid develops early (stages 11–13) and is followed by the posterior communicating (stage 14), basilar and vertebral (stage 16), anterior, middle, and posterior cerebral (stage 17), and finally the anterior communicating (stage 21), thereby completing the circulus arteriosus (Figs. 19-17 and 21-20). Initially the posterior communicating is an important channel, and its distal end constitutes the stem of the posterior cerebral. It supplies the hindbrain until the vertebral system is completed and the basilar artery becomes dominant. The hypoglossal artery disappeared after stage 15, and the stapedial artery likewise at about stage 20, whereas the trigeminal artery is still present.

The main channels of the venous system correspond to the reconstructions of a stage 21 (24 mm) embryo shown by Padget (1957). The cavernous sinus is not yet present. The beginning development of the superior sagittal sinus is shown in Figure 23-9. Bilateral foramina for emissary veins are present in the parietal part of the chondrocranium. The capsuloparietal foramen constantly contains a vein that connects the transverse sinus to the external surface of the chondrocranium. A bilateral emissary foramen in the occipital contains a vein that connects the sigmoid sinus with the external surface. Reconstruction and further details: Müller and O'Rahilly (1980).

Fig. 23-30.

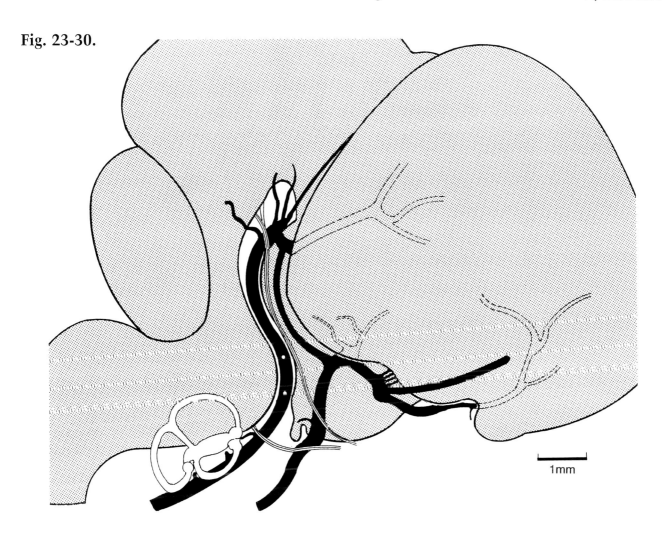

1mm

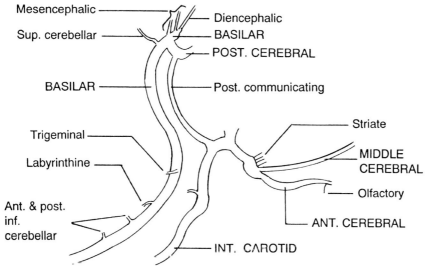

Mesencephalic ———————— Diencephalic

Sup. cerebellar ———————— BASILAR

——— POST. CEREBRAL

BASILAR ———————— Post. communicating

Striate

Trigeminal ———————— MIDDLE
CEREBRAL

Labyrinthine ————————

——— Olfactory

Ant. & post.
inf.
cerebellar

——— ANT. CEREBRAL

——— INT. CAROTID

335

The Spinal Cord in the Embryonic Period

Both the brain and the spinal cord are modifications of a continuous neural tube, so that, although this book is on the brain, it is appropriate to provide a summary of the development of the spinal cord.

The alar and basal laminae of the neural tube (Fig. 6-3) are separated by the sulcus limitans. The alar laminae, essentially afferent in function, are united by the roof plate, whereas the basal laminae, essentially efferent (the Bell–Magendie "law"), are joined by the floor plate, which is induced by the notochord. At 6 weeks the spinal cord shows ventricular, intermediate, and marginal layers, and all the spinal nerves are present (stage 17).

The following sequence of appearance has been found in the human embryo (Marti et al., 1987): (1) cells of the floor plate, (2) motor neurons, which arise in rostrocaudal and ventrodorsal gradients; (3) cells of the nucleus proprius, and (4) sensory neurons (for pain afferents) in the substantia gelatinosa. Motor neurons, the first neural cells to show expression of neuronal antigens, present synapses very early, namely at stage 15 (Okado, 1981). Synapses between primary afferents and interneurons of the substantia gelatinosa also appear early (stage 17). The first movements observed ultrasonically (Okado, 1981; de Vries, 1992) occur at about $5\frac{1}{2}$ postfertilizational weeks (probably stage 16).

The trigeminospinal tract enters the cervical region of the cord already at 6 weeks (stage 17), the dorsal funiculus is prominent, and the tractus solitarius soon reaches the thoracic region (stage 19). By the end of the embryonic period (stage 23), the funiculi gracilis et cuneatus, medial lemniscus, corticopinal tracts, and lateral spinothalamic tract are present (Müller and O'Rahilly, 1990a).

At this time the spinal cord still extends as far as the caudal end of the vertebral column (O'Rahilly, Müller, and Meyer, 1980, Fig. 4). Subsequently some dedifferentiation takes place caudally and the spinal cord "ascends" to a lumbar level during the first half of prenatal life, reaching L3 at birth and generally L1 or L2 in the adult. The disproportion in growth between the spinal cord and the vertebral column results in the characteristically increasing obliquity of the roots of the spinal nerves from lower cervical to coccygeal; those of L2 to Co. 1 constitute the cauda equina.

Comments on Neuroteratology (Stage 23)

An embryo of 8 postfertilizational weeks is less than half the length of an adult thumb, but already possesses several thousand named structures, practically any of which may be subject to developmental deviations. The embryonic period proper, which has been studied in much greater detail than the fetal, is particularly important because, during that time, the vast majority of congenital anomalies make their appearance.

Neuroschisis.   The claim that "neural clefts (neuroschisis)" existed in 100 of more than 200 Carnegie embryos from stage 10 to stage 23 (Padget, 1970) has not been substantiated (O'Rahilly and Müller, 1988).

Medulloblastoma.   The external granular layer of the cerebellum, which appears at this stage and disappears within 1–2 years after birth, is generally believed to be the origin of so-called medulloblastoma, most instances of which occur in the vermis.

Spina bifida occulta   is normal at this time. It is important to keep in mind that before ossification of the spinous processes has taken place, a normal spina bifida occulta may be said to be present throughout the length of the vertebral column. This is the condition at birth. In the lumbosacral region it continues into childhood, and in part of the sacrum it persists in about one-fifth to one-quarter of adults.

337

Trimester 1,
Postembryonic Phase

The most noticeable external changes in the fetus are (1) the union of the cerebellar halves and the definition of the vermis, (2) the increasing concealment of the diencephalon and mesencephalon, and (later on) of a part of the cerebellum, by the cerebral hemispheres, (3) further approach of the frontal and temporal poles around the insula, which becomes increasingly buried by opercula, (4) the appearance of sulci on the hemispheric surface at about the middle of prenatal life, and (5) the decreasing conspicuousness of the flexures, although the longitudinal axis of the cerebral hemispheres is set obliquely in relation to the brain stem throughout life (i.e., the "forebrain angle" is greater than a right angle). The "C-shaped structures" are listed with Figure 24-5.

Although this book is concerned primarily with the embryonic period, the fetal period is summarized in several chapters in order to provide some degree of continuity between the embryonic and the postnatal brain. The subdivision is based on trimesters because a morphological staging system is not available for the fetal period. Further information concerning the fetal brain is available in such books as those by Barbé (1938), Fontes (1944), Lemire et al. (1975), and Gilles et al. (1983), and in the useful atlas by Feess-Higgins and Larroche (1987).

Trimester 1: Early Postembryonic Phase

Approximately 30–50 mm in Greatest Length
Approximately 8–9 Postfertilizational Weeks

The period from 8 to 9 weeks, i.e., the week following the embryonic period, is exemplified here mainly by three fetuses: 27.5, 33, and 42 mm GL. It has already been pointed out that morphology and not size is the criterion for staging, and this atlas includes an embryo of 33 mm as well as a fetus of 27.5 mm. It has been mentioned also that a staging system is not (yet) available for the fetal period, and proposals so far have been based on age and fetal length, which do not provide (morphological) stages.

Although fusion of the medial walls of the cerebral hemispheres does not occur during the embryonic period, the events during the fetal period are not as clear. Fusion was denied by Hochstetter (1929), whereas others have supported fusion "between the banks of the median groove" formed in the floor of the longitudinal fissure "by the infolding of the lamina reuniens of His" (Rakic and Yakovlev, 1968). The cavum septi pellucidi has been described as arising "as a pocket between the walls of the infolded primordium hippocampi and bridged by the corpus callosum" (Rakic and Yakovlev, 1968). Moreover, according to the same authors, "the pocket is open at first" into the longitudinal fissure, but later becomes "sealed by the rostrum of corpus callosum." Others, however, believe that the cavum "is formed by necrosis within the massa commissuralis and never was open to the subarachnoid space" (Lemire et al., 1975, who, in their Fig. 16-4, show the sharply decreasing incidence of the cavum during the first 6 months after birth).

At the end of the embryonic period proper the spinal cord still reaches to the caudal end of the vertebral column (O'Rahilly, Müller, and Meyer, 1980, Fig. 4). Some dedifferentiation then takes place caudally and the spinal cord "ascends" to a lumbar level during the first half of prenatal life.

Figures 24-1 to 24-5 are from a fetus of 33 mm (CEC 5852, silver-impregnated). In contrast to stage 23, the external capsule is now present and the olivary nucleus has five components.

Fig. 24-1. 33 mm. Lateral view showing the cranial nerves. The brain is still as compact as in stage 23. Most of the hemispheric surface is neopallial. The lateral olfactory tract is indicated. In the cerebellum, the germinal layer covers only a part of the flocculonodular primordium, as is also the case in stage 23. Olivo-arcuate migratory material is shown by stippling. The ganglia are identified in the key drawing.

340

Fig. 24-1.

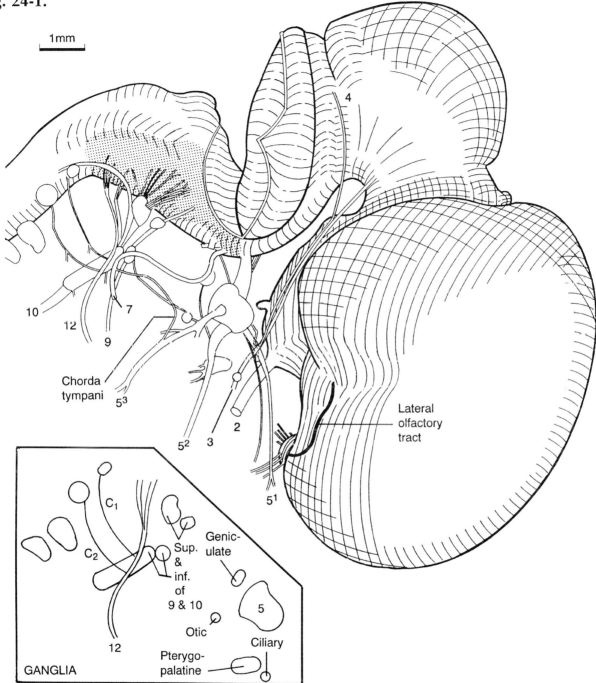

1mm

10

12

9

7

Chorda
tympani

5^3

5^2 3   2

5^1

Lateral
olfactory
tract

4

GANGLIA

C_1

C_2

Sup.
&
inf.
of
9 & 10

Genic-
ulate

5

Otic

12

Ciliary

Pterygo-
palatine

Fig. 24-2. Graphic reconstruction from sagittal sections to show a median view of the brain at 33 mm (CEC 5852). The asterisk marks the junction with the spinal cord. The commissural plate is now impressive. The rostral part of the roof of the third ventricle is folded. The entrance of the lateral prosencephalic fasciculus (*Stammbündel*) into the diencephalon is shown, as is the stria terminalis arching over it at the di-telencephalic border. Three nuclear areas (stippled) are beginning to be outlined in the thalamus. (See also Fig. 24-3.) The thalamostriatal and striatothalamic fibers are connected mostly with what may later become the dorsomedial nucleus. The facial colliculus (arrow) is noticeable on the floor of the rhombencephalon. The central stem of the chondrocranium (hatched) has been included, as well as the left optic nerve and the eye.

Fig. 24-2.

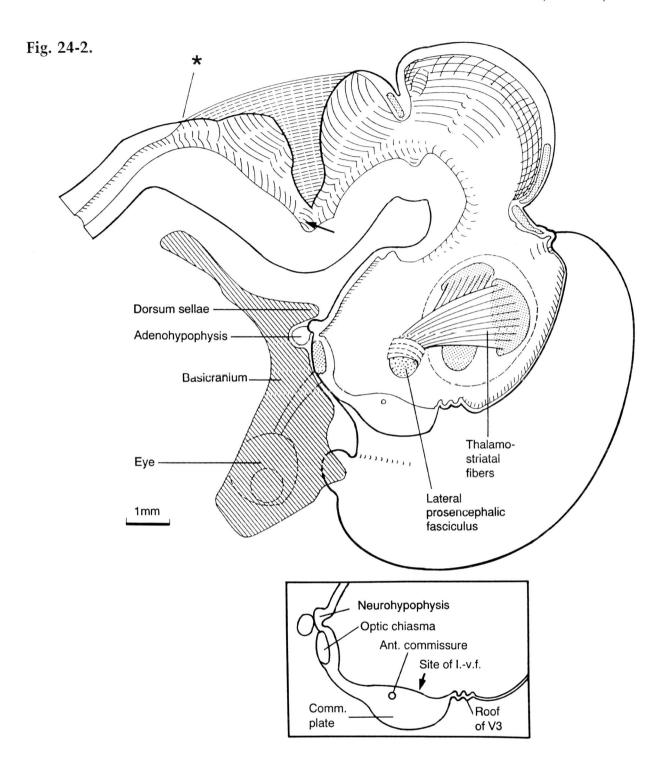

Dorsum sellae

Adenohypophysis

Basicranium

Eye

1mm

Thalamo-
striatal
fibers

Lateral
prosencephalic
fasciculus

Neurohypophysis

Optic chiasma

Ant. commissure

Site of I.-v.f.

Comm.
plate

Roof
of V3

Fig. 24-3. 33 mm. Projection of diencephalic tracts. The entrance of the *Stammbündel* (Fig. 24-2) has not been included. The dorsal thalamus (stippled) takes up almost half of the medial surface. Some of the diencephalic nuclei are shown (hatched). The subthalamic and entopeduncular nuclei, and the globus pallidus externus, are clearly identifiable but have not been represented in the reconstruction. The preoptico-hypothalamotegmental tract is indicated by a dagger. The accessory optic tract ends in the region of the subthalamic nucleus, as described by Gilbert (1935) and Cooper (1946b), although the fibers in the adult are connected to the mesencephalic lateral and dorsal terminal nuclei (Fredericks et al., 1988). From Müller and O'Rahilly (1990b).

Fig. 24-4. 33 mm. Schematic presentation of the inferior olivary nucleus. In addition to the accessory olivary nucleus (medial to the hypoglossal nerve) and the principal olivary nucleus (lateral to the hypoglossal nerve) seen in stage 23, further subdivisions can now be distinguished: (1) the medial accessory olivary nucleus, a rostral part with tall cells; (2) a mediocaudal portion consisting of medium-sized cells related to internal arcuate fibers; (3) probably the caudal medial accessory nucleus, a group between the first two and containing small cells; (4) probably the dorsal accessory nucleus, situated dorsolaterally and containing small cells; and (5) the main nucleus, the most voluminous part, which consists of tall cells. Projections to the cerebellum were present already in stage 23 (Fig. 23-28D). The olivocerebellar fibers join the inferior cerebellar peduncle. The olivoarcuate migratory area (stippled in Figure 24-1) is still present. In cross sections the migrating cells are seen as superficial and intermediate strands, and the cellular axes are arranged tangentially. From Müller and O'Rahilly (1990c).

Fig. 24-3.

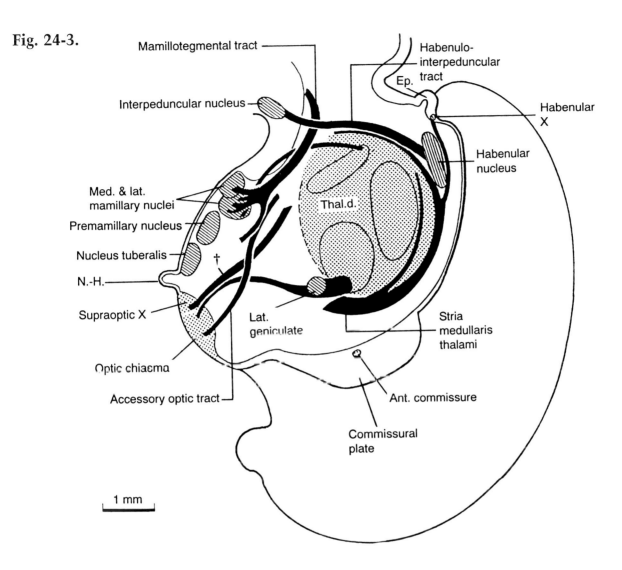

Mamillotegmental tract

Habenulo-
interpeduncular
tract

Ep.

Interpeduncular nucleus

Habenular
X

Habenular
nucleus

Med. & lat.
mamillary nuclei

Thal.d.

Premamillary nucleus

Nucleus tuberalis

†

N.-H.

Supraoptic X

Lat.
geniculate

Stria
medullaris
thalami

Optic chiasma

Accessory optic tract

Ant. commissure

Commissural
plate

1 mm

Fig. 24-4.

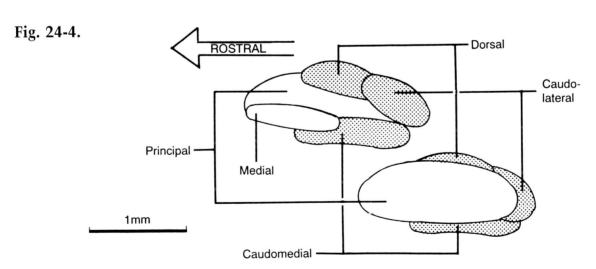

ROSTRAL

Dorsal

Caudo-
lateral

Principal

Medial

Caudomedial

1mm

C-Shaped Structures. Associated with the growth of the relatively fixed corpus striatum and the expansion of the cerebral hemispheres in a curved direction to form the temporal lobes, a number of structures develop in a C-shaped manner. These include (1) the frontal, parietal, and temporal lobes; (2) the limbic lobe (cingulate and parahippocampal gyri); (3) the lateral ventricle (anterior horn, central part, and inferior horn); (4) the hippocampus and dentate gyrus, the rostral portions of which are found later merely as a remnant termed the indusium griseum; (5) the corpus callosum, which halts (as the splenium) without descending into the temporal lobe; (6) the caudate nucleus (head, body, and tail); (7) the fornix (columns, body, and crura) and its continuation, the fimbria, and (8) the choroid plexus and the choroid fissure through which it passes.

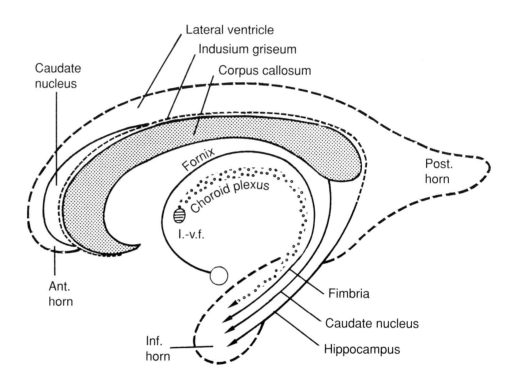

Fig. 24-5. 33 mm. Lateral view showing the ventricles. Some recesses are well formed, e.g., the supramamillary and the inframamillary, whereas others, e.g., the suprapineal, are not clear. The long cavity of the isthmus is narrowing because of the growth of the cerebellum, but it still extends into a well-developed isthmic recess.

Fig. 24-5.

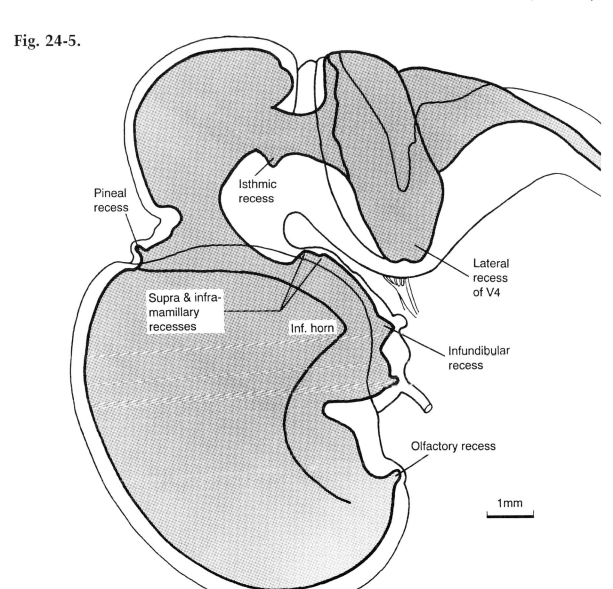

Pineal recess

Isthmic recess

Lateral recess of V4

Supra & infra-mamillary recesses

Inf. horn

Infundibular recess

Olfactory recess

1mm

Figures 24-6 to 24-11 are from a fetus of 27.5 mm (CEC 10287, silver-impregnated). The brain is slightly more developed than that of the 33 mm fetus; e.g., the cortical plate now extends to the occipital pole, and the brain is no longer as compact. Additional features include the external capsule, the hippocampal sulcus, and choroid villi in the roof of the third ventricle. The photomicrographs from this fetus are oriented so that the rostral end is uppermost. The levels of the sections are indicated in two key drawings in Figures 24-6 and 24-8. Figures 24-6 to 24-8 show a lateral view, with bars representing 0.15 mm. Figures 24-9 to 24-11 show a medial view, with bars representing 0.2 mm.

Fig. 24-6. 27.5 mm. The cerebral cortex. The cortical plate is present on the surface of the entire neopallium and is thickest (approximately 12 rows of cells) mostly where it began in stage 21: in the lateral wall opposite the lateral ventricular eminence (Fig. 24-7). The subpial layer occupies approximately half the thickness of the cortical plate, which is relatively less than in stage 23. The subplate is at least twice the thickness of the cortical plate, which is substantially greater than in stage 23. This is based on an increase of fibers, some of which lead to the lateral prosencephalic fasciculus (Fig. 24-8). Synapses in early fetuses are present above and below the cortical plate, but never within it (Molliver et al., 1973). The key drawing is a graphic reconstruction.

Fig. 24-6.

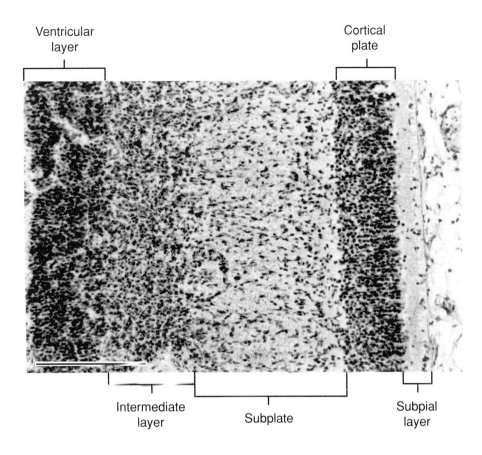

Ventricular layer   Cortical plate

Intermediate layer   Subplate   Subpial layer

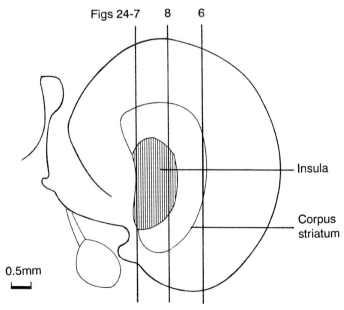

Figs 24-7   8   6

Insula

Corpus striatum

0.5mm

Fig. 24-7. 27.5 mm. The corpus striatum, internal capsule, and adjacent structures. The claustrum is well developed, and a clear connection with the ventricular layer of the olfactory area still exists (Fig. 24-11). The external capsule has appeared. Fibers of the internal capsule are seen to reach the diencephalon through the hemispheric stalk, which is delimited by the sulcus terminalis. The key drawing shows the area included in the photomicrograph. The ventricular eminences are said to expand to about 10 times the maximum thickness observed in other regions of the CNS during the second month, but reach their peak only at the middle of prenatal life (Rakic and Sidman, 1982). Their growth is supported by the striatal arteries (Nelson, et al., 1991), which mature earlier than the arteries of the cerebral wall, that is, they develop a muscularis between 20 and 22 weeks. The ventricular layer contains a network of vessels that possess no muscularis at any age. The regression of the ventricular layer is accompanied by a regression of the capillaries (Nelson et al., 1991).

Fig. 24-7.

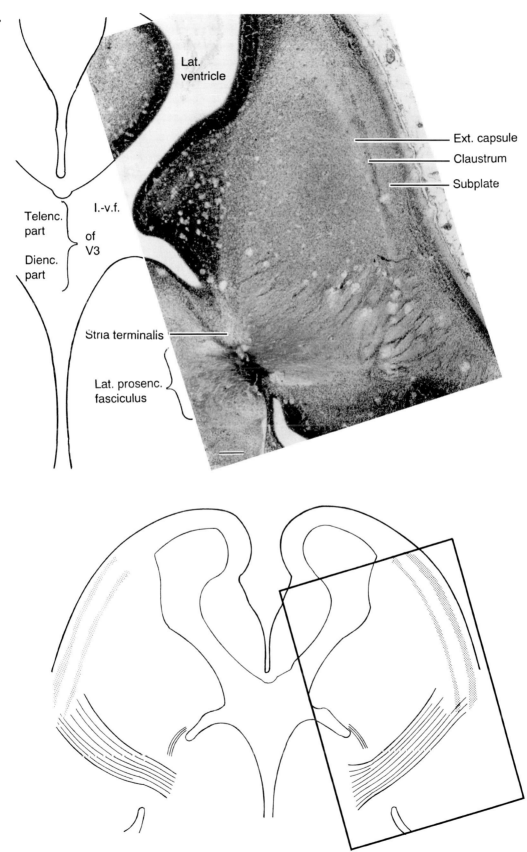

Lat. ventricle

Ext. capsule

Claustrum

Subplate

Telenc. part

Dienc. part

l.-v.f. of V3

Stria terminalis

Lat. prosenc. fasciculus

Fig. 24-8. 27.5 mm. An enlargement of the internal capsule at a more dorsal level. Figure 24-7 shows the arrival and origin of the fibers in the subplate. The key drawing is a graphic reconstruction.

Pain Pathways. It is commonly stated that the thalamocortical constituents develop before their corticothalamic counterparts of the internal capsule. They may, however, develop simultaneously (in rodents).

Receptors, such as those in the skin, appear during the embryonic period, as do also interneurons in the substantia gelantinosa of the spinal cord. Moreover, the spinothalamic tract and thalamocortical fibers are identifiable later in the embryonic period (stages 22 and 23 in the authors' observations). Corticothalamic fibers are probably present early in the fetal period. Thalamocortical fibers form temporary synapses in the cortical subplate during trimester 2 and penetrate the cortical plate in trimester 3, at which time thalamic inputs reach the somatosensory cortex. The functional significance of these immature pathways is not clear, and it is possible that information concerning pain is transferred differently before and after birth. Myelination, however, is not necessary for pain either before or after birth. It may be concluded that, although nociperception (the actual perception of pain) awaits the appearance of consciousness, nociception (the experience of pain) is present some time before birth. In the absence of disproof, it is merely prudent to assume that pain can be experienced even early in fetal life (Dr. J. Wisser, Zürich).

Fig. 24-8.

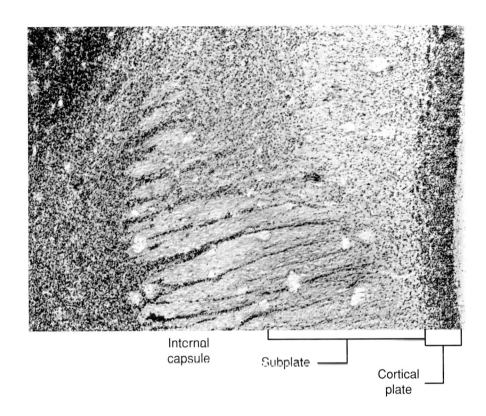

Internal
capsule

Subplate

Cortical
plate

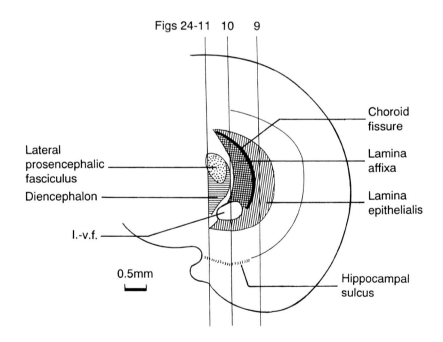

Figs 24-11   10   9

Lateral
prosencephalic
fasciculus

Diencephalon

l.-v.f.

0.5mm

Choroid
fissure

Lamina
affixa

Lamina
epithelialis

Hippocampal
sulcus

353

Fig. 24-9. 27.5 mm. The hippocampus is clearly recognizable because of its thinner ventricular layer, which is contiguous to the lamina epithelialis. The third ventricle is visible below, and its folded roof seems to show the beginning development of choroid villi. The thick fiber bundle on each side of the roof area is the stria medullaris thalami. The choroid plexuses of the lateral ventricles are well shown.

Fig. 24-10. 27.5 mm. The hippocampus more ventrally has joined the prosencephalic septum. The hippocampal sulcus has appeared and is contiguous to the rhinal sulcus, as shown in the key drawing with Figure 24-8. The falx cerebri is evident. The lateral ventricles are seen to be continuous with the cavity of the telencephalon medium, which in turn blends with the third ventricle between the thalami. See also Figure 24-7. The sulcus terminalis lies between the ventricular eminence and the dorsal thalamus.

Fig. 24-9.

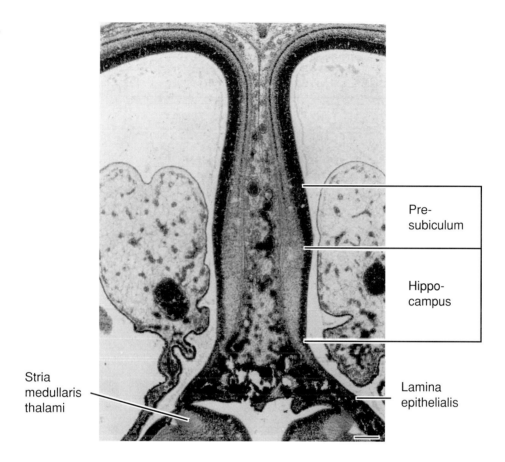

Pre-subiculum

Hippo-campus

Stria
medullaris
thalami

Lamina
epithelialis

Fig. 24-10.

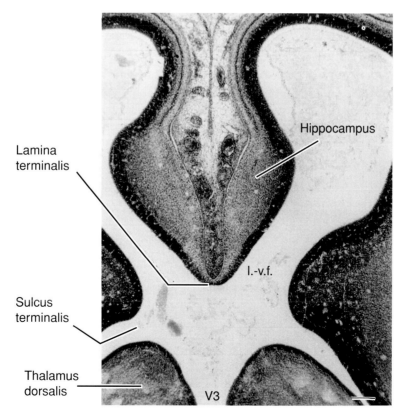

Hippocampus

Lamina
terminalis

l.-v.f.

Sulcus
terminalis

Thalamus
dorsalis

V3

355

Fig. 24-11. 27.5 mm. The dorsal portions of the olfactory bulbs are separated from the prosencephalic septum by the rhinal sulcus. The olfactory ventricles are evident. The falx cerebri has developed in the loose tissue of the subarachnoid space. Dark-appearing tissue emanating from the ventricular layer of the right-hand olfactory bulb leads to the claustrum.

The transient subpial granular layer, which appears before the end of trimester 1, seems to arise from the same area as the claustrum (Fig. 22-12). Two streams of cells have been observed at 14 weeks: one from the medial and the other from the lateral angle of the subventricular layer of the olfactory bulb (Gadisseux et al., 1992). The cells form a continuous lamina of unknown significance within the primordial plexiform layer, but the sheet has almost completely disappeared at birth.

The nucleus basalis (of Meynert) develops during the fetal period. Cholinesterase-reactive fibers arising from it are distributed to the neocortex and the limbic cortex by the end of trimester 2 (Kostović, 1986).

Fig. 24-11.

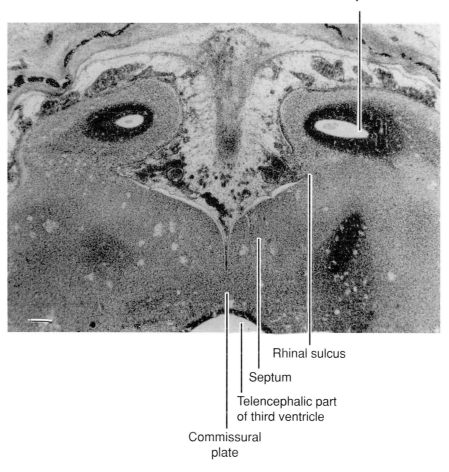

Olfactory ventricle

Rhinal sulcus

Septum

Telencephalic part
of third ventricle

Commissural
plate

Figures 24-12 to 24-14 are from a fetus of 42 mm (CEC 886), which was studied by Streeter (1918), Hines (1922), and Padget (1948, 1957). In Figure 24-12 and in subsequent illustrations, an orientation more similar to that of the adult is shown; i.e., the cerebral hemispheres have been "lifted" into a more horizontal position and the brain stem is almost vertical.

Fig. 24-12. 42 mm. Lateral view, based on a solid (Born) reconstruction. The membranous labyrinth has been added. The insula is becoming deeper. The interval between the diencephalon and the rhombencephalon is wider than in stage 23, and the pontine flexure is less marked. Parts of the diencephalon, as well as the mesencephalon, still remain uncovered by the cerebral hemispheres. The (caudal) mesencephalic *Blindsack* is visible. The intraventricular part of the cerebellum lies within the fourth ventricle and the extraventricular portion is subdivided by the posterolateral fissure.

Fig. 24-13. 42 mm. The brain *in situ*. The face is positioned more or less vertically to allow easier comparison with the adult. The head is less spherical than in stage 23, and its rostrocaudal axis is lengthening. This seems to allow more space for the brain, which is now less compact. From O'Rahilly, Müller, and Bossy (1986). Padget (1948, Fig. 21) reconstructed the arteries of this fetus.

Planes have been added to show that prenatally a transverse plane through the trunk does not correspond to the orbitomeatal plane in the adult, which is accepted as the horizontal standard. Similarly, coronal planes are not comparable.

Fig. 24-12.

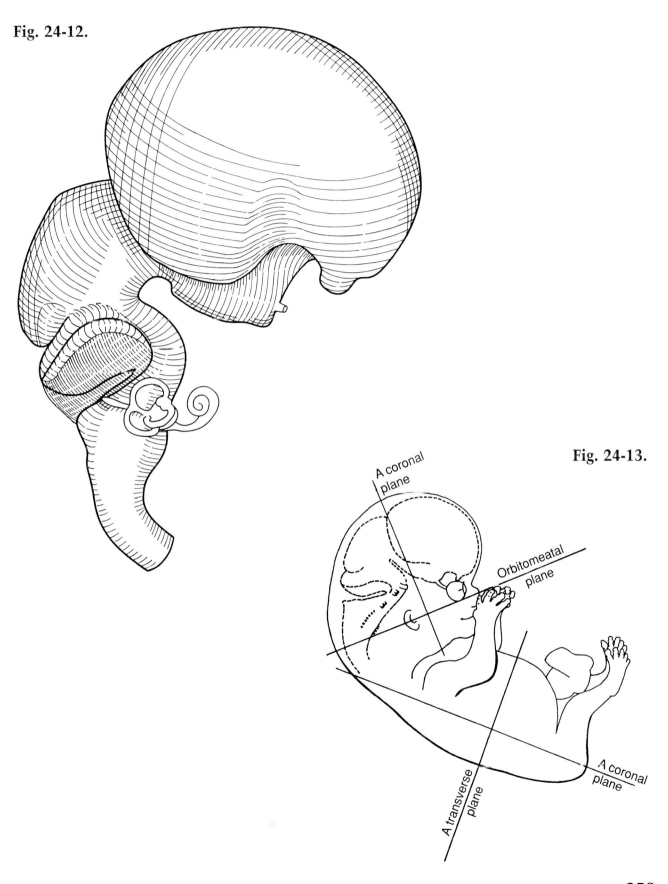

Fig. 24-13.

A coronal plane

Orbitomeatal plane

A transverse plane

A coronal plane

Fig. 24-14. 42 mm (CEC 886). Median view.

(**A**) The prosencephalic septum is relatively reduced in its rostrocaudal extent. The paraphysis is inconspicuous compared with that of stage 23. The dorsal thalamus now extends over half of the lateral diencephalic wall. The marginal ridge between the dorsal and ventral thalami is no longer clear, although the sulcus medius is visible (Fig. 24-21). The posterior commissure and the commissure of the superior colliculi are separated. The floor of the mesencephalon has become greatly thickened by an increase in ascending and descending fibers. The isthmic groove, formerly the isthmic recess, is scarcely visible. The rostrocaudal extent of the fourth ventricle is relatively less. The ventral thalamus becomes so reduced that the former dorsal thalamus, now termed merely the thalamus, borders directly on the subthalamus, as established by Richter (1965) using excellent fetal preparations.

(**B**) The overlapping of the left cerebral hemisphere on the left half of the diencephalon. The hippocampus, the dentate area, the area epithelialis, and the choroid fissure are shown as if the prosencephalon were transparent. The lamina affixa is cross-hatched. The olfactory bulb is no longer directed caudally, a change that is perhaps related to a rostral extension of the nasal cavities (Hochstetter, 1919). In slightly older fetuses the olfactory bulb grows rostrally and becomes thinner and longer, concomitant with the lengthening of the frontal part of the cerebral hemisphere. The site of the entrance of the lateral prosencephalic fasciculus into the diencephalon is stippled. Based partly on Hines (1922). The levels of two sections, Figures 24-20 and 24-21, are indicated. Three-dimensional reconstructions, prepared ultrasonically, of the ventricles *in vivo* in fetuses of 38 or 40 mm are illustrated by Blaas et al. (1995, 1998).

Fig. 24-14.

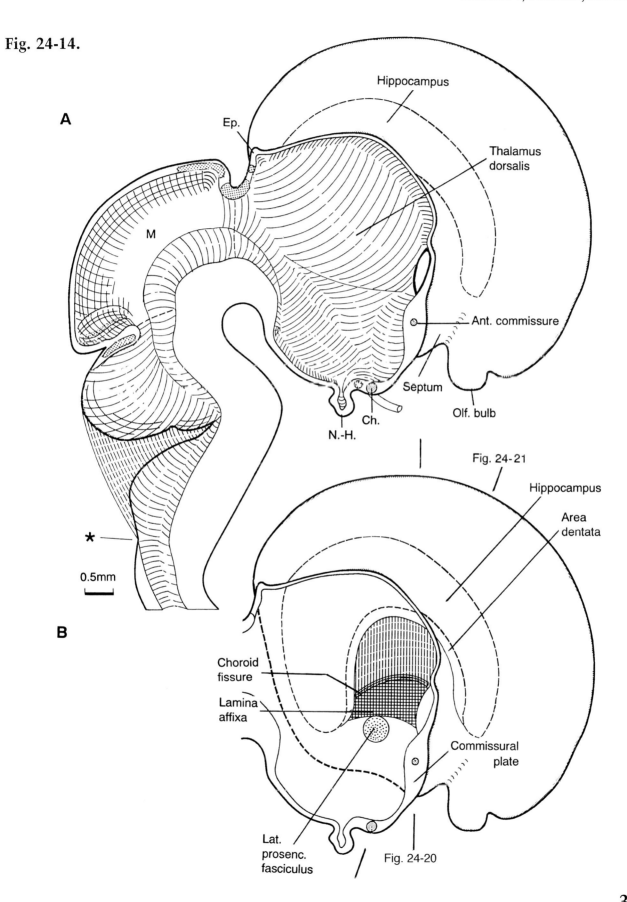

A

Hippocampus

Ep.

Thalamus
dorsalis

M

Ant. commissure

Septum

Olf. bulb

Ch.

N.-H.

*

0.5mm

B

Fig. 24-21

Hippocampus

Area
dentata

Choroid
fissure

Lamina
affixa

Commissural
plate

Lat.
prosenc.
fasciculus

Fig. 24-20

Fig. 24-15. Topographical changes in the cerebellum of the first trimester. The flocculonodular lobe (or vestibulocerebellum), shown here by stippling, is the archicerebellum, which is formed differently from the rest of the vermis and is considered by some not to belong to the cerebellum *sensu stricto.* Both the vermis and the hemispheres will contribute to the paleocerebellum (or spinocerebellum) and the neocerebellum (or corticopontocerebellum).

(**A**) At stage 20 (CEC 966) the floccular region begins to become tilted from a rostrolateral to an occipitolateral position. The internal cerebellar swellings are well separated. The mesencephalon is still relatively small.

(**B**) At 9 weeks (42 mm, CEC 886) the flocculonodular lobe is pointed in an occipital direction. An increase in the size of the internal swellings (at 50 mm according to Hochstetter) is leading to the formation of a single intraventricular thickening ("*Verschmelzung der innereren Kleinhirn-wülste*"). Soon (at about 63 mm) the external swellings also begin to increase in bulk.

(**C**) and (**C′**) At 13 weeks (95 mm, CEC 146) several folia and fissures can be distinguished in the vermis.

(**D**) and (**D′**) At 14 weeks (120 mm) the beginning of trimester 2, the cerebellum resembles that of the adult. The median aperture in the (horizontally hatched) roof of the fourth ventricle is shown in black in D and by an open arrow in D′. At this time the dentate nucleus contains bipolar cells; the characteristic five types of cell are present at the end of trimester 2, and dendritic proliferation has been observed early in trimester 3 (Hayaran et al., 1992).

Abbreviations: 1, fissura prima; 2, fissura secunda; P-L, posterolateral fissure. B and C are based on reconstructions in Streeter (1912, where No. 86, 30 mm, is given incorrectly instead of No. 886, 42 mm). D is modified from Kollmann, Hochstetter, Streeter, and other sources.

Fig. 24-15.

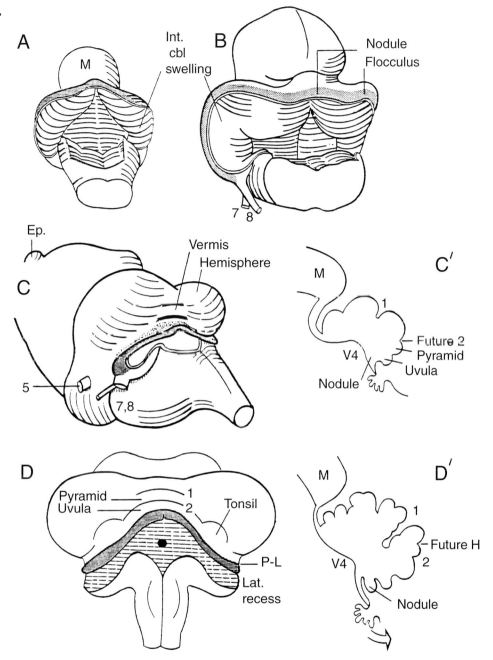

Fig. 24-16. 46 mm (CEC 1630). A nearly median section. The dorsal thalamus, which appears dark because it is cut at the level of the ventricular layer, is well shown. It is separated from the ventral thalamus by a band of gray material, which is probably the tract of the zona intrathalamica. When the individual thalamic nuclei are said to appear depends on the criteria selected, and these are mainly the establishment of cell-poor boundaries and the presence of nerve fibers, followed by differentiation into nuclear groups. Further information: Dekaban (1954), Fabiani and Barontini (1956), Yamadori (1965). The lateral geniculate body shows lamination during trimester 2. The pulvinar, which begins to develop at the commencement of trimester 2, is derived mainly from the medial ventricular eminence and grows greatly during the second half of prenatal life. Migrating cells from the medial ventricular eminence cover the fetal corpus striatum adjacent to the sulcus terminalis (constituting the "corpus gangliothalamicum" of Rakic and Sidman, 1969) and are said to participate in the formation of other thalamic nuclei (Letinić and Kostović, 1997).

The epiphysis cerebri, the posterior commissure, and the commissure of the superior colliculi are all recognizable. The three subdivisions of the axis (termed X, Y, and Z by O'Rahilly, Müller, and Meyer, 1983, in their account of the occipitocervical region) are evident. A key drawing is provided.

Fig. 24-16.

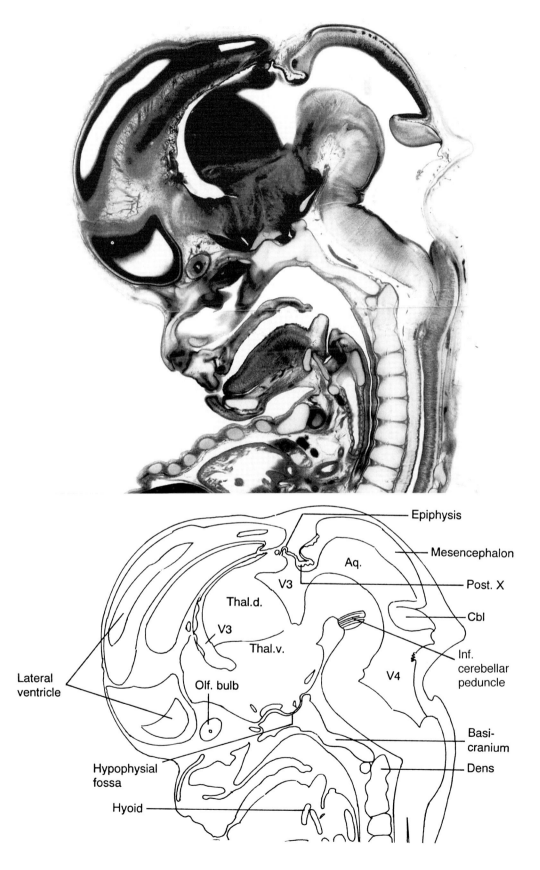

Epiphysis

Mesencephalon

Aq.

V3

Post. X

Thal.d.

Cbl

V3

Thal.v.

Inf.
cerebellar
peduncle

Lateral
ventricle

Olf. bulb

V4

Basi-
cranium

Hypophysial
fossa

Dens

Hyoid

Fig. 24-17. 42 mm. A dorsal view of the brain with parts of the hemispheres removed. The external capsule, which is not clearly distinguishable in stage 23, is now visible. This instructive view, which shows a number of important relationships, is based on Kollmann (1907).

Fig. 24-17.

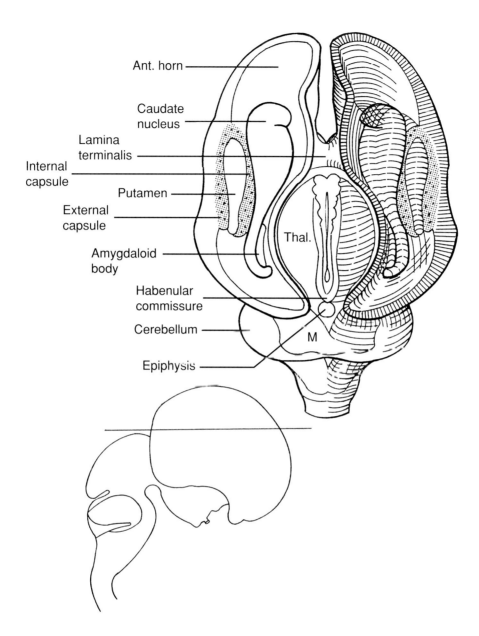

Ant. horn

Caudate
nucleus

Lamina
terminalis

Internal
capsule

Putamen

External
capsule

Amygdaloid
body

Habenular
commissure

Cerebellum

Epiphysis

Thal.

M

Fig. 24-18. 42 mm. A lateral view of the exposed basal nuclei, choroid fissure, and internal and external capsules. The part of the cerebral hemisphere that has been removed here is indicated by a dotted line in Figure 24-21. Based on Kollmann (1907), with some corrections.

Fig. 24-18.

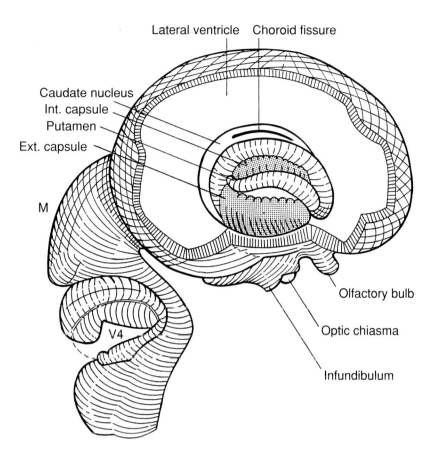

Lateral ventricle   Choroid fissure

Caudate nucleus
Int. capsule
Putamen
Ext. capsule

M

V4

Olfactory bulb

Optic chiasma

Infundibulum

Fig. 24-19. A sagittal section at 40 mm (CEC 6658). The relatively great size of the choroid plexus is noticeable. The key shows the hippocampal thickening. (The cortical plate is present in the other areas of the hemispheres.) The dorsal thalamus is closely related to the ventricular eminences. Thalamocortical fibers are already numerous, although the thalamic nuclei have yet to form. The habenulo-interpeduncular and mamillotegmental tracts can be followed to the mesencephalic tegmentum. The decussation of the trochlear nerves is identifiable in the isthmus. The internal cerebellar swelling is large. The rhombic lip can be seen here and again further caudally at the end of the medulla oblongata.

Fig. 24-19.

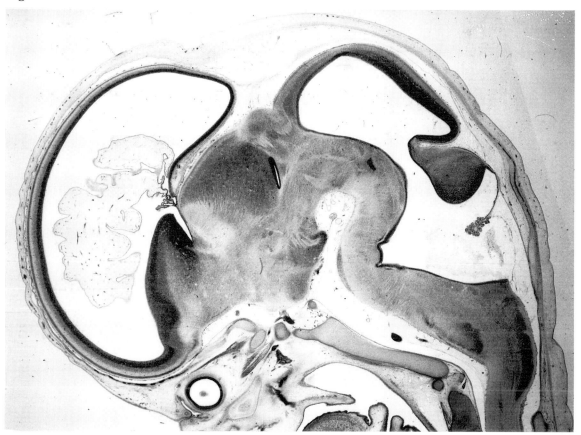

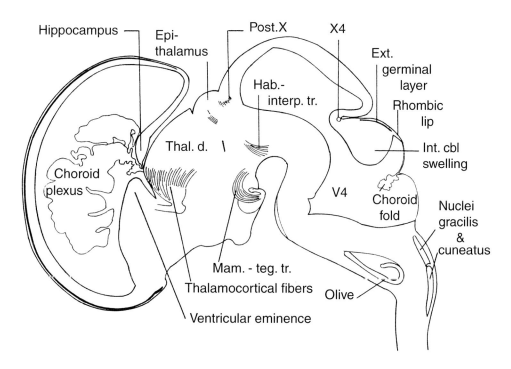

Hippocampus
Epi-thalamus
Post.X
X4
Ext. germinal layer
Rhombic lip
Hab.- interp. tr.
Thal. d.
Int. cbl swelling
Choroid plexus
V4
Choroid fold
Nuclei gracilis & cuneatus
Mam. - teg. tr.
Thalamocortical fibers
Olive
Ventricular eminence

371

Fig. 24-20.   50 mm. A coronal section showing the anterior commissure, the caudate nucleus, the internal capsule, and the putamen. Based on a photomicrograph in Feess-Higgins and Larroche (1987).

Fig. 24-21.   37 mm. A coronal section showing the interventricular foramina and a number of important relationships. Based on an excellent photomicrograph in Richter (1965). The dotted line indicates the part of the cerebral hemisphere removed in Figure 24-18.

Cholinesterase-reactive fibers from the nucleus basalis complex are distributed widely to the neocortex and limbic cortex by the end of trimester 2 (Kostović, 1986).

Fig. 24-20.

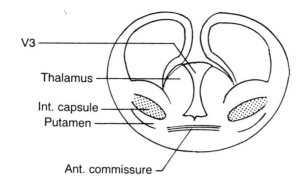

V3

Thalamus

Int. capsule

Putamen

Ant. commissure

Fig. 24-21.

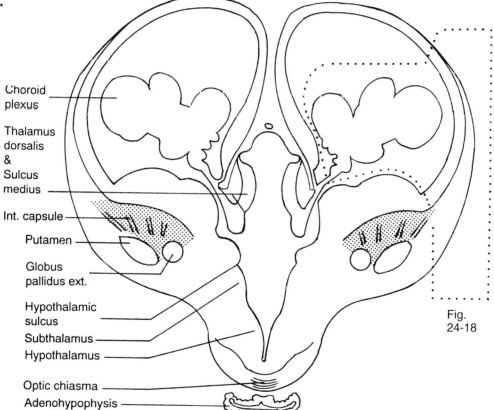

Choroid plexus

Thalamus dorsalis & Sulcus medius

Int. capsule

Putamen

Globus pallidus ext.

Hypothalamic sulcus

Subthalamus

Hypothalamus

Optic chiasma

Adenohypophysis

Fig. 24-18

373

Fig. 24-22. The arterial system at 42 mm (CEC 886). The internal carotid artery is shown in black, and the basilar by horizontal hatching.

(**A**) Left lateral view. The various vessels are identified in the inset: the three cerebral arteries (A.C., M.C., P.C.), the anterior and posterior choroid (A.chor., P.chor.), the posterior communicating (P.co.), superior cerebellar (Sup.cbl), and the anterior and posterior inferior cerebellar arteries (AICA, PICA).

(**B**) Basal view. "The arteries resemble the adult conformation . . . at about 40 mm" (Padget, 1957). In both views the choroid plexuses of the lateral and fourth ventricles are included.

These drawings are based on graphic reconstructions made by Padget (1948), whose work should be studied for further details. The venous system at 40 mm has been illustrated by Padget (1957, Fig. 13), according to whom "the adult pattern of most venous sinuses and cerebral veins can be recognized" by 80 mm, although "several important anastomoses typical of adult sinuses usually do not appear until after birth."

Fig. 24-22.

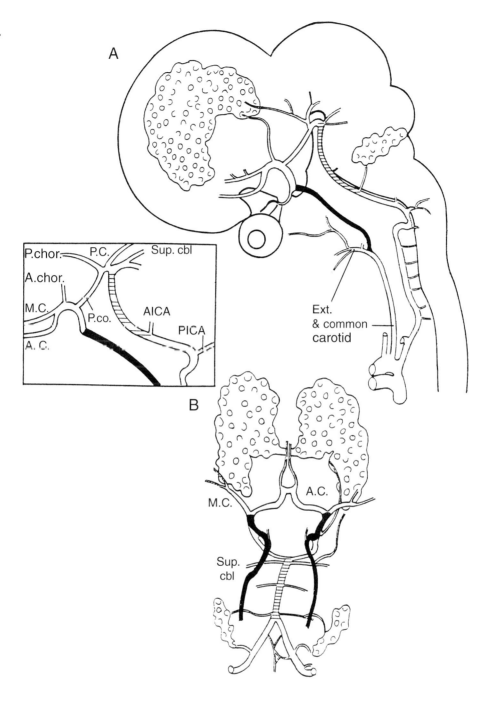

Trimester 1: Later Postembryonic Phase

Approximately 50–100 mm in Greatest Length
Approximately 9–13 Postfertilizational Weeks

Mathematical and hormonal criteria have been used (by Guyot) to indicate an important step in fetal development when the GL is approximately 90 mm at some 90 postfertilizational days.

Fig. 24-23. 75 mm (approximately 12 weeks). This is a horizontal section through the interventricular foramina. The longitudinal fissure is evident rostrally, and the tectum caudally. Many features are already arranged more or less as in the adult, e.g., the sequence of corpus striatum, internal capsule, thalamus, and third ventricle, as well as the sequence of lateral and medial geniculate bodies, and tectum. The aqueduct is still relatively large, and the corpus callosum is still limited to the rostral region. Several structures show the characteristic C-shaped disposition; e.g., the lateral ventricle, hippocampus, and caudate nucleus are each sectioned twice. The lateral ventricle (shown also in the upper right-hand drawing) is sectioned in its anterior and inferior horns. The key drawings are at 88 mm (left) and 78 mm (right). The section is based on a photomicrograph in Feess-Higgins and Larroche (1987), and the outline of the lateral ventricle is after Westergaard (1971).

A basal view of the brain at 68 mm (about 11 weeks) is shown in Figure 25-6B.

Details of the medial surface of the prosencephalon at 80 mm are presented in Figure 26-2A.

Fig. 24-23.

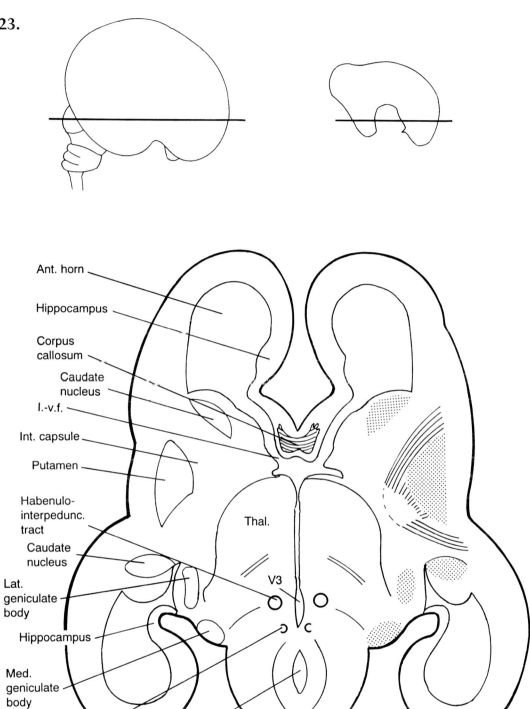

Ant. horn

Hippocampus

Corpus callosum

Caudate nucleus

I.-v.f.

Int. capsule

Putamen

Habenulo-interpedunc. tract

Caudate nucleus

Lat. geniculate body

Hippocampus

Med. geniculate body

Post. commissure

Aqueduct

Tectum

Thal.

V3

Fig. 24-24. Median sections through the brain stem at (**A**) 54 mm (10 postfertilizational weeks), (**B**) 68 mm (11 weeks), and (**C**) 80 mm (12 weeks).
A sequence of six key features is numbered; these were distinguishable already at 6 weeks (Fig. 17-6, key), the main difference being that the anterior commissure and the corpus callosum had not yet become differentiated within the commissural plate. The sequence continues to be evident later in the fetal period (Fig. 25-2) and in the adult. The mesocoelic recess, which is shallow in A, is indicated by an asterisk. Based on Hochstetter (1929).

Fig. 24-24.

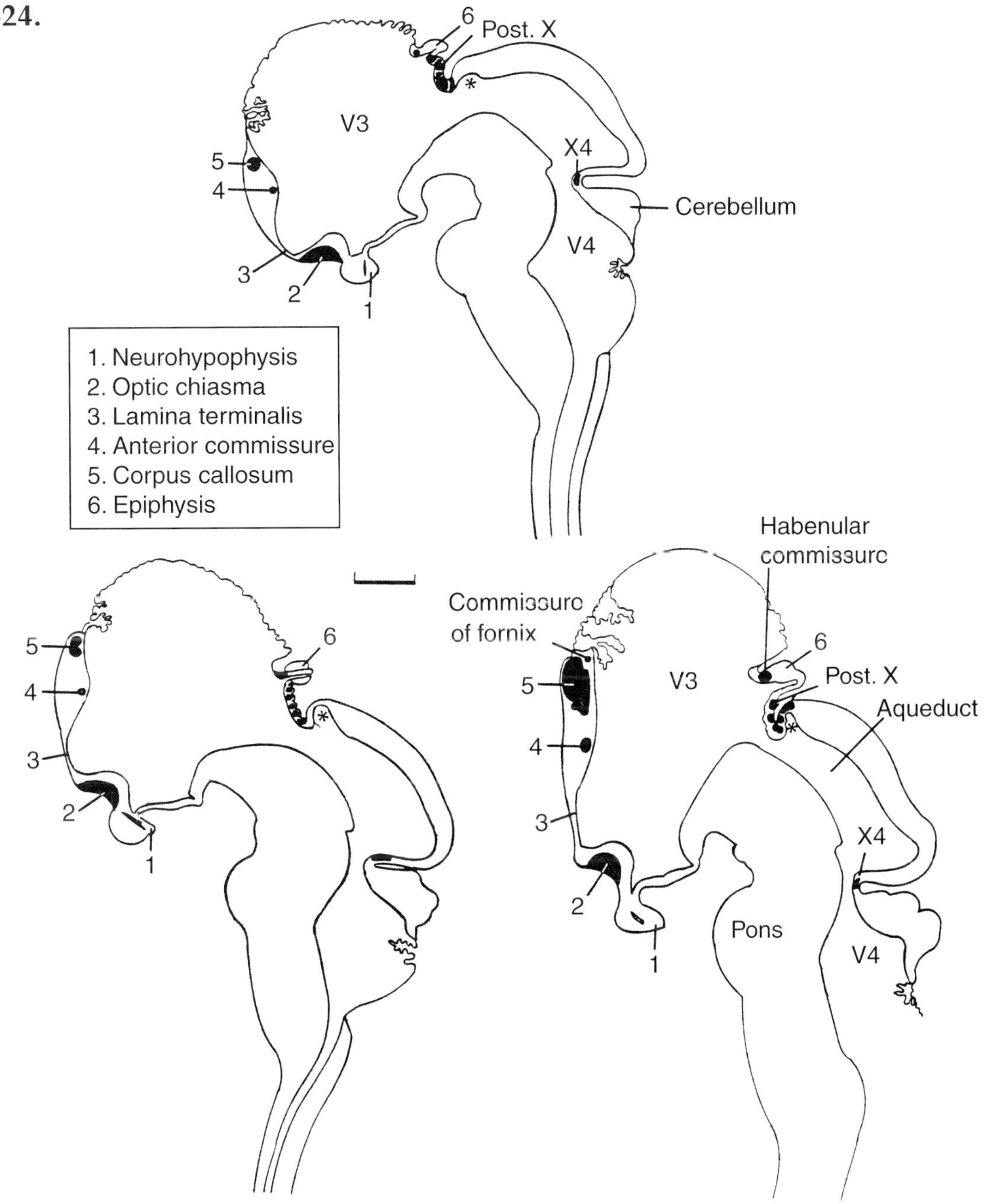
6
Post. X
V3
X4
5
4
Cerebellum
V4
3
2
1
1. Neurohypophysis
2. Optic chiasma
3. Lamina terminalis
4. Anterior commissure
5. Corpus callosum
6. Epiphysis
Habenular commissure
Commissure of fornix
Aqueduct
Pons

Fig. 24-25. 100 mm (approximately 13 weeks). This is a median section at the end of trimester 1. The medial surface of the left cerebral hemisphere is stippled. The corpus callosum is still small, so that the roof of the third ventricle is exposed at the bottom of the longitudinal fissure. The pineal region and its associated recesses and commissures are well developed. The aqueduct is still relatively wide. (A graph of its cross-sectional area correlated with age is given by Lemire et al., 1975, p. 98.) The vermis is small. (The number of folia seen in the vermis increases greatly during trimesters 2 and 3, as shown in a graph by Lemire et al., 1975, p. 150.) The tegmental portion of the brain stem is voluminous. Although the forebrain is at an angle (of approximately 116°) with the brain stem, the flexures characteristic of the embryonic period proper have now become difficult to detect. The parts marked a and b are described with Figure 26-2. The section of the brain stem is based on Hochstetter (1919), and the inset showing the lateral ventricle is from a cast by Day (1959).

Details of the medial surface of the prosencephalon at 95 mm are given in Figure 26-2B.

The distribution of the facial nerve at 80 mm has been illustrated by Gasser (1967), who also showed it at what were considered to be stages 13, 14, 18, 19, 21, and 22.

Fig. 24-25.

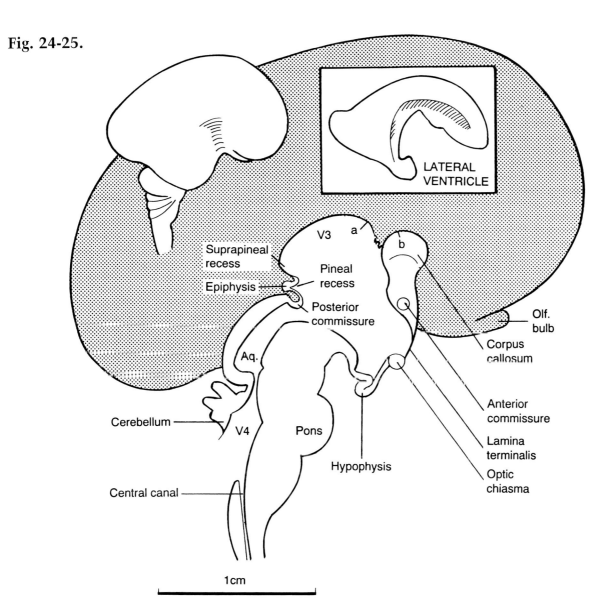

LATERAL VENTRICLE

V3
a
b
Suprapineal recess
Pineal recess
Epiphysis
Posterior commissure
Olf. bulb
Corpus callosum
Aq.
Anterior commissure
Cerebellum
V4
Pons
Lamina terminalis
Central canal
Hypophysis
Optic chiasma

1cm

Fig. 24-26. 95 mm (approximately 13 weeks). Anteromedial view of some major fiber tracts. The right half of the brain stem has been preserved intact. In the rostral part of the telencephalon everything has been removed except the fiber tracts, thereby exposing the corpus callosum, the column and commissure of the fornix, two divisions of the anterior comissure, and the internal capsule, which last subdivides the corpus striatum into the caudate and lentiform nuclei. On the left side of the brain, the connection from the stria terminalis to the anterior commissure is shown. Various features are identified in the key drawing. Based on Streeter in Keibel and Mall (1912).

The development of the fornix can be summarized as follows. The earliest components of the fornix, present already at stage 20, are the precommissural fibers from the septal nuclei to the (as yet poorly developed) hippocampus (Fig. 20-10). Early in the fetal period (at about 9–11 weeks) the columns arise as connections between the hippocampal system and the mamillary nuclei (Figs. 25-1 and 26-3B). The commissure of the fornix develops as the corpus callosum becomes identifiable (55 mm, 10 weeks, Rakic and Yakovlev, 1968; 105 mm, 13 weeks, Hochstetter, 1929).

Fig. 24-26.

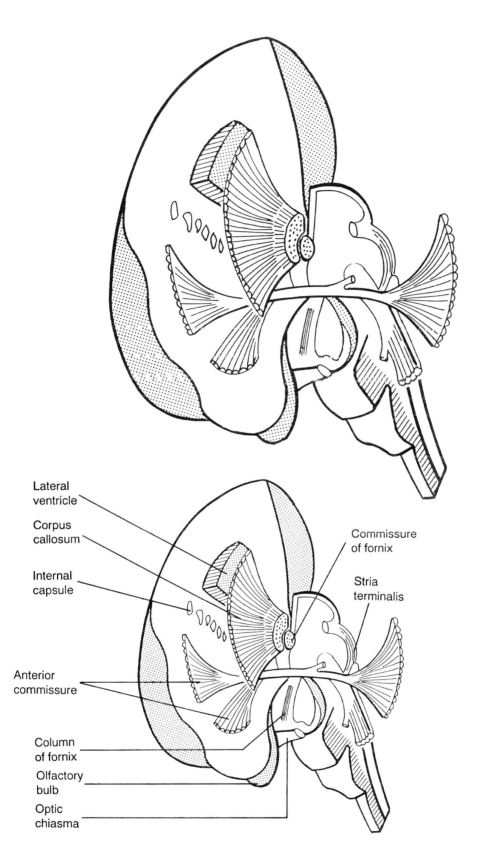

Lateral
ventricle

Corpus
callosum

Internal
capsule

Commissure
of fornix

Stria
terminalis

Anterior
commissure

Column
of fornix

Olfactory
bulb

Optic
chiasma

Fig. 24-27. Outlines of the cerebral hemisphere at 25, 38, 53, 68, and 96 mm, drawn to the same scale, showing the considerable enlargement from the end of the embryonic period proper. The lowermost drawing presents the entire brain at 25 mm (cf. Figs. 22-1 and 22-2). The uppermost drawing shows the brain *in situ* at 31 mm (stage 23, CEC 9226) in almost natural size. The main and the lowermost drawings are based on Hochstetter (1919).

Fig. 24-27.

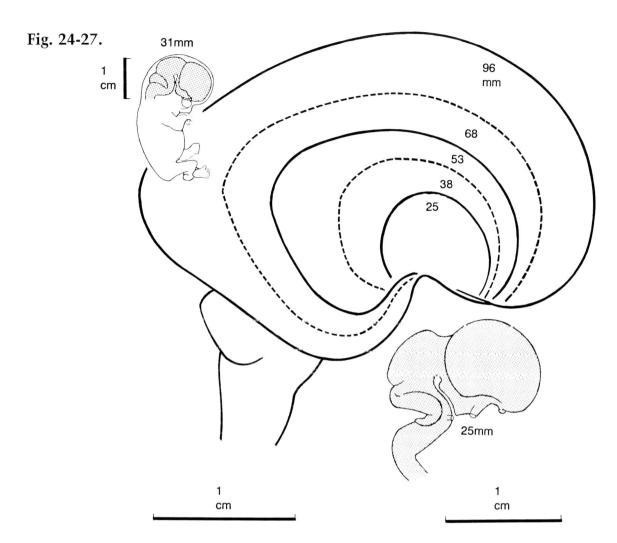

31mm

1 cm

96 mm

68

53

38

25

25mm

1 cm

1 cm

Comments on Neuroteratology

Anencephaly develops successively as (1) cerebral dysraphia (see stages 11 and 13), (2) exencephaly (see stage 22; a good example at 35 mm has been illustrated by Hunter, 1934), and (3) degeneration of the exposed brain throughout the fetal period. Phase 3 is believed to be brought about by partial or complete exposure of the uncovered brain to amniotic fluid for prolonged periods (Lemire et al., 1977). This secondary degeneration of a well-developed brain affects mainly those parts that are situated rostral to the medulla oblongata. Interesting clinical studies of anencephaly have been published by André-Thomas and de Ajuriaguerra (1959).

Precision

Anencephaly, hydrocephaly, and similar terms refer to the condition, whereas the designations anencephalus, hydrocephalus, etc. are restricted to individually afflicted fetuses or infants.

Trimester 2

Approximately 100–250 mm in Greatest Length
Approximately 13–26 Postfertilizational Weeks

Sulci begin to appear on the surface of the cerebral hemisphere at about the middle of prenatal life. The data of Larroche have been schematized by Lemire et al. (1975, pp. 235 and 236) and further details are given by Gilles, et al. (1983, pp. 96–99). The progression is well displayed in a series of photographs in Feess-Higgins and Larroche (1987, pp. 14 and 15). Cerebral asymmetry is present at the latest during trimester 2. The maturation of the fetal brain can be correlated with the microscopical development of the renal glomeruli (Dorovini-Zis and Dolman, 1977). Synapses increase significantly in number at the beginning of trimester 2 (Kostović and Rakic, 1990). Electrical activity can be detected in the hippocampal region and in the diencephalon.

The supracallosal portion of the hippocampus begins to regress early in trimester 2 and later becomes the indusium griseum. At about the same period, the characteristic interlocking C formation of the hippocampus and the dentate gyrus becomes noticeable, at approximately 150 mm.

The crura cerebri, although identifiable during trimester 1, have become prominent bundles on the ventral surface of the midbrain by the middle of prenatal life.

Myelination, as detected by light microscopy, begins in the CNS at about 20 weeks; by electron microscopy, evidence in the spinal cord can be found late in trimester 1. The data of Yakovlev and LeCours have been schematized by Lemire et al. (1975, pp. 44–46), and numerous tables and graphs are provided by Gilles et al., (1983, Chapter 12). The pyramidal tracts do not begin to be myelinated until shortly before birth, although myelinated fibers

387

are present at the level of the pyramidal decussation by the middle of prenatal life (Woźniak and O'Rahilly, 1982).

A solid reconstruction of a brain at 145 mm has been illustrated by Velasco-Villamar (1967).

A basal view of the brain at 150 mm (about 17 weeks) is shown in Figure 25-6.

Functional cortical innervation of spinal gray matter is probably in place by 22–26 postfertilizational weeks (Dr. G.J. Clowry, Newcastle-upon-Tyne, personal communication, 1998).

Fig. 25-1. Approximately 230 mm (about 24–26 weeks). This horizontal section is taken near the end of trimester 2. It resembles very closely a corresponding section through the adult brain, except for the almost total absence of sulci and gyri. Moreover, the insula is not yet buried by its opercula. The level of the section is that of the interthalamic adhesion and the epiphysis cerebri. (The interthalamic adhesion appears at about the junction of trimesters 1 and 2, and disappears at approximately 40–60 years of age, as shown in a graph in Lemire et al., 1975, p. 179). The third ventricle is sectioned twice, as is also the caudate nucleus. The anterior and posterior horns of each lateral ventricle are evident. Also shown are the pulvinar (a), the habenula (b), and the suprapineal recess (c). The section is based on a photomicrograph in Feess-Higgins and Larroche (1987), and the upper drawing showing the ventricular system is after Kier (1977).

For a long period, the cerebral wall is irrigated by blood vessels that consist of simple endothelial channels. A vascular network within the cortex develops between 22 and 24 weeks. A muscularis is acquired only near term and postnatally (Nelson et al., 1991). The right lateral view of the ventricular system illustrated in an inset shows the triangular part of the lateral ventricle, where the inferior and posterior horns diverge. This part is frequently referred to in radiology as the atrium, and its floor is the collateral trigone.

Fig. 25-1.

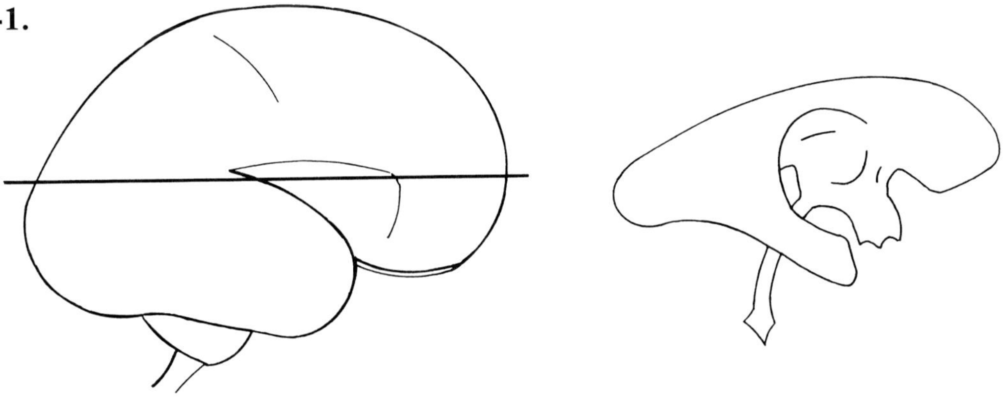

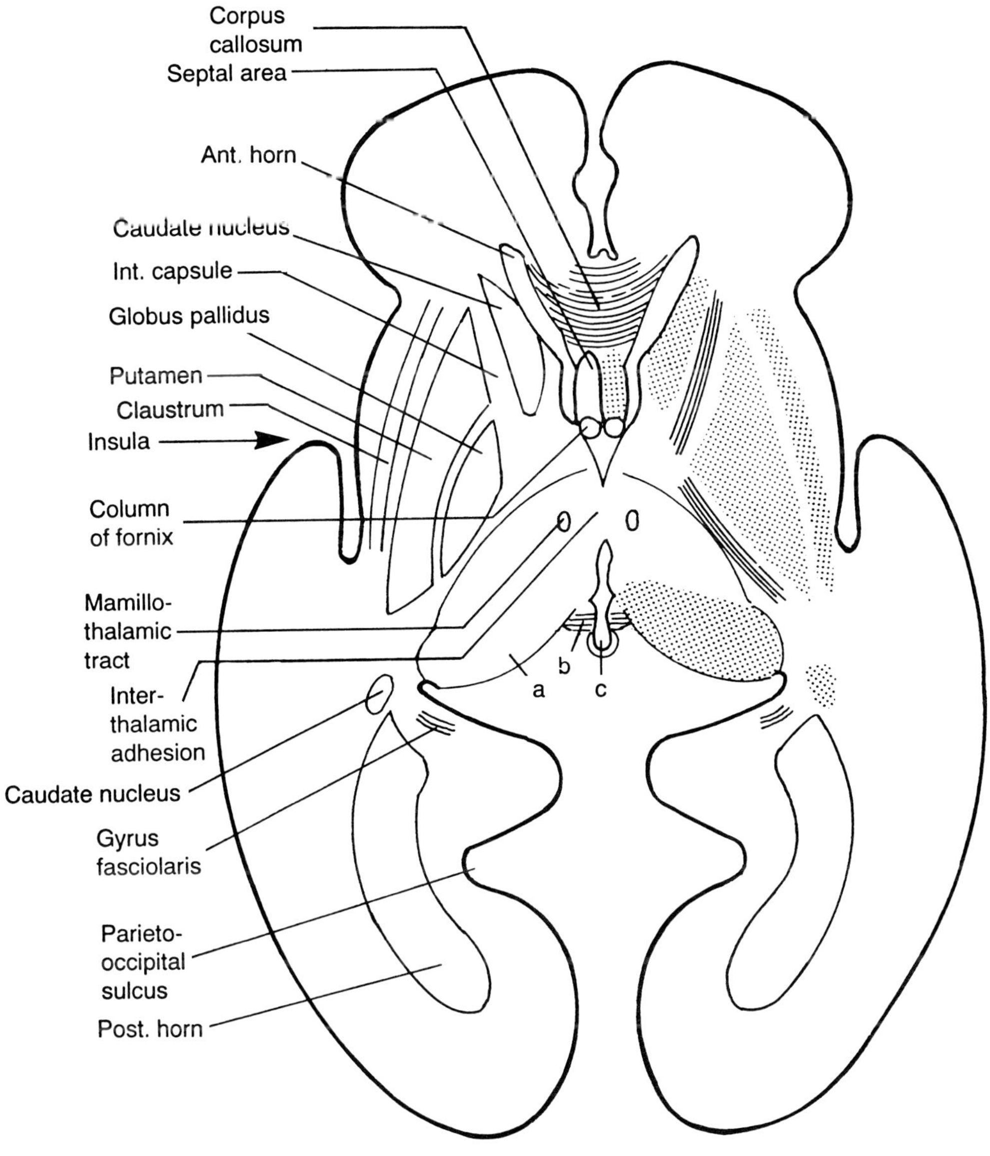

Corpus
callosum

Septal area

Ant. horn

Caudate nucleus

Int. capsule

Globus pallidus

Putamen

Claustrum

Insula

Column
of fornix

Mamillo-
thalamic
tract

Inter-
thalamic
adhesion

Caudate nucleus

Gyrus
fasciolaris

Parieto-
occipital
sulcus

Post. horn

Fig. 25-2.   Median sections: (**A**) and (**B**) at about 100 mm (13 weeks) and (**C**) at 125 mm (15 weeks). A sequence of six features, already visible earlier (Fig. 24-24) and readily seen in the adult, is numbered. The trunk of the corpus callosum becomes elongated within a few days (compare A with B) and the genu is well developed in C. The mesocoelic recess, which has become very deep in C, is indicated by an asterisk. A more complete view of the brain at 100 mm is shown in Figure 24-25. Based on Hochstetter (1929). Bars: 2 mm.

Because the trunk of the corpus callosum is sometimes found in the absence of a genu, it has been proposed by Kier and Truwit (1996) that the first part of the corpus callosum to become visible is the front portion of the trunk, which then develops bidirectionally, thereby forming the genu and the splenium. The genu was found always to project in front of a reference line from the mamillary body through the anterior commissure and corpus callosum. Their interpretation is shown below.

(**A**) 13 weeks (105 mm), (**B**) 15 weeks (125 mm), and (**C**) adult. A and B are modified from Hochstetter. Darker stippling, trunk. Lighter stippling, genu. a, anterior commissure. m, mamillary body.

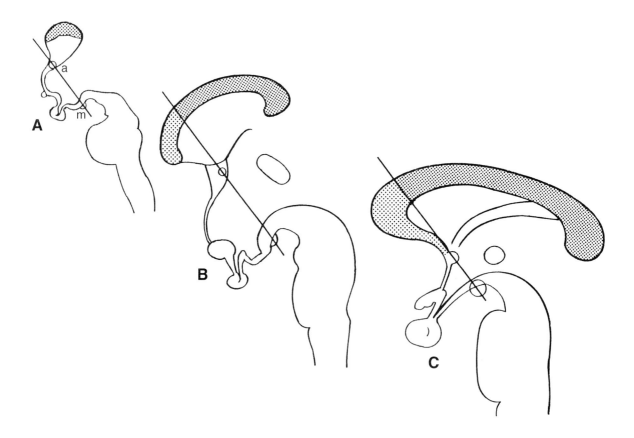

Fig. 25-2.

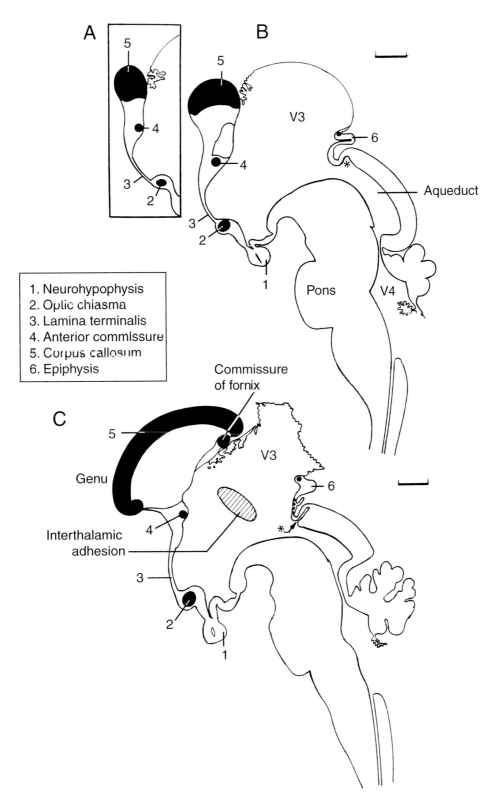

A

B

V3

6

Aqueduct

Pons

V4

1. Neurohypophysis
2. Optic chiasma
3. Lamina terminalis
4. Anterior commissure
5. Corpus callosum
6. Epiphysis

Commissure
of fornix

C

Genu

Interthalamic
adhesion

V3

6

Fig. 25-3. Magnetic resonance images (MRI) of a postmortem brain at approximately 16 postfertilizational weeks. (**A**) The lateral and third ventricles are readily identifiable. The bilateral prominences below the thalami are the cerebral peduncles. The hippocampal region is also visible, adjacent to the inferior horn of the lateral ventricle. (**B**) In addition to the posterior horns of the lateral ventricles, the vermis and medulla oblongata can be seen, and between them the fourth ventricle. Small projections adjacent to the cerebellum are cranial nerves 7 and 8. Courtesy of Martha C. Ballesteros, M.D., Miami Beach, Florida, from Hansen et al. (1993).

Fig. 25-3.

A

B

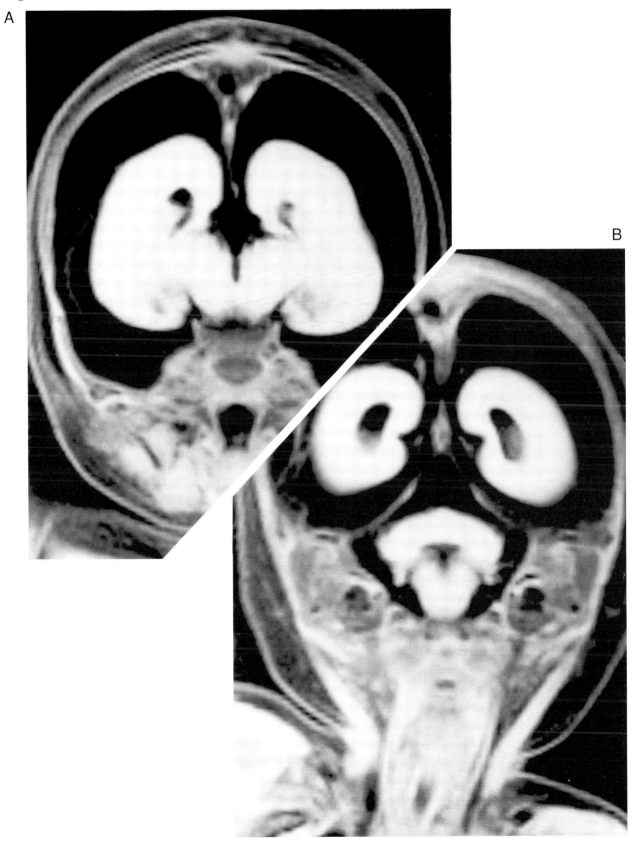

Fig. 25-4. A comparison of coronal sections at (**A**) 20 mm (stage 20, 7 weeks, CEC 462) and (**B**) 240 mm (approximately 24–28 weeks), at the junction of trimesters 2 and 3. Section B1 is slightly anterior to section B2. A comparison between the embryonic and the fetal sections indicates the further development after 7 weeks. Some of the fetal features are already foreshadowed even at 8 weeks (stage 23). The most striking difference is in the corpus callosum, which, after 100 mm, extends rapidly in a caudal direction, thereby covering the roof of the third ventricle. Hence, during the embryonic period, the longitudinal fissure leads directly onto the roof of the third ventricle, whereas beginning in trimester 2, the fissure becomes blocked below by the corpus callosum.

Another very important feature is the descent of the fibers of the internal capsule. They traverse the region of the ventricular eminences at the end of the embryonic period, and during the fetal period (B, open arrow) they pass first between two telencephalic structures, the putamen and the caudate nucleus, and then between two diencephalic components, the globus pallidus and the thalamus. Even in the adult brain, slight histological (vascular) differences can be seen between the two telencephalic elements and the two diencephalic constituents, emphasizing their different prosencephalic origins.

At least two subcortical afferent systems are said to "wait" in the subplate in the second half of trimester 2: thalamocortical fibers and basal forebrain fibers (Kostović et al., 1992b). Shortly thereafter, thalamocortical fibers penetrate the cortical plate, where intensive synaptic formation is occurring (Kostović et al., 1992b). The first sign of the nucleus basalis complex has been shown by cholinesterase reactivity at the beginning of the fetal period, and reactive bundles develop also (Kostović, 1986).

TABLE 25-1. Relationships of Internal Capsule in the Fetus and in the Adult

Laterally		Medially
Telencephalon: Putamen	Internal capsule	Telencephalon: Caudate nucleus
Diencephalon: Globus pallidus		Diencephalon: Thalamus and Subthalamus

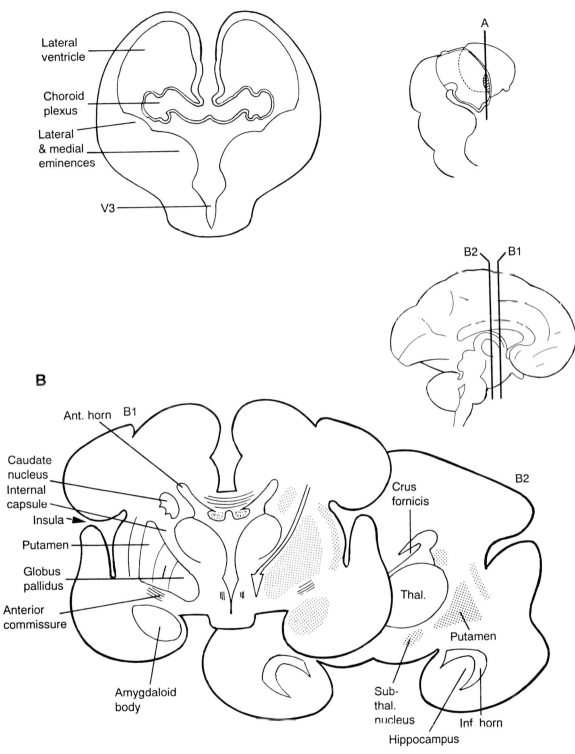

Fig. 25-4. **A**

B

395

The Hippocampal Formation

The dentate gyrus, the hippocampus, the subiculum, and the parahippocampal gyrus (entorhinal area) are conveniently grouped as the hippocampal formation.

The hippocampus was probably first observed by Achillini of Bologna (1463–1512). It was named by Aranzi (Arantius) of Bologna (1530–1589), who described it as "a raised, partially attached, whitish substance" showing "an uneven, bent form that resembles the appearance of a hippocampus, that is, a sea-horse." The name is an example of *Witz der Namengebung* (Burdach). The alternative name Cornu Ammonis, now avoided as are other eponyms, was used by Winslow (1669–1760) because of a supposed resemblance to the curling horn of a ram, which was the crest of the Egyptian deity Ammon.

The name Cornu Ammonis gave rise to the abbreviation CA and the structure was divided by Lorente de Nó into CA1 to CA4; CA4 is now frequently included in CA3. Although the preferred term is hippocampus, the abbreviation CA can still be used (as proposed here) for Cellular Areas 1 to 4. In a different system, five hippocampal fields are designated H1 to H5.

The embryonic development of the hippocampus and dentate gyrus has already been illustrated in Figures 15-6, 16-7B, C, 16-17, 18-3, 20-10, 21-15, and 23-22.

Fig. 25-5. Development of the hippocampal formation.
(**A**) and (**B**) During trimester 1. The embryonic development is characterized mainly by cellular production and migration (Table 25-2). The rostral, middle, and occipital regions are alike before the appearance of the corpus callosum. Here the occipital (retrocommissural) part is represented.
(**A**) A horizontal section at 49 mm ($9\frac{1}{2}$ weeks), at the level of the insula. The rectangle indicates the portion (at 44 mm) shown in A'.
(**A'**) A structure resembling cortex represents the future pyramidal layer of the hippocampus. The marginal layer of the dentate area is very broad.
(**B**) A horizontal section at 85 mm (12 weeks). The pyramidal layer (hippocampal plate) is continuous with the dentate primordium and with the cortical plate. The rectangle indicates the portion (at 56 mm) shown in B'.
(**B'**) A stream of migrating cells leads from the ventricular layer to the dentate primordium. The hippocampal sulcus is evident. The **C**urved, **C**ellular **A**reas, CA 1–3, are marked. The fimbria has appeared and is well delineated near the dentate area.
A and B are modified from drawings, and A' and B' are based on photomicrographs, in Humphrey (1965).

Fig. 25-5.

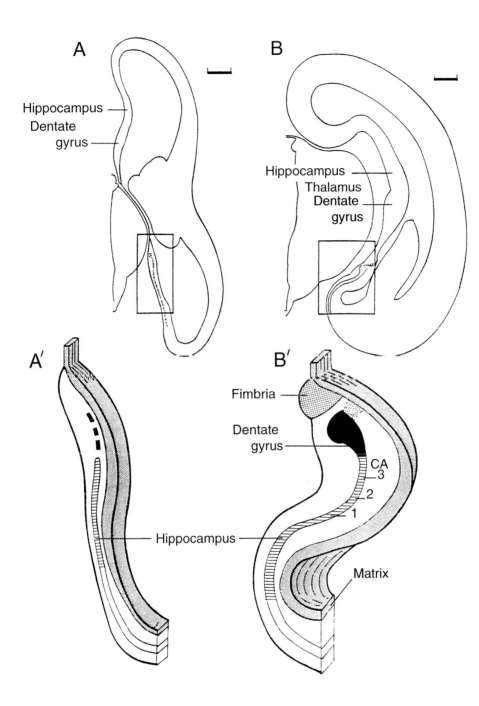

Fig. 25-5, continued.   Development of the hippocampal formation.

(**C**) and (**D**) Development of the hippocampal formation during trimester 2. Cellular production and migration continue. As the corpus callosum develops, the more rostral parts of the hippocampal primordium regress. The formation, which became curved and multilayered in trimester 1, becomes S-shaped and then rolled during trimester 2.

(**C**) A coronal section at 150 mm (17 weeks). The width of the pyramidal layer in CA1 narrows progressively from the subiculum towards CA2 to CA4. Its cells are small and immature. Three layers can be identified already in the dentate gyrus. The dentate area presents a wide marginal layer, the subiculum is double-layered, and the entorhinal cortex is bipartite.

(**D**) At 203 mm (21 weeks). The pyramidal layer is still populated with mostly immature neurons, as is also the dentate gyrus. Fibers connecting the entorhinal cortex, hippocampus, and subiculum are present by about 19 weeks, and connections between other subdivisions of the hippocampal formation may be established about one week later. Connections with the neocortex, however, are still only beginning at 22 weeks (Hevner and Kinney, 1996).

(**E**) Summary of the change in shape from 9 weeks to curved and multilayered at 10 weeks, S-shaped at 17 weeks, and infolded at 21 weeks.

(**F**) The hippocampal formation of the adult. C and D are drawn from photomicrographs in Arnold and Trojanowski (1996).

Stippling, fimbria. Black, dentate gyrus. Horizontal hatching, hippocampus. The subiculum and the parahippocampal gyrus are left white.

398

Fig. 25-5.

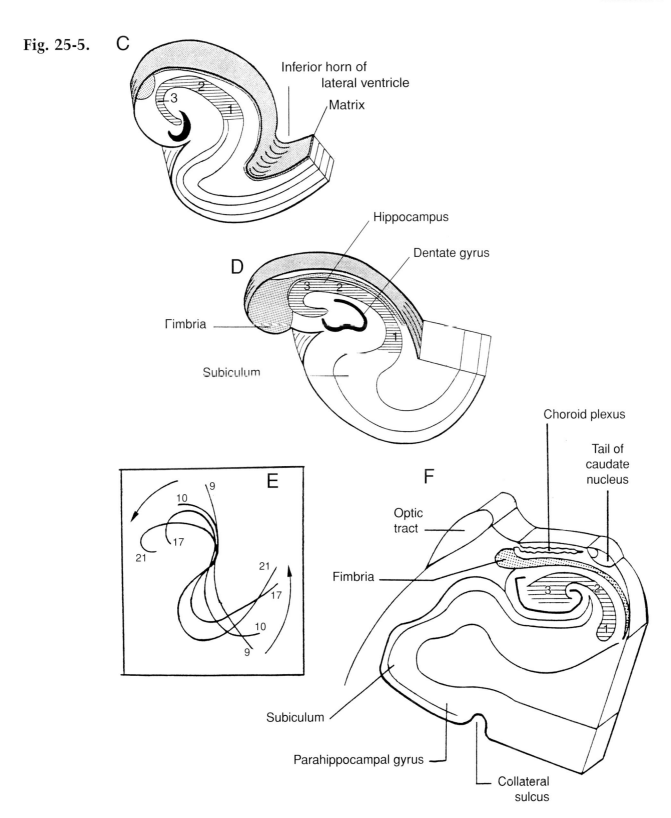

C

Inferior horn of lateral ventricle

Matrix

Hippocampus

Dentate gyrus

D

Fimbria

Subiculum

E

Choroid plexus

Tail of caudate nucleus

Optic tract

F

Fimbria

Subiculum

Parahippocampal gyrus

Collateral sulcus

Fig. 25-6. A comparison of basal views of the brain at (**A**) 31 mm (stage 23, CEC 9226, 8 weeks), (**B**) 68 mm (11 weeks), (**C**) ca 130 mm (ca. 15 weeks), (**D**) ca. 210 mm (22 weeks). The inferior views illustrate the development of some of the olfactory structures (olfactory bulb and tracts in white in A to C). Already at 8 weeks (A) the lateral olfactory tract (striae laterales or gyrus olfactorius lateralis), which had formed by stage 17, reaches the area of the amygdaloid nuclei (although mitral cells are not yet present in the olfactory bulb). A medial olfactory tract (striae mediales or gyrus olfactorius medialis) is shown in B and C. (Those fibers also are already present at stage 17.) The striae are sometimes termed gyri because they are covered by a small amount of gray matter. The lateral olfactory tract reaches the temporal lobe and is continued by the gyrus ambiens (C). The changing relationship of the olfactory structures can be studied further in views by Macchi (1951). The optic nerves, chiasma, and tracts in A to C are shown in black, as is also the trigeminal nerve.

View A is based on Müller and O'Rahilly (1990b), B is after Hochstetter (1919), C is after Kollmann's *Handatlas der Entwicklungsgeschichte des Menschen* and Corning's *Lehrbuch der Entwicklungsgeschichte des Menschen*, D is by courtesy of Marvin D. Nelson, M.D., Children's Hospital, Los Angeles.

Fig. 25-6.

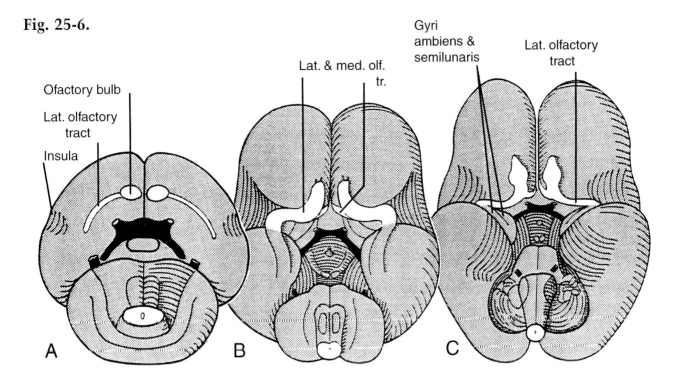

Ofactory bulb

Lat. olfactory tract

Insula

A

Lat. & med. olf. tr.

B

Gyri ambiens & semilunaris

Lat. olfactory tract

C

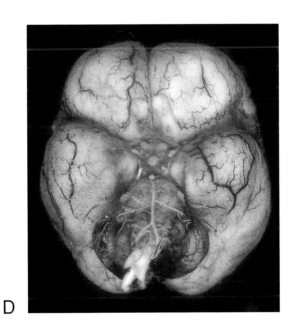

D

401

TABLE 25-2. Summary of Development of Hippocampal Formation

A. Embryonic Period

Fig.	Hippocampus	Dentate Area	Fibers
15-6	Hippocampal thickening on both sides of lamina terminalis		
16-7B,C	Hippocampal thickening extends from future frontal to future temporal pole.		
16-17	Thickening is accompanied by a cell-free marginal layer		
18-3	Hippocampal primordium has grown and reaches forebrain septum	Dentate area is a small rim intercalated between hippocampal thickening and area epithelialis.	
18-5	Rostral and temporal parts are alike		
20-10			Hippocamposeptal and pre-commissural fibers
21-15	Thin sheath of marginal cells appears opposite hippocampal thickening	Migrating cells form primordium of dentate area	
23-22	About 5 rows of scattered marginal cells		

B. Fetal Period

GL (mm)	Weeks	Hippocampus	Dentate Gyrus	Fibers
32	8		Migrating cells	Fimbria
44	9	Distinct pyramidal layer. CA 1–3 distinguishable	Patches of cells (Fig. 25-5A′)	Columns of fornix
49	$9\frac{1}{2}$	H1, H2, and H3 can be distinguished		
50–83	$9\frac{1}{2}$–12	Marginal cells in marginal layer		
56	10		Spherical cell mass (Fig. 25-5B′). Fimbriodentate sulcus	Hippocampal commissure
61	10		Polymorphic and granular layers	Alveus forming
65	$10\frac{1}{2}$	Marginal layer with Cajal–Retzius cells		
79–85	12		Granular layer more distinct and clearly separated from H3	Alveus complete
120	14	Involution complete; hippocampal matrix wider than subicular		
150	17	Fig. 25-5C		Formation of synapses mainly in marginal layer
200	21	Fig. 25-5D; ventricular layer seems to be exhausted		Connections in subdivisions of hippocampus by 20 weeks
≥300	32–45	Hippocampus has grown in volume; walls of hippocampal sulcus are fused; molecular layer still has some Cajal–Retzius cells		
Newborn		Hippocampal surface only one-third of adult area		

Sources: A: based on authors' research. B: based on data from various authors, including Humphrey (1965), Rakic and Yakovlev (1968), Kahle (1969), Bogolepova (1995), Hevner and Kinney (1996), and Bogolepova (1997).

Comments on Neuroteratology

Agenesis of the corpus callosum, a complete or partial lack of callosal fibers between the cerebral hemispheres, is discovered usually as an accidental finding. The anterior commissure may be enlarged, providing supplementary neocortical interconnections. It is assumed that the condition arises in the commissural plate, the callosal component of which may fail to develop or may not grow caudally. At least some instances may represent a failure of commissuration rather than an agenesis. Defects of the corpus callosum and the adjacent region are considered by some to be types of cerebral dysraphia.

Trimester 3 and the Newborn

Approximately 250–335 mm in Greatest Length
**Approximately 26 Postfertilizational
Weeks to Birth**

The sulci and gyri increase rapidly in number during trimester 3, although they are not quite as numerous as in the adult. Their sequential appearance is listed in Table 26-1 (p. 420).

The duration of prenatal life is generally about 38 postfertilizational weeks, the mean being 264 days. The range 35 to 40 postfertilizational weeks is considered to indicate an infant at "term." Commonly used figures at birth are about 335 mm for the greatest length (exclusive of the lower limbs) and about 500 mm for the crown–heel length. The biparietal diameter is approximately 95 mm and the head circumference is of the order of 350 mm. The body weight at birth varies from 2500 to 4000 g or more, with an average of about 3350 g. The brain weight, which also varies considerably, ranges from about 300 to 400 g at birth and continues to increase rapidly up to the fourth year, more slowly up to the twelfth year.

A useful general summary of the central nervous system in the newborn has been provided by Robinson and Tizard (1965). An important account of the brain stem of two newborns was published by Sabin (1900, cf. Fig. 26-6B). It contains precise drawings of two series of sections: 22 coronal and 27 transverse. See also Sabin (1901, 1902). Photomicrographs and drawings of the motor cortex of a newborn have been published by Marín-Padilla and Marín-Padilla (1982) and by Marín-Padilla (1992).

Fig. 26-1. Medial view of the right half of a brain at about 28 postfertilizational weeks. The corpus callosum, which has become elongated and curved, shows the rostrum, genu, trunk, and splenium. The maximum splenial thickness at about this time has been found to be greater in female fetuses in one study (de Lacoste et al., 1986) but not in another (Clark et al., 1989). The asterisk indicates the parieto-occipital sulcus. Bar: 10 mm. From Kier and Truwit (1996). Courtesty of E. Leon Kier, M.D., Yale University School of Medicine.

Precision

It is incorrect to refer to the trunk of the corpus callosum as its body, because the entire structure is a body, Latin *corpus.* Moreover, the central part of the lateral ventricle is not a body because all parts of the ventricle are cavities.

Fig. 26-1.

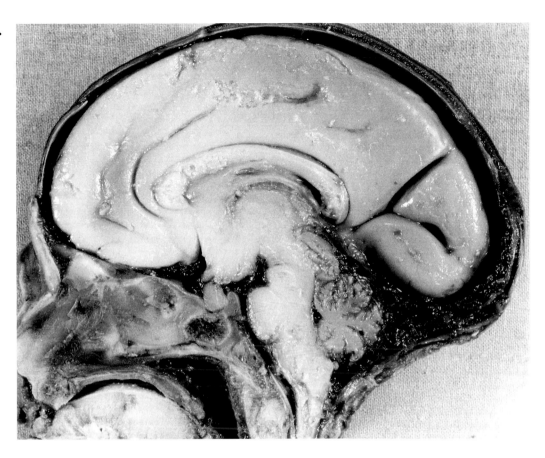

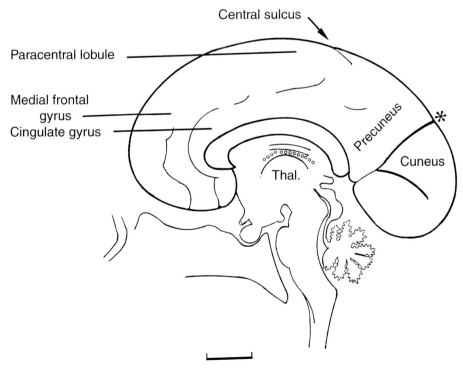

Fig. 26-2. A comparison of the medial surface of the forebrain at (**A**) 80, (**B**) 95, (**C**) 150, and (**D**) approximately 265 mm. The left thalamus has been sectioned sagittally (horizontal lines). In A, B, and C the entire brain stem has been removed, whereas in D it has been sectioned transversely at the level of the midbrain and its caudal portion has been eliminated. The considerable increase in length of the corpus callosum (shown in black) after 100 mm can readily be appreciated by comparing B and C. In D the corpus callosum shows clearly the rostrum, genu, central part, and splenium. The commissural plate beneath the corpus callosum becomes attenuated (C) to form the septum pellucidum. The cavum septi pellucidi, which may perhaps develop by necrosis within the commissural plate, becomes obliterated posteriorly before birth and anteriorly shortly after birth, but persists in about one fifth of adults as shown in a graph in Lemire et al. (1975, p. 264). The hippocampus is stippled. Modified from models in Keibel and Mall (1912).

The upper right-hand drawings show schematically the arrangement of the pia mater over the corpus callosum at 100 mm, 170 mm, and at birth. As the corpus callosum grows posteriorly, a pial layer (b) is reflected backwards over the original layer (a), so that a double fold is formed. This is the velum interpositum, between the two layers of which blood vessels can pass forward beneath the corpus callosum, through the transverse fissure (asterisk). These vessels contribute to the tela choroidea of the third ventricle.

Probably the most valuable treatise on the cerebral hemispheres during the fetal period is that by Kahle (1969), because, unlike more recent accounts, it is based on a series of careful graphic reconstructions. Studies of the fetal cerebral cortex, in continuity with those of Conel on the newborn, and on the postnatal cortex of 1 to 6 years, have been published by Rabinowicz (1986, for references). Useful photomicrographs, drawings, and measurements of neocortical areas during the fetal period have been published by Marín-Padilla (1970, 1988a, and 1992).

The subplate of the primary visual cortex disappears during the last prenatal weeks, whereas that of the prefrontal cortex persists as long as 6 months after birth (Kostović and Rakic, 1990). The changes include relocation of fibers in the cortical plate, incorporation of subplate neurons in the gyral white matter, and cell death. Postnatally, cortico-cortical and association fibers continue to grow, and overproduction of dendritic spines as well as excessive synaptogenesis have been recorded.

408

Fig. 26-2.

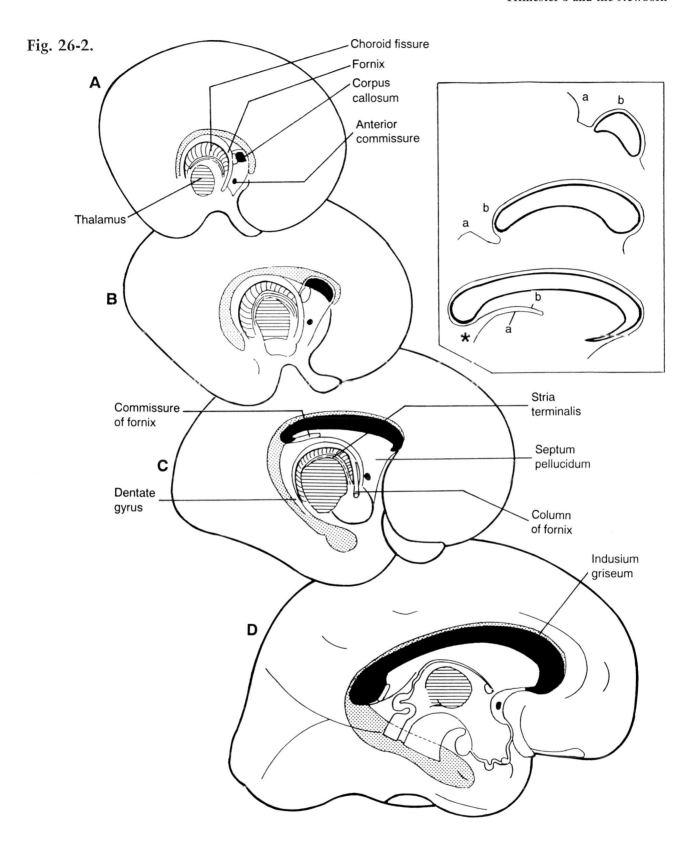

Fig. 26-3. (**A**) Lateral view and (**B**) medial view of the brain around the time of birth, at 335 mm GL, 490 mm CH, biparietal diameter 94 mm, occipitofrontal diameter 108 mm, head circumference 355 mm, body weight 3,340 g, and fresh brain weight 403 g. The pattern of sulci and gyri is essentially similar to that of the adult. The names given here apply to the gyri. Arrows indicate the central and parieto-occipital sulci. Abbreviations: F1, 2, 3, superior, middle, and inferior frontal gyri, T1, 2, 3, superior, middle, and inferior temporal gyri; a., angular gyrus; s., supramarginal gyrus. Based on photographs in Feess-Higgins and Larroche (1987).

Fig. 26-3.

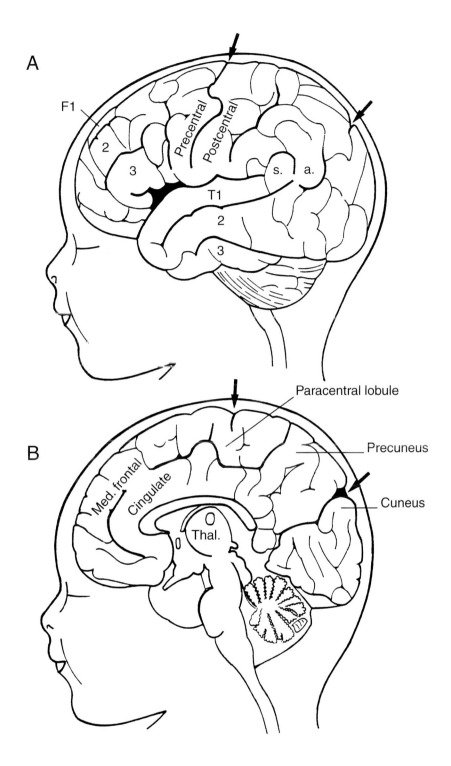

A

F1

2

3

Precentral

Postcentral

s.   a.

T1

2

3

B

Med. frontal

Cingulate

Thal.

Paracentral lobule

Precuneus

Cuneus

Fig. 26-4. The brain around the time of birth: (**A**) superior view, (**B**) left lateral view, and (**C**) medial view. Courtesy of Marvin D. Nelson, M.D., and Floyd H. Gilles, M.D., Children's Hospital, Los Angeles.

Fig. 26-4.

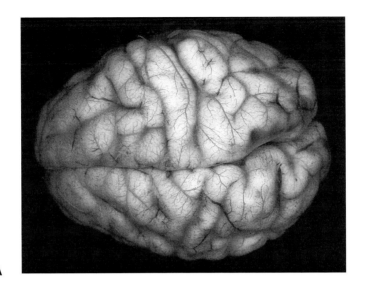

A

B

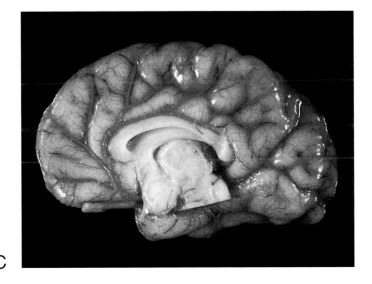

C

Figure 26-5. The histological differentiation of the cerebellum.

(**A**) The ventricular layer provides cells that migrate externally: piriform (Purkinje) cells (arrow) and cells for the deep nuclei. The external germinal layer, which began to form at the end of the embryonic period, continues to receive cells from the rhombic lip.

(**B**) Near the end of the fetal period, cells from the external germinal layer migrate internally (open arrow) and form the internal granular layer and basket cells.

(**C**) In the adult, one piriform (Purkinje) cell is shown with its dendrites and axon. The external germinal layer disappears after birth.

The ventricular and external germinal layers, as well as the deep nuclei, are stippled. Based on Jakob (1929).

Homeobox genes are believed to be involved in the initial development of the external germinal layer, and interaction with glial fibers is necessary for the internal cellular migration. Cell proliferation in the external germinal layer is the main cause of the increase in the cerebellar surface.

Piriform cells are generated at the beginning of the fetal period (Rakic and Sidman, 1970) and their characteristic shape is attained by the middle of prenatal life. Their maturation continues after birth (Zecevic and Rakic, 1976). Modified radial glial cells known as Bergmann cells are necessary for the migration of the piriform cells (Choi and Lapham, 1980).

Photomicrographs of the fetal cerebellum have been published by Rakic and Sidman (1970), Zecevic and Rakic (1976), and Choi and Lapham (1980).

Fig. 26-5.

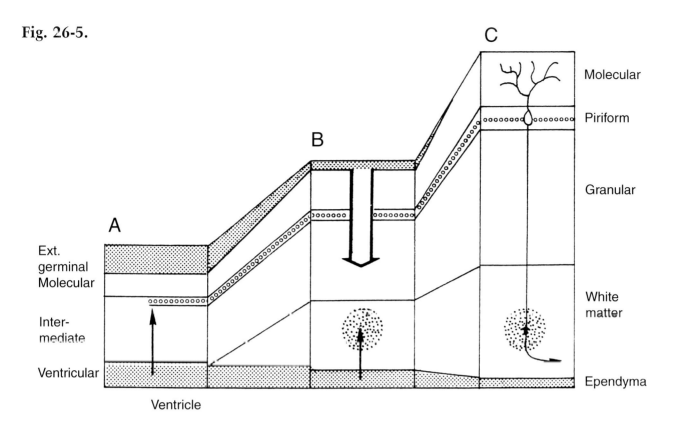

Fig. 26-6. Dorsal views of the rhombencephalon (**A**) at 8 postfertilizational weeks (stage 23: cf. Figs. 23-27 and 23-28), and (**B, C**) in two different reconstructions from the newborn. The arrangement of the nuclei and tracts, as well as the location of the rhombencephalic nuclei at 8 weeks, are very similar to those in the newborn. The striking resemblance between the rhombencephalon of the newborn and that of the embryo at 8 weeks is based on the circumstance that the fundamental organization of the rhombencephalon is attained much earlier than that of other parts of the brain. The sensory nuclei are shown by small open circles, the somatic efferent nuclei in bold stippling, and the visceral efferent nuclei are hatched. Figure 26-6B is based on a reconstruction by Sabin (1901). Figure 26-6C is after Hikji (1933). The neurons in the nucleus of the tractus solitarius are still immature at birth (Denawit-Saubié et al., 1994).

Fig. 26-6.

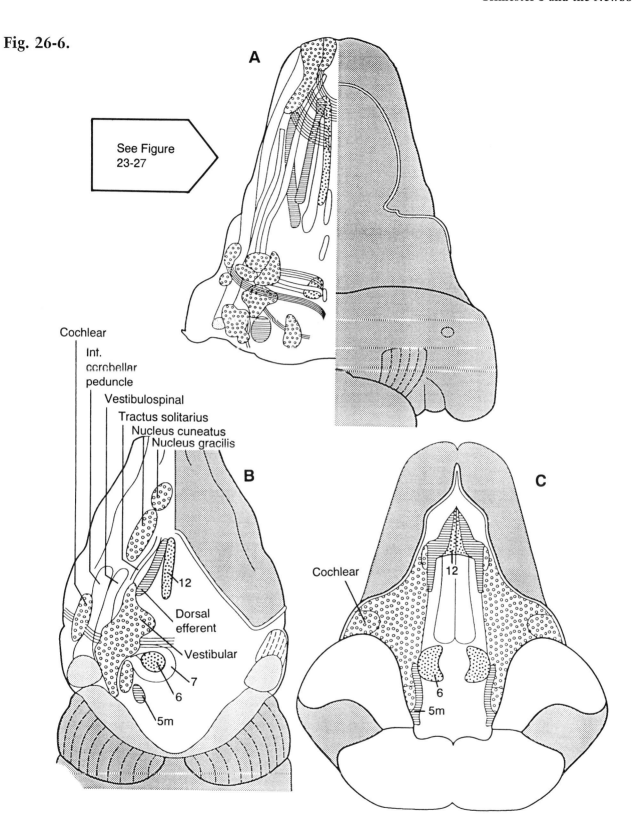

See Figure
23-27

A

Cochlear
Int.
cerebellar
peduncle
Vestibulospinal
Tractus solitarius
Nucleus cuneatus
Nucleus gracilis

B

12
Dorsal
efferent
Vestibular
7
6
5m

Cochlear

C

12
6
5m

Fig. 26-7. (**A**) and (**B**) The arterial system of the newborn. The internal carotid artery is shown in black, and the basilar by horizontal hatching. The choroid plexuses of the lateral and fourth ventricles are included. The vessels marked are the three cerebral arteries (A.C., M.C., P.C.), the posterior communicating (P. co.), the anterior choroidal (A. chor.), the superior cerebellar (Sup. cbl), and the anterior and posterior inferior cerebellar arteries (AICA, PICA). The asterisk indicates the hypophysis. The posterior communicating is relatively large prenatally and in the newborn. In the adult, however, the blood flow in the posterior cerebral (initially merely a collateral branch of the posterior communicating) has been transferred from the carotid to the basilar system. These drawings are based on graphic reconstructions made by Padget (1948), whose work should be studied for further details. The venous system has been illustrated by Padget (1957, Fig. 17).

Fig. 26-7.

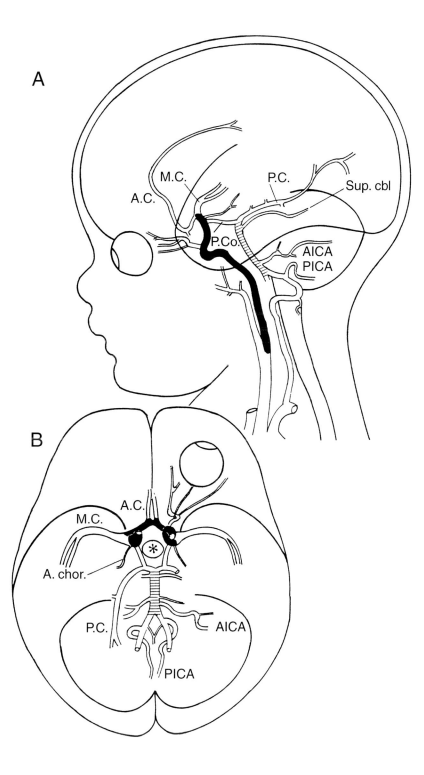

A

B

TABLE 26-1. Sequence of Appearance of Sulci and Gyri in the Cerebral Hemispheres

Post-fertilizational weeks	Sulci	Gyri
8–13	Longitudinal & transverse fissures Lateral & callosal sulci	
14–17	Parieto-occipital, cingulate, calcarine, circular, & olfactory	Cingulate & gyrus rectus
18–21	Central, collateral, & sup. temporal	Sup. temporal & parahippocampal
22–25	Precentral, postcentral, sup. frontal, inf. temporal, intraparietal, & lat. occipital	Precentral, postcentral, sup. & middle frontal, middle temporal, sup. & inf. parietal lobules, sup. & inf. occipital, cuneus, med. occipitotemporal, & lingual
26–29	Inf. frontal & occipitotemporal	Inf. temporal, pars triangularis of inf. frontal, supramarginal & angular, transverse temporal, med. & lat. orbital, & lat. occipitotemporal
30–33	Middle frontal & middle temporal	Paracentral lobule
34–37	Various secondary & tertiary sulci	Ant. & post. orbital

Source: Modified from Chi, Dooling, and Gilles (1977).

CHAPTER 27

Early Postnatal Life

A few examples of magnetic resonance imaging serve to illustrate the increasing degree of myelination. Postnatal myelination in the central nervous system has been studied extensively by Brody and Kinney and their colleagues (Brody et al., 1987; Kinney et al., 1988).

Figure 27-1

(**A**) A boy at 14 postnatal days, showing the myelin in the thalamic region, brain stem, and cerebellum.

(**B**) A girl at 20 postnatal days. The hypophysis, optic chiasma and tracts, and mamillary bodies (superimposed) are clearly visible, as are the corpus callosum, epiphysis, tectum, tentorium cerebelli, and fourth ventricle.

Fig. 27-1.

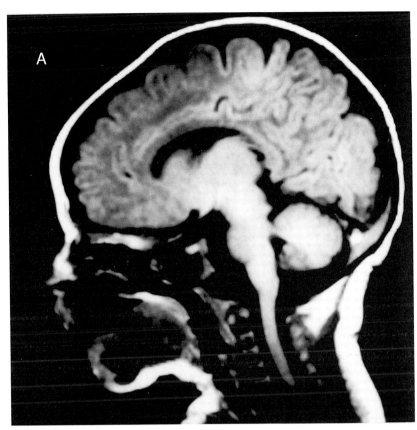

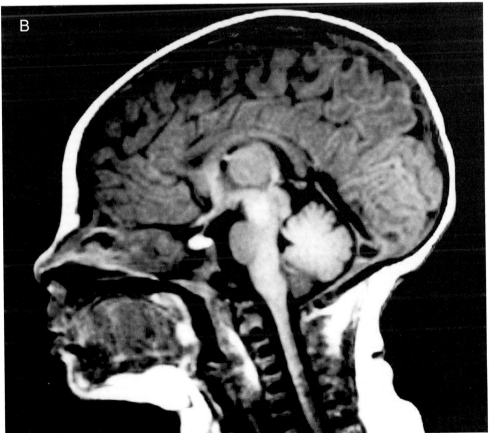

Figure 27-1. *continued.*

(C) At 3 years, most of the adult features are already clearly visible. Structures seen more readily in this image include the septum pellucidum, the aqueduct, and the spheno-occipital joint. In the cerebellum the fissura prima, the nodule, and the tonsil are distinguishable. (From O'Rahilly and Müller, 1996a.)

(D) A coronal view at 2 postnatal months, showing myelination bilaterally in the white matter of the cerebellum.

(E) At 4 years, showing the considerable advance in myelination, e.g., in the corona radiata, corpus callosum, fornices, thalami, colliculi, arbor vitae of the cerebellum, and cerebellar peduncles. The lateral, third, and fourth ventricles are distinguishable, as are also the tentorium cerebelli and the cerebellar folia.

A–E, courtesy of Marvin D. Nelson, M.D., Children's Hospital, Los Angeles.

Fig. 27-1.

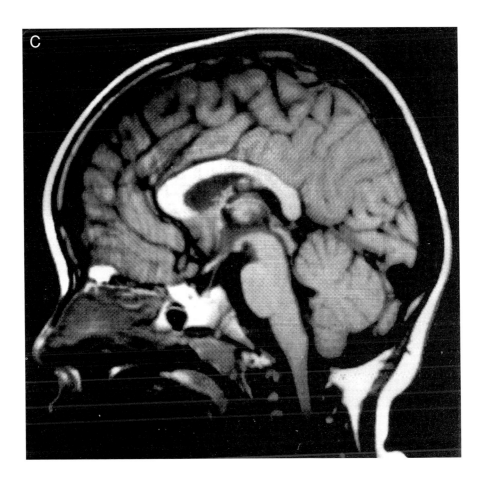

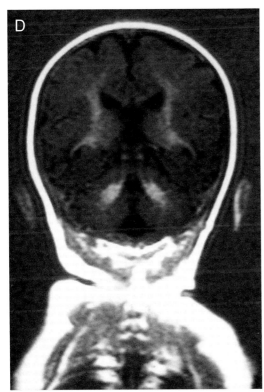

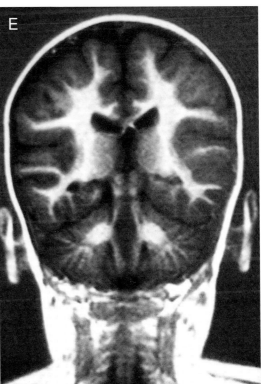

Bibliography

The references provided here are almost entirely limited to studies of normal *human* prenatal development. Only a few references to neuroteratological conditions are included.

Adelmann, H.B. 1966 *Marcello Malpighi and the Evolution of Embryology.* Cornell University Press, Ithaca, NY.

Alcolado, R., Weller, R.O., Parrish, E.P., and Garrod, D. 1988 The cranial arachnoid and pia mater in man. Neuropathol. Appl. Neurobiol., 14:1–17.

Alexandre, J.-H., and Pineau, H. 1970 Détermination de la taille assise et de l'âge des anencéphales. Arch. Anat. Cytol. Pathol., 18:265–270.

André-Thomas, and de Ajuriaguerra, A. 1959 Etude anatomo-clinique de l'anencéphalie. In G. Heuyer, M. Feld, and J. Gruner (eds.), *Malformations congénitales du cerveau.* Masson, Paris, pp. 207–267.

Andy, O.J., and Stephan, H. 1968 The septum in the human brain. J. Comp. Neurol., 133:383–409.

Ariëns Kappers, C.U. 1932 Principles of development of the nervous system (neurobiotaxis). In W. Penfield (ed.), *Cytology and Cellular Pathology of the Nervous System,* Vol. 1. Hoeber, New York, pp. 73–89.

Ariëns Kappers, J. 1955 The development of the paraphysis cerebri in man with comments on its relationship to the intercolumnar tubercle and its significance for the origin of cystic tumors in the third ventricle. J. Comp. Neurol., 102:425–509.

Ariëns Kappers, J. 1966 Strukturelle und funktionelle Änderungen im telencephalen Plexus chorioideus des Menschen während der Ontogenesese. Wiener Z. Nervenheilk. Grenzgeb., Suppl. 1:30–48.

Arnold, S.E., and Trojanowski, J.Q. 1996 Human fetal hippocampal development: I. Cytoarchitecture, myeloarchitecture, and neuronal morphologic features; II. The neuronal cytoskeleton. J. Comp. Neurol., 367:274–292, 293–307.

Augustine, J.R. 1996 Circuitry and functional aspects of the insular lobe in primates including humans. Brain Res. Rev., 22:229–244.

Barbé, A. 1938 *Recherches sur l'embryologie du système nerveux central de l'homme.* Masson, Paris.

Bartelmez, G.W. 1923 The subdivisions of the neural folds in man. J. Comp. Neurol. 35:231–295.

Bartelmez, G.W., and Dekaban, A.S. 1962 The early development of the human brain. Contrib. Embryol. Carnegie Inst., 37:13–32.

Bartelmez, G. W., and Evans, H.M. 1926 Development of the human embryo during the period of somite formation. Contrib. Embryol. Carnegie Inst., 17:1–67.

Blaas, H.-G., Eik-Nes, S.H., Berg, S., et al. 1998 In-vivo three-dimensional ultrasound reconstructions of embryos and early fetuses. Lancet, 352:1182–1186.

Blaas, H.-G., Eik-Nes, S.H., Kiserud, T., et al. 1995 Three-dimensional imaging of the brain cavities in human embryos. Ultrasound Obstet. Gynecol., 5:228–232.

Bogolepova, I.N. 1995 Ontogenesis of cytoarchitecture of human hippocampus. Acta Anat., 152: 260 (abstract).

Bogolepova, I.N. 1997 The limbic system as a model of cytoarchitectonical changes in the developing brain. In S. U. Dani, A. Hori, and G. F. Walter (eds.), Principles of Neural Aging, Elsevier, Amsterdam.

Borkowski, W.J., and Bernstine, R.L. 1955 Electroencephalography of the fetus. Neurology (N.Y.), 5:362–365.

Bossy, J. 1966 Diverticule télencéphalique de la région du neuropore antérieur chez un embryon humain de 35 mm V.C. Bull. Assoc. Anat. (Nancy), 50:200–210.

Bossy, J. 1980 Development of olfactory and related structures in staged human embryos. Anat. Embryol., 161:225–236.

Bossy, J., Godlewski, G., and Maurel, J.C. 1976 Etude de l'asymétrie droite–gauche du planum temporale chez le foetus humain. Bull. Assoc. Anat. (Nancy), 60/169:253–258.

Brana, C., Charron, G., Aubert, D., et al. 1995 Ontogeny of the striatal neurons expressing neuropeptide genes in the human fetus and neonate. J. Comp. Neurol., 360:488–505.

Brana, C., Caille, I., Pellevoisin, C., et al. 1996 Ontogeny of the striatal neurons expressing the D1 dopamine receptor in human. J. Comp. Neurol., 370:23–34.

Brocklehurst, G. 1969 The development of the human cerebrospinal fluid pathway with particular reference to the roof of the fourth ventricle. J. Anat., 105:467–475.

Brody, B.A., Kinney, H.C., Kloman, A.S., and Gilles, F.H. 1987 Sequence of central nervous system myelination in human infancy: I. An autopsy study of myelination. J. Neuropathol. Exp. Neurol., 46:283–301.

Brown, J.W. 1990 Prenatal development of the human nucleus ambiguus during the embryonic and early fetal periods. Am. J. Anat., 189:267–283.

Brun, A. 1965 The subpial granular layer of the foetal cerebral cortex in man. Its ontogenesis and significance in congenital cortical malformations. Acta Pathol. Microbiol. Scand., Suppl. 179, 13:1–98.

Butler, H., and Juurlink, B.H.J. 1987 An Atlas for Staging Mammalian and Chick Embryos. CRC Press, Boca Raton, FL.

Chi, J.G., Dooling, E.C., Gilles, F.H. 1977 Gyral development of the human brain. Ann. Neurol., 1:86–93.

Choi, B.H. 1987 Cortical dysplasia associated with massive ectopia of neurons and glial cells within the subarachnoid space. Acta Neuropathol., 73:105–109.

Choi, B.H., 1988 Developmental events during the early stages of cerebral cortical neurogenesis in man. Acta Neuropathol., 75:441–447.

Choi, B.H. 1994 Role of the basement membrane in neurogenesis and repair of injury in the central nervous system. Microsc. Res. Tech., 28:193–203.

Choi, B.H., and Lapham, W. 1980 Evolution of Bergmann glia in developing human fetal cerebellum: A Golgi electron microscopic and immuno-fluorescent study. Brain Res., 190:369–383.

Clark, S., Kraftsik, R., van der Loos, H., and Innocenti, G.M. 1989 Forms and measures of adult and developing human corpus callosum: is there sexual dimorphism? J. Comp. Neurol., 280:213–230.

Cleland, J. 1883 Contribution to the study of spina bifida, encephalocele, and anencephalus. J. Anat. Physiol., 17:257–292.

Conklin, J.L. 1968 The development of the human fetal adenohypophysis. Anat. Rec., 160:79–91.

Cooper, E.R.A. 1946a The development of the human red nucleus and corpus striatum. Brain, 69:34–44.

Cooper, E.R.A. 1946b Accessory optic tracts in the human fetus. Brain, 69:45–49.

Crawford, J.D., Cadera, W., and Vilis, T. 1991 Generation of torsional and vertical eye position signals by the interstitial nucleus of Cajal. Science, 252:1551–1553.

Crosby, C.E. Humphrey, T., and Lauer, E.W. 1962 *Correlative Anatomy of the Nervous System.* Macmillan, New York.

Crosby, R.W., and Cody, J. 1991 *Max Brödel, the Man Who Put Art into Medicine.* Springer, New York.

Danı, S.U., Hori, A., and Walter, G.F. (eds.) 1997 *Principles of Neural Aging.* Elsevier, Amsterdam.

Dart, R.A. 1924 The anterior end of the neural tube and the anterior end of the body. J. Anat., 58:181–205.

Day, R.W. 1959 Casts of foetal lateral ventricles. Brain, 82:109–115.

Dekaban, A.S. 1954 Human thalamus: II. Development of the human thalamic nuclei. J. Comp. Neurol, 100:63–97.

Dekaban, A.S. 1963 Anencephaly in early human embryos. J. Neuropathol. Exp. Neurol., 22:533–548.

Dekaban, A.S., and Bartelmez, G.W. 1964 Complete dysraphism in 14 somite human embryo. Am. J. Anat., 115:27–41.

DeMyer, W. 1975 Median facial malformations and their implications for brain malformations. Birth Defects, XI:155–181.

DeMyer, W. 1987 Holoprosencephaly (cyclopia-arhinencephaly). In P.J. Vinken, G.W. Bruyn, and H.L. Klawans (eds.), *Handbook of Clinical Neurology.* Vol. 6, Elsevier, Amsterdam. Revised Series, pp. 225–244.

Denawit-Saubié, M., Kalia, M., Pierrefiche, O., et al. 1994 Maturation of brain stem neurons involved in respiratory rhythmogenesis: Biochemical, bioelectrical and morphological properties. Biol. Neonate, 65:171–175.

Dorovini-Zis, K., and Dolman, C.L. 1977 Gestational development of brain. Arch. Pathol. Lab. Med., 101:192–195.

Dunn, H.L. 1921 The growth of the central nervous system in the human fetus. J. Comp. Neurol., 33:405–491.

Essick, C.R. 1912 The development of the nuclei pontis and the nucleus arcuatus in man. Am. J. Anat., 13:25–54.

Fabiani, F., and Bartonini, F. 1956 I primi stadi ontogenetici del talamo ottico umano. Rass. Studi Psichiat., 45:1184–1154.

Feess-Higgins, A., and Larroche, J.-C. 1987 *Le développement du cerveau foetal humain. Atlas anatomique.* INSERM-CNRS, Masson, Paris.

Fontes, V. 1944 *Morfologia do cortex cerebral (desenvolvimento).* Instituto de Antonio Aurélio da Costa Ferreira, Lisbon.

Fredericks, C.A., Giolli, R.A., Blanks, R.H.I., and Sadun, A.A. 1988 The human accessory optic system. Brain Res., 454:116–122.

429

Freed, C.R., Breeze, R.E., Rosenberg, N.L., et al. 1992 Survival of implanted fetal dopamine cells and neurologic improvement 12 to 46 months after transplantation for Parkinson's disease. New Engl. J. Med., 327:1549–1555.

Freeman et al. 1991, is already in first edition.

Freeman, T.B., Sanberg, P.R., and Isacson, O. 1995 Development of the human striatum. Implications for fetal striatal transplantation in the treatment of Huntington's disease. Cell Transplant., 4:539–545.

Freeman, T.B., Spence, M.S., Boss, B.D., et al. 1991 Development of dopaminergic neurons in the human substantia nigra. Exp. Neurol., 113:344–353.

Friant, M. n.d. *Anatomie comparée du cerveau.* Prisma, Paris.

Fujimoto, E., Miki, A., and Mizoguti, H. 1989. Histochemical study of the differentiation of microglial cells in the developing human cerebral hemispheres. J. Anat., 166:253–264.

Gadisseux, J.-F., Goffinet, A.M., Lyon, G., and Evrard, P. 1992 The human transient subpial granular layer: an optical, immunohistochemical, and ultrastructural analysis. J. Comp. Neurol., 324:94–114.

Gardner, E., O'Rahilly, R., and Prolo, D. 1975 The Dandy–Walker and Arnold–Chiari malformations. Arch. Neurol., 32:393–407.

Gasser, R.F. 1967 The development of the facial nerve in man. Ann. Otol., 76:37–56.

Gérard, M., Abitbol, A.-L. Delezoide, J.L., et al. 1995 PAX-genes expression during human embryonic development, a preliminary report. C.R. Acad. Sci., 318:57–66.

Geschwind, N.W., and Galaburda, A.M. 1985 Cerebral lateralization: biological mechanisms, associations, and pathology. Arch. Neurol., 42:428–459, 521–552, 634–654.

Gilbert, M.S. 1935 The early development of the human diencephalon. J. Comp. Neurol., 62:81–115.

Gilbert, P.W. 1957 The origin and development of the human extrinsic ocular muscles. Contrib. Embryol. Carnegie Inst., 34:59–78.

Gilles, F.H., Leviton, A., and Dooling, E.C. 1983 *The Developing Human Brain.* Wright-PSG, Boston.

Gilles, F.H., Nelson, M.D., and Gonzalez-Gomez, I. 1992 Human telencephalic angiogenesis: an update. In K. Fujisawa and Y. Morimatsu (eds.), *Development and Involution of Neurones.* Japan Science Society Press, Tokyo, pp. 31–41.

Hansen, P.E., Ballesteros, M.C., Soila, K., et al. 1993 MR imaging of the developing brain: Part 1. Prenatal development. RadioGraphics, 13:21–36.

Hayaran, A., Wadhwa, S., and Bijlani, V. 1992 Cytoarchitectural development of the human dentate nucleus: a Golgi study. Dev. Neurosci, 14:181–194.

Hevner, R.F., and Kinney, H.C. 1996 Reciprocal entorhinal–hippocampal connections established by human fetal midgestation. J. Comp. Neurol., 372:384–394.

Heuser, C.H., and Corner, G.W. 1957 Developmental horizons in human embryos. Description of age group X, 4 to 12 somites. Contrib. Embryol. Carnegie Inst., 36:29–39.

Hewitt, W. 1958 The development of the human caudate and amygdaloid nuclei. J. Anat., 92:377–382.

Hikij, K. 1933 Zur Anatomie des Bodens der Rautengrube beim Neugeborenen. Anat. Anz., 75:406–442.

Hines, M. 1922 Studies in the growth and differentiation of the telencephalon in man. The fissura hippocampi. J. Comp. Neurol., 34:73–171.

His, W. 1890 Die Entwickelung des menschlichen Rautenhirns vom Ende des ersten bis zum Beginn des dritten Monats: I. Verlängertes Mark. Abh. KS Gesellsch. Wissensch., 29:3–74.

His, W. 1895 Die anatomische Nomenclatur. Nomina anatomica. Arch. Anat. Physiol., Anat. Abth., Suppl., 1–183.

His, W. 1904 *Die Entwickelung des menschlichen Gehirns während der ersten Monate. Untersuchungsergebnisse.* Hirzel, Leipzig.

Hochstetter, F. 1913 Über die Entwickelung der Plexus chorioidei der Seitenkammern des menschlichen Gehirns. Anat. Anz., 45:225–238.

Hochstetter, F. 1919 *Beiträge zur Entwicklungsgeschichte des menschlichen Gehirns.* I. Teil. Deuticke, Vienna.

Hochstetter, F. 1923 *Beiträge zur Entwicklungsgeschichte des menschlichen Gehirns. II. Teil. 1. Lieferung. Die Entwicklung der Zirbeldrüse.* Deuticke, Vienna.

Hochstetter, F. 1929 *Beiträge zur Entwicklungsgeschichte des menschlichen Gehirns. II. Teil, 3. Lieferung. Die Entwicklung des Mittel- und Rautenhirns.* Deuticke, Vienna.

Hochstetter, F. 1934 Über die Entwicklung und Differenzierung der Hüllen des Rückenmarkes beim Menschem. Morphol. Jahrb., 74:1–104.

Hochstetter, F. 1939 Über die Entwicklung und Differenzierung der Hüllen des menschlichen Gehirnes. Morphol. Jahrb., 83:359–494.

Hochstetter, F. 1954 Über die Herstellung besonders instruktiver Lichtbilder der Körperoberfläche von Keimlingen. Ciba-Symposium, 2:52–57.

Hoving, E.W. 1993 Frontoethmoidal Encephaloceles. A Study of Their Pathogenesis. Doctoral dissertation, Rijksuniversiteit Groningen, The Netherlands. 175 pp.

Humphrey, T. 1965 The development of the human hippocampal formation correlated with some aspects of its phylogenetic history. In R. Hassler and H. Stephan (eds.), *Evolution of the Forebrain.* Thieme, Stuttgart.

Humphrey, T. 1968 The development of the human amygdala during early embryonic life. J. Comp. Neurol., 132:135–165.

Hunter, R.H. 1934 Extroversion of the cerebral hemispheres in a human embryo. J. Anat., 59:82–85.

Inke, G., and Palkovits, M. 1963 Die embryonale Entwicklung des Subcommissuralkomplexes (Subcommissuralorgan und seine Komponenten) beim Menschen. Anat. Anz., 113:240–254.

Jacobs, M.J. 1970 The development of the human motor trigeminal complex and accessory facial nucleus and their topographic relations with the facial and abducens nuclei. J. Comp. Neurol., 138:161–194.

Jakob, A. 1929 Das Kleinhirn. In W. von Möllendorff (ed.), *Handbuch der mikroskopischen Anatomie des Menschen,* Vol. 4 (1). Springer, Berlin. pp. 674–916.

Johnston, J.B. 1909 The morphology of the forebrain vesicle in vertebrates. J. Comp. Neurol., 19:457–539.

Kahle, W. 1956 Zur Entwicklung des menschlichen Zwischenhirns. Dtsch. Z. Nervenheilk., 175:259–318.

Kahle, W. 1969 Die Entwicklung der menschlichen Grosshirnhemisphäre. Schriftenr. Neurol., 1:1–116.

Kehrli, P., Maillot, C., and Wolff Quenot, M.J. 1995 Les gaines des nerfs crâniens dans la paroi latérale de la loge parasellaire. Neurochirurgie, 41:403–412.

Keibel, F., and Mall, F.P. 1912 *Manual of Human Embryology,* Vol. 2. Lippincott, Philadelphia.

431

Kier, E.L. 1977 The cerebral ventricles: a phylogenetic and ontogenetic study. Radiology of the skull and brain. Anat. Pathol., 3:2787–2914.

Kier, E.L., and Truwit, C.L. 1996 The normal and abnormal genu of the corpus callosum: an evolutionary, embryologic, anatomic, and MR analysis. Am J. Neuroradiol., 17:1631–1641.

Kinney, H.C., Brody, B.A., Kloman, A.S., and Gilles, F.H. 1988 Sequence of central nervous system myelination in human infancy. J. Neuropathol. Exp. Neurol., 47:217–234.

Kostović, I. 1986 Prenatal development of nucleus basalis complex and related fiber systems in man: a histochemical study. Neuroscience, 17:1047–1077.

Kostović, I., and Rakic, P. 1990 Developmental history of the transient subplate zone in the visual and somatosensory cortex of the macaque monkey and human brain. J. Comp. Neurol., 297:441–470.

Kostović, I., Knežević, S., Wisnieswski, H.M., and Spilich, G.J. (eds.) 1992a Neurodevelopment, Aging and Cognition. Birkhäuser, Boston.

Kostović, I., Petanjek, Z., Delalle, I., and Judas, M. 1992 Developmental reorganization of the human association cortex during perinatal and postnatal life. In I. Kostović, S. Knežević, H.M. Wisniewski, and G. J. Spilich (eds.), Neurodevelopment, Aging and Cognition. Birkhäuser, Basel.

Kuhlenbeck, H. 1973 The Central Nervous System of Vertebrates. Overall Morphologic Pattern, Vol. 3, Part II. Karger, Basel, pp. 1–768.

Kuhlenbeck, H. 1977 The Central Nervous System of Vertebrates. Derivatives of the Prosencephalon: Diencephalon and Telencephalon. Vol. 5, Part I, Karger, Basel, pp. 461–888.

Kuhlenbeck, H. 1978 The Central Nervous System of Vertebrates. Mammalian Telencephalon, Vol. 5, Part II. Karger, Basel, pp. 1–478.

deLacoste, M.-C., Holloway, R.L., and Woodward, D.J. 1986 Sex differences in the fetal human corpus callosum. Hum. Neurobiol., 5:93–96.

Larroche, J.-C. 1981 The marginal layer in the neocortex of a 7-week-old human embryo. Anat. Embryol. (Berlin), 162:301–312.

Larroche, J.-C., and Houcine, O. 1982 Le néo-cortex chez l'embryon et le foetus humain. Apport du microscope électronique et du Golgi. Reprod. Nutr. Dev., 22:163–170.

Larroche, J-C., and Jardin, L. 1985 Cited by Marín-Padilla (1988a).

Larsell, O. 1947 The development of the cerebellum in man in relation to its comparative anatomy. J. Comp. Neurol., 87:85–129.

Lemire, R.J., Beckwith, J.P., and Warkany, J. 1978 Anencephaly. Raven Press, New York.

Lemire, R.J., Shepard, T.H., and Alvord, E.C. 1965 Caudal myeloschisis (lumbosacral spina bifida cystica) in a five millimeter (Horizon XIV) human embryo. Anat. Rec., 152:9–16.

Lemire, R.J., Loeser, J.D., Leech, R.W., and Alvord, E.C. 1975 Normal and Abnormal Development of the Human Nervous System. Harper & Row, Hagerstown, MD.

Letinič, K., and Kostović, I. 1997 Transient Fetal structure, the gangliothalamic body, connects telencephalic germinal zone with all thalamic regions in the developing human brain. J. Comp. Neurol., 384:373–395.

Macchi, G. 1951 The ontogenetic development of the olfactory telencephalon in man. J. Comp. Neurol., 95:245–305.

Marín-Padilla, M. 1970 Prenatal and early postnatal ontogenesis of the human motor cortex. A Golgi study: 1. The sequential development of the cortical layers. Brain Res., 23:167–183.

Marín-Padilla, M. 1978 Dual origin of the mammalian neocortex and evolution of the cortical plate. Anat. Embryol. (Berlin), 152:109–126.

Marín-Padilla, M. 1983 Structural organization of the human cerebral cortex prior to the appearance of the cortical plate. Anat. Embryol. (Berlin), 168:21–40.

Marín-Padilla, M. 1985 Early vascularization of the embryonic cerebral cortex: Golgi and electron microscopic studies. J. Comp. Neurol., 241: 237–249.

Marín-Padilla, M. 1988a Early ontogenesis of the human cerebral cortex. Cerebral Cortex, 7:1–34.

Marín-Padilla, M. 1988b Embryonic vascularization of the mammalian cerebral cortex. Cerebral Cortex, 7:479–509.

Marín-Padilla, M. 1991 Cephalic axial skeletal–neural dysraphic disorders: embryology and pathology. Can. J. Neurol. Sci., 18:153–169.

Marín-Padilla, M. 1992 Ontogenesis of the pyramidal cells of the mammalian neocortex and developmental cytoarchitectonics: a unifying theory. J. Comp. Neurol., 321:223–240.

Marín-Padilla, M. 1995 Prenatal development of fibrous (white matter), protoplasmic (gray matter), and layer I astrocytes in the human cerebral cortex. a Golgi study. J. Comp. Neurol., 357:554–572.

Marín-Padilla, M., and Marín-Padilla, M.T. 1982 Origin, prenatal development and structural organization of layer I of the human cerebral (motor) cortex. Anat. Embryol. (Berlin), 164:161–206.

Markowski, J. 1922 Entwicklung der Sinus durae matris und der Hirnvenen des Menschen. Bull. Int. Acad. Polon. Sci. Lett. (Suppl), pp. 1–269.

Marti, E., Gibson, S.J., Polak, J.M., et al. 1987 Ontogeny of peptide- and amine-containing neurones in motor, sensory and autonomic regions of rat and human spinal cord, dorsal root ganglia and rat skin. J. Comp. Neurol., 266:332–359.

McConnell, S.K., Ghosh, A., and Shatz, C.J. 1989 Subplate neurons pioneer the first axon pathway from the cerebral cortex. Science, 245:978–982.

Molliver, M.E., Kostović, I., and van der Loos, H. 1973 The development of synapses in cerebral cortex of the human fetus. Brain Res., 50:403–407.

Mrzijak, L., Uylings, H.B.M., Kostović, I., van Eden, C.G. 1988 Prenatal development of neurons in the human prefrontal cortex: I. A qualitative study. J. Comp. Neurol., 271:355–386.

Müller, F., and O'Rahilly, R. 1980 The human chondrocranium at the end of the embryonic period proper, with particular reference to the nervous system. Am. J. Anat., 159:33–58.

Müller, F., and O'Rahilly, R. 1983 The first appearance of the major divisions of the human brain at stage 9. Anat. Embryol., 168:419–432.

Müller, F., and O'Rahilly, R. 1984 Cerebral dysraphia (future anencephaly) in a human twin embryo at stage 13. Teratology, 30:167–177.

Müller, F., and O'Rahilly, R. 1985 The first appearance of the neural tube and optic primordium in the human embryo at stage 10. Anat. Embryol., 172:157–169.

Müller, F., and O'Rahilly, R. 1986a The development of the human brain and the closure of the rostral neuropore at stage 11. Anat. Embryol. (Berlin), 175:205–222.

Müller, F., and O'Rahilly, R. 1986b Somitic–vertebral correlation and vertebral levels in the human embryo. Am. J. Anat., 177:1–19.

433

Müller, F., and O'Rahilly, R. 1987 The development of the human brain, the closure of the caudal neuropore, and the beginning of secondary neurulation at stage 12. Anat. Embryol., 176:413–430.

Müller, F., and O'Rahilly, R. 1988a The development of the human brain from a closed neural tube at stage 13. Anat. Embryol., 177:203–224.

Müller, F., and O'Rahilly, R. 1988b The first appearance of the future cerebral hemispheres in the human embryo at stage 14. Anat. Embryol., 177:495–511.

Müller, F., and O'Rahilly, R. 1988c The development of the brain, including the longitudinal zoning in the diencephalon at stage 15. Anat. Embryol. (Berlin), 179:55–71.

Müller, F., and O'Rahilly, R. 1989a The human brain at stage 16, including the initial evagination of the neurohypophysis. Anat. Embryol. (Berlin), 179:551–569.

Müller, F., and O'Rahilly, R. 1989b The human brain at stage 17, including the appearance of the future olfactory bulb and the first amygdaloid nuclei. Anat. Embryol. (Berlin), 179:353–369.

Müller, F., and O'Rahilly, R. 1989c Mediobasal prosencephalic defect, including holoprosencephaly and cyclopia, in relation to the development of the human forebrain. Am. J. Anat., 185:391–414.

Müller, F., and O'Rahilly, R. 1990a The human brain at stages 18–20, including the choroid plexuses and the amygdaloid and septal nuclei. Anat. Embryol., 182:285–306.

Müller, F., and O'Rahilly, R. 1990b The human brain at stages 21–23, with particular reference to the cerebral cortical plate and to the development of the cerebellum. Anat. Embryol., 182:375–400.

Müller, F., and O'Rahilly, R. 1990c The human rhombencephalon at the end of the embryonic period proper. Am. J. Anat., 189:127–145.

Müller, F., and O'Rahilly, R. 1991 Development of anencephaly and its variants. Am. J. Anat., 190:193–218.

Müller, F., and O'Rahilly, R. 1994 Occipitocervical segmentation in staged human embryos. J. Anat., 185:251–258.

Müller, F. and O'Rahilly, R. 1997a Development of the human central nervous system. In S.U. Dani, A. Hori, and G.F. Walter (eds.), *Principles of Neural Aging.* Elsevier, Amsterdam, pp. 175–191.

Müller, F., and O'Rahilly, R. 1997b The timing and sequence of appearance of neuromeres and their derivatives in staged human embryos. Acta Anat., 158:83–99.

Müller, F., O'Rahilly, R., and Tucker, J.A. 1981 The human larynx at the end of the embryonic period proper: I. The laryngeal and infrahyoid muscles and their innervation. Acta Otolaryngol. (Stockholm), 91:323–336.

Müller, F., O'Rahilly, R., and Tucker, J.A. 1985 The human larynx at the end of the embryonic period proper: 2. The laryngeal cavity and the innervation of its lining. Ann. Otol. Rhinol. Laryngol. (Stockholm), 94:607–617.

Nelson, M.D., Gonzalez-Gomez, I., and Gilles, F.H. 1991 The search for human telencephalic ventriculofugal arteries. Am. J. Neuroradiol., 12:215–222.

Okado, N. 1981 Onset of synapse formation in the human spinal cord. J. Comp. Neurol., 201:211–219.

O'Rahilly, R. 1965 The optic, vestibulocochlear, and terminal-vomeronasal neural crest in staged human embryos. In J.W. Rohen (ed.) *Second Symposium on Eye Structure.* Schattauer, Stuttgart, pp. 557–564.

O'Rahilly, R. 1966 The early development of the eye in staged human embryos. Contrib. Embryol. Carnegie Inst., 38:1–42.

O'Rahilly, R. 1968 The development of the epiphysis cerebri and the subcommissural complex in staged human embryos. Anat. Rec., 160:488–489.

O'Rahilly, R. 1975 The prenatal development of the human eye. Exp. Eye Res., 21:93–112.

O'Rahilly, R. 1983 The timing and sequence of events in the development of the human endocrine system during the embryonic period proper. Anat. Embryol., 166:439–451.

O'Rahilly, R. 1983 The timing and sequence of events in the development of the human eye and ear during the embryonic period proper. Anat. Embryol. (Berlin), 168:87–99.

O'Rahilly, R. 1988 One hundred years of human embryology. Issues Rev. Teratol., 4:81–128.

O'Rahilly, R. 1996 Making planes plain. Clin. Anat., 10:128–129.

O'Rahilly, R., and Gardner, E. 1979 The initial development of the brain. Acta Anat., 104:123–133.

O'Rahilly, R., and Müller, F. 1981 The first appearance of the human nervous system at stage 8. Anat. Embryol. (Berlin), 163:1 13.

O'Rahilly, R., and Müller, F. 1984a Embryonic length and cerebral landmarks in staged human embryos. Anat. Rec., 209.265–271.

O'Rahilly, R., and Müller, F. 1984b The early development of the hypoglossal nerve and occipital somites in staged human embryos. Am. J. Anat., 169:237–257.

O'Rahilly, R., and Müller, F. 1985 The origin of the ectodermal ring in staged human embryos of the first 5 weeks. Acta Anat., 122:145–157.

O'Rahilly, R., and Müller, F. 1986 The meninges in human development. J Neuropathol. Exp. Neurol., 45:588–608.

O'Rahilly, R., and Müller, F. 1987a *Developmental Stages in Human Embryos Including a Revision of Streeter's "Horizons" and a Survey of the Carnegie Collection.* Carnegie Institution of Washington, Washington, DC, Publication No. 637.

O'Rahilly, R., and Müller, F. 1987b The developmental anatomy and histology of the human central nervous system. In P.J. Vinken, G.W. Bruyin, and H.L. Klawans (eds.), *Handbook of Clinical Neurology.* Elsevier, Amsterdam.

O'Rahilly, R., and Müller, F. 1988 "Neuroschisis" in human embryos. Teratology, 38:189.

O'Rahilly, R., and Müller, F. 1989a Bidirectional closure of the rostral neuropore in the human embryo. Am. J. Anat., 184:259–268.

O'Rahilly, R., and Müller, F. 1989b Interpretation of some median anomalies as illustrated by cyclopia and symmelia. Teratology, 40:409–421.

O'Rahilly, R., and Müller, F. 1990 Ventricular system and choroid plexuses of the human brain during the embryonic period proper. Am. J. Anat., 189:285–302.

O'Rahilly, R., and Müller, F. 1994 Neurulation in the normal human embryo. In *Neural Tube Defects,* Ciba Foundation Symposium No. 181. Wiley, Chichester.

O'Rahilly, R., and Müller, F. 1996a The nervous system. In O'Rahilly and Müller (eds.), *Human Embryology and Teratology,* 2nd ed., Wiley-Liss, New York, pp. 361–416.

O'Rahilly, R., and Müller, F. 1996b Prenatal development of the brain. In I. Timor-Tritsch A. Monteagudo, and H.L. Cohen (eds.), *Ultrasonography of the Prenatal and Neonatal Brain.* Appleton & Lange, East Norwalk, CT, pp. 1–10.

O'Rahilly, R., and Müller, F. 1999 A summary of the initial development of the human nervous system. Teratol., in press.

O'Rahilly, R., Müller, F., and Bossy, J. 1986 Atlas des stades du développement des formes extérieures de l'encéphale chez l'embryon humain. Arch. Anat. Histol. Embryol., 69:3–39.

O'Rahilly, R., Müller, F., and Bossy, J. 1990 Atlas des stades du développement de l'encéphale chez l'embryon humain étudié par des reconstructions graphiques du plan médian. Arch. Anat. Histol. Embryol., 72:3–34.

O'Rahilly, R., Müller, F., Hutchins, G.M., and Moore, G.W. 1984 Computer ranking of the sequence of appearance of 100 features of the brain and related structures in staged human embryos during the first 5 weeks of development. Am. J. Anat., 171:243–257.

O'Rahilly, R., Müller, F., Hutchins. G.M., and Moore, G.W. 1987 Computer ranking of the sequence of appearance of 73 features of the brain and related structures in staged human embryos during the sixth week of development. Am. J. Anat., 180:69–86.

O'Rahilly, R., Müller, F., Hutchins, G.M., and Moore, G.W. 1988 Computer ranking of the sequence of appearance of 40 features of the brain and related structures in staged human embryos during the seventh week of development. Am. J. Anat., 182:295–317.

O'Rahilly, R., Müller, F., and Meyer, D.B. 1980 The human vertebral column at the end of the embryonic period proper: 1. The column as a whole. J. Anat., 131:565–575.

O'Rahilly, R., Müller, F., and Meyer, D.B. 1983 The human vertebral column at the end of the embryonic period proper: 2. The occipitocervical region. J. Anat., 136:181–195.

O'Rahilly, R., Müller, F., and Meyer, D.B. 1990a The human vertebral column at the end of the embryonic period proper: 3. The thoracicolumbar region. J. Anat., 168:81–93.

O'Rahilly, R., Müller, F., and Meyer, D.B. 1990b The human vertebral column at the end of the embryonic period proper: 4. The sacrococcygeal region. J. Anat., 168:95–111.

Orts Llorca, F. 1977 Morfogenesis de los tuberculos mamilares ("Corpora mamillaria"). Arch. Neurobiol. (Madrid), 40:139–164.

Padget, D.H. 1948 The development of the cranial arteries in the human embryo. Contrib. Embryol. Carnegie Inst., 32:205–261.

Padget, D.H. 1957 The development of the cranial venous system in man, from the viewpoint of comparative anatomy. Contrib. Embryol. Carnegie Inst., 36:79–140.

Padget, D.H. 1970 Neuroschisis and human embryonic maldevelopment. J. Neuropathol. Exp. Neurol., 29:192–216.

Pearson, A.A. 1941 The development of the nervus terminalis in man. J. Comp. Neurol., 75:39–66.

Pearson, A.A. 1946 The development of the motor nuclei of the facial nerve in man. J. Comp. Neurol., 85:461–476.

Peter, K., Wetzel, G., and Heiderich, F. 1938 *Handbuch der Anatomie des Kindes.* Bergmann, Munich.

Rabinowicz, T. 1986 The differentiated maturation of the cerebral cortex. In F. Falkner and J.M. Tanner (eds.), *Human Growth,* 2nd ed. Plenum, New York, pp. 385–410.

Rager, G. 1972 Die Entstehung der Insel (*Insula Reilii*) beim menschlichen Embryo. Z. Morphol. Anthropol., 64:245–278.

Raimondi, A.J., Sato, K., and Shimoji, T. 1984 *The Dandy–Walker Syndrome.* Karger, Basel.

Rakic, P. 1965 Mesocoelic recess in the human brain. Neurology, 15: 708–715.

Rakic, P. 1974 Embryonic development of the pulvinar-LP complex in man. In I.S. Cooper, M. Riklan, and P. Rakic (eds.), *The Pulvinar-LP Complex.* Thomas, Springfield, IL, pp. 3–35.

Rakic, P. 1984 Organizing principles for development of primate cerebral cortex. In S.C. Sharma (ed.), *Organizing Principles of Neural Development.* Plenum, New York, pp. 21–48.

Rakic, P. 1991 Development of the Primate cerebral cortex. In M. Lewis (ed.), *Child and Adolescent Psychiatry.* Williams & Wilkins, Baltimore, pp. 11–28.

Rakic, P., and Sidman, R.L. 1969 Telencephalic origin of pulvinar neurons in the fetal human brain. Z. Anat. Entwicke., 129:53–82.

Rakic, P., and Sidman, R.L. 1970 Histogenesis of cortical layers in human cerebellum, particularly the lamina dissecans. J. Comp. Neurol., 139: 473–500.

Rakic, P., and Yakovlev, P.I. 1968 Development of the corpus callosum and cavum septi in man. J. Comp. Neurol., 132:45–72.

Retzius, G. 1896 *Das Menschenhirn. Studien in der makroskopischen Morphologie,* 2 volumes. Norstedt, Stockholm.

Rhodes, R.H. 1979 A light microscopic study of the developing human neural retina. Am. J. Anat. 154:195–209.

Richter, E. 1965 Die Entwicklung des Globus pallidus und des Corpus subthalamicum. Monogr. Gesamtgeb. Neurol. Psychiat, (Berlin), 108:1–132.

Robinson, R.J., and Tizard, J.P.M. 1965 The central nervous system in the new-born. Br. Med. Bull., 22:49–55.

Ruano Gil, D. 1965 Grave malformacion encefalica (encefalosquisis) en un embrion humano da 10.25 mm con un humano gemelo normal. An. Desarrollo, 13:149–160.

Sabin, F.R. 1900 A model of the medulla oblongata, pons and midbrain of a newborn babe. Johns Hopkins Hosp. Rep., 9:925–1023.

Sabin, F.R. 1901 *An Atlas of the Medulla and Midbrain.* Friedenwald, Baltimore.

Sabin, F.R. 1902 A note concerning the model of the medulla, pons and midbrain of a new-born babe as reproduced by F. Ziegler. Anat. Anz., 22:281–289.

Schachenmayr, W., and Friede, R.I. 1978 The origin of subdural neomembranes: I. Fine structure of the dura–arachnoid interface in man. Am. J. Pathol., 92:53–68.

Sensenig, E.C. 1951 The early development of the meninges of the spinal cord in human embryos. Contrib. Embryol. Carnegie Inst., 34:45–157.

Sharp, J.A. 1959 The junctional region of cerebral hemisphere and third ventricle in mammalian embryos. J. Anat., 93: 159–168.

Shiota, K. 1991 Development and intrauterine fate of normal and abnormal human conceptuses. Congenital Anomalies, 31:67–80.

Shuangshoti, S., and Netsky, M.G. 1966 Histogenesis of choroid plexus in man. Am. J. Anat., 118:283–315.

437

Sidman, R.L., and Rakic, P. 1982 Development of the human central nervous system. In W. Haymaker and R.E. Adams (eds.), *Histology and Histopathology of the Nervous System*. Thomas, Springfield, IL, pp. 3–145.

Siebert, J.R., Cohen, M.M., Sulik, K.K., Shaw, C.-M., and Lemire, R.J. 1990 *Holoprosencephaly. An Overview and Atlas of Cases*. Wiley-Liss, New York.

Smith, T.D., Siegel, M.I., Mooney, M.P., et al. 1997 Prenatal growth of the human vomeronasal organ. Anat. Rec., 248:447–455.

Streeter, G.L. 1912 The development of the nervous system. In F. Keibel and F.P. Mall (eds.), *Manual of Human Embryology*, Vol. 2. Lippincott, Philadelphia, pp. 1–156.

Streeter, G.L. 1915 The development of the venous sinuses of the dura mater in the human embryo. Am. J. Anat., 18:145–178.

Streeter, G.L. 1918 The developmental alterations in the vascular system of the brain of the human embryo. Contrib. Embryol. Carnegie Inst., 8:5–38.

Streeter, G.L. 1919 Factors involved in the formation of the filum terminale. Am. J. Anat., 25:1–11.

Streeter, G.L. 1927 Archetypes and symbolism. Science, 65:405–412.

Tanimura, T., Nelson, T., Hollingworth, R.R., and Shepard, T.H. 1971 Weight standards for organs from early fetuses. Anat. Rec., 171:227–236.

Tiedemann, F. 1816 *Anatomie und Bildungsgeschichte des Gehirns im Foetus des Menschen*. Steinische Buchhandlung, Nürnberg.

Tiedemann, F. 1823 *Anatomie du cerveau, contenant l'histoire de son développement dans le foetus*. Baillière, Paris.

Toledano, A. 1992 Evolution of cholinergic cortical innervation after nbM lesioning (an experimental Alzheimer model). In I. Kostović, S. Knežević, H.M. Wisniewski, and G.J. Spilich (eds.), *Neurodevelopment, Aging and Cognition*. Birkhäuser, Basel.

Turkewitsch, N. 1933 Die Entwicklung der Zirbeldrüse beim Menschen. Morphol. Jahrb., 72:379–345.

Turkewitsch, N. 1935 Die Entwicklung des Aquaeductus cerebri des Menschen. Morphol. Jahrb., 76:421–447.

Velasco-Villamar, I. 1967 Sobre la organización del allocortex diagonalis. An. Anat. (Zaragoza), 16:109–179.

Verney, C., Zecevic, N., Nikolic, B., et al. 1991 Early evidence of catecholaminergic cell groups in 5- and 6-week-old human embryos using tyrosine hydroxylase and dopamine-β-hydroxylase immunocytochemistry. Neurosci. Lett., 131:121–124.

Verney, C., Milosevic, A., Alvarez, C., and Berger, B. 1993 Immunocytochemical evidence of well-developed dopaminergic and noradrenergic innervations in the frontal cerebral cortex of human fetuses at midgestation. J. Comp. Neurol., 336:331–344.

de Vries, D.J.I.P. 1992 The first trimester. In J.G. Nijhuis (ed.), *Fetal Behaviour*. Oxford University Press, Oxford, pp. 19–50.

Westergaard, E. 1971 The lateral cerebral ventricles of human foetuses with a crown–rump length of 26–178 mm. Acta Anat., 79:409–421.

Wilson, J.T. 1937 On the nature and mode of origin of the foramen of Magendie. J. Anat., 71:423–436.

Windle, W.F. 1970 Development of neural elements in human embryos of four to seven weeks gestation. Exp. Neurol. (Suppl. 5), 28:44–83.

Woźniak, W., and O'Rahilly, R. 1980 The times of appearance and the developmental sequence of the cranial parasympathetic ganglia in staged human embryos. Anat. Rec., 196:255A–256A.

Woźniak, W., and O'Rahilly, R. 1982 An electron microscopic study of myelination of pyramidal fibres at the level of the pyramidal decussation in the human fetus. J. Hirnforsch., 23:331–342.

Yamadori, T. 1965 Die Entwicklung der Thalamuskerne mit ihren ersten Fasersystemen bei menschlichen Embryonen. J. Hirnforsch., 7:393–413.

Zecevic, N., and Milosevic, A. 1997 Initial development of γ-aminobutyric acid immunoreactivity in the human cerebral cortex. J. Comp. Neurol., 380:495–506.

Zecevic, N., and Rakic, P. 1976 Differentiation of Purkinje cells and their relationship to other components of developing cerebellar cortex in man. J. Comp. Neurol., 167:27–48.

Zecevic, N., and Verney, C. 1995 Development of the catecholamine neurons in human embryos and fetuses, with special emphasis on the innervation of the cerebral cortex. J. Comp. Neurol., 351:509–535.

Computer Ranking of the Sequence of Appearance of Features of the Brain

Stage	7	8	9	10	11	12	13	14	15	Total
Total number	7	32	3	21	24	36	44	56	40	263
Good quality	7	21	3	12	18	22	20	36	26	165
Silver-treated	0	0	0	0	1	2	5	5	5	18
Greatest length (mm)	0.3–0.7	0.4–1.5	1.4 ± 0.5	2.1 ± 0.2	3.4 ± 0.2	3.6 ± 0.1	4.9 ± 0.1	6.6 ± 0.2	7.4 ± 0.3	
Age (weeks)	3		3½	4			4½		5	
1. Neural groove		5/19	+	+	+	+	+	+	+	
2. Otic disc/groove/pit		1/21	+	+	+	+	+	+	+	
3. Neural groove closes				9/12	+	+	+	+	+	
4. Optic sulcus				6/12	+	+	+	+	+	
5. Optic vesicle					16/18	+	+	+	+	
6. Entire notochord					5/18	17/17	+	+	+	
7. Rostral neuropore closes					4/18	+	+	+	+	
8. Otocyst						19/22	+	+	+	
9. Adenohypophysial pocket						18/21	+	+	+	
10. Ganglia of 5 and 7 are compact						15/19	+	+	+	
11. Rhombencephalic marginal layer						15/16	+	+	+	
12. Root of fourth ventricle is thin					1/18	16/19	+	+	+	
13. Caudal neuropore closes					0/17	13/22	+	+	+	
14. Hypoglossal roots appear						3/22	+	+	+	
15. Lens disc							+	+	+	
16. Intramedullary roots 5 and 7							13/13	35/35	+	
17. Intramedullary roots 9–11							12/12	34/34	+	
18. Nucleus of lateral longitudinal fasciculus							+	35/35	+	
19. Nucleus of 3							19/20	35/35	+	
20. Nucleus of 4							15/19	34/35	+	
21. Vestibular ganglion							12/19	33/35	25/25	
22. Endolymphatic appendage							11/20	33/35	+	
23. Ventral longitudinal fasciculus							7/12	32/35	+	
24. Lateral longitudinal fasciculus							4/4	4/4	22/22	
25. Terminal-vomeronasal crest							+	+	+	
26. Mesencephalic marginal layer							+	+	+	
27. Migration in alar plate of rhombomere 1							18/20	35/35	+	
28. Loose cells in chiasmatic plate							9/13	25/27	+	
29. Hypothalamic cell cord							9/20	+	+	
30. Fibers in vestibular ganglion							8/16	35/35	+	
31. Occipital dermatomes disappear							12/18	28/33	+	
32. Rhombencephalic ventral commissure							6/17	25/27	+	
33. Optic cup							5/20	34/36	+	
34. Spinal tract of 5							4/14	31/34	+	
35. Spinal tract of 7 and 8							3/13	30/34	+	
36. Medial longitudinal fasciculus							7/15	27/36	+	
37. Area of epiphysis cerebri							3/19	30/32	+	
38. Superior glossopharyngeal ganglion is compact							5/20	28/34	+	
39. Migration in marginal layer of retina							3/20	28/33	+	
40. Lamina terminalis is thin							1/20	30/35	25/25	
41. Perinotochordal mesenchyme is dense								31/36	+	
42. Loose cells in tectum mesencephali								29/34	25/25	
43. Cervical dorsal funiculus								27/33	+	
44. Hypoglossal roots are united								23/34	25/25	
45. Terminal-vomeronasal crest reaches telencephalon							5/17	20/35	24/26	
46. Dorsal funiculus reaches C 2								20/31	25/25	
47. Marginal layer in hippocampus							1/19	14/27	19/19	
48. Intra-isthmic root of 4								11/24	25/25	
49. Oculomotor fibers leave mesencephalon							1/20	16/33	25/25	

The period covered is from stage 8 (probably about 23 days) to stage 19 (6½ weeks). Based on 467 embryos. Corrected and modified from O'Rahilly, Müller, Hutchins, and Moore (1984, 1987, 1988). The ages are postfertilizational. Cranial nerves are indicated by Arabic numerals.

442

Stage	13	14	15	16	17	Total
Total number			40	56	44	140
Good quality			26	39	32	97
Silver-treated			5	3	5	13
Greatest length (mm)			7.4±0.3	9.3±1.5	12.6±1.2	
Age (weeks)			5	$5\frac{1}{2}$	6	
50. Amygdaloid part of basal nuclei		14/27	21/22	+		
51. Lens vesicle separated from surface ectoderm		13/36	+	+	+	
52. Fibers of 8 (vestibular) to otic vesicle		11/27	24/24	+	+	
53. Preoptico-hypothalamic tract		13/25	23/24	+	+	
54. 6 leaves rhombencephalon		10/34	24/25	+	+	
55. Common afferent tract	0/14	6/34	25/26	+	+	
56. Future cerebral hemispheres		11/28	25/26	+	+	
57. Habenular nucleus			24/25	37/37	+	
58. Future primordial plexiform layer in future cerebral hemispheres			23/24	+	+	
59. Dorsal roots of C N 1 and 2 contain nerve fibers	0/17	11/30	24/26	+	+	
60. Dorsolateral nucleus of 5		9/29	22/24	+	+	
61. Retinal pigment			20/23	+	+	
62. Utriculo-endolymphatic fold			21/25	I	+	
63. Ventral roots of C N 1 and 2 contain nerve fibers	1/15	14/34	21/26	+	+	
64. Decussation of mesencephalic root of 5			8/11	24/24	+	
65. Preoptic sulcus		12/16	6/12	17/17	I	
66. Decussation of 4		2/34	21/24	37/39	+	
67. Nasal pit		2/35	20/26	+	+	
68. Fibers in amygdaloid part of basal nuclei			11/15	35/35	+	
69. Nerve fibers in habenular nucleus			19/24	31/33	+	
70. Ventral thalamus and subthalamus are loose peripherally			10/18	36/36	+	
71. Trochlear fibers leave isthmus rhombencephali		0/34	9/13	35/37	+	
72. Zona limitans intrathalamica			7/12	17/17	+	
73. Mesencephalic root of 5			9/21	27/28	+	
74. Basilar artery		2/26	13/18	28/34	+	
75. Basement membranes (adenohypophysis and hypothalamus) are in contact	13/20	15/30	8/25	+	+	
76. Interpeduncular nucleus			11/16	25/31	24/25	
77. Decussation of superior colliculi		0/32	7/15	30/35	21/21	
78. Nucleus of mamillary body			16/24	28/36	+	
79. Dorsolateral nucleus of 9		3/23	9/26	29/35	+	
80. Rostral olfactory elevation			7/19	4/4	29/30	
81. Caudal olfactory elevation			0/16	34/34	30/30	
82. Cells of cochlear ganglion are different from those of vestibular ganglion		0/34	10/20	25/30	21/28	
83. Rostrolateral groove of vestibular pouch			3/9	14/21	+	
84. Hypothalamotegmental tract		2/34	4/13	12/22	26/27	
85. Supramamillary commissure			6/13	13/27	22/24	
86. Medial forebrain bundle			3/10	10/13	23/23	
87. Basal nuclei protrude into ventricle				36/37	+	
88. Caudolateral groove of vestibular pouch			2/9	21/25	+	
89. Crossed tectobulbar tract				29/31	28/28	
90. Sulcus limitans hippocampi			3/16	25/34	23/24	
91. Area epithelialis			6/20	22/33	26/27	
92. Ventrolateral and dorsolateral nuclei of 10				30/32	28/28	
93. Tractus solitarius separates from common afferent tract			4/24	24/37	+	
94. Hippocampal thickening			2/16	23/33	31/31	
95. Common afferent tract reaches more rostrally than entrance of 5				29/29	+	
96. Atrial fossa of otic vesicle			2/14	16/30	31/31	
97. Olfactory fibers enter telencephalon			3/16	17/32	+	

443

Stage	13	14	15	16	17	Total
Total number			40	56	44	140
Good quality			26	39	32	97
Silver-treated			5	3	5	13
Greatest length (mm)			7.4±0.3	9.3±1.5	12.6±1.2	
Age (weeks)			5	$5\frac{1}{2}$	6	
98. Mamillotegmental tract			11/23	13/31	28/31	
99. Dorsolateral nucleus of 7		0/24	4/26	22/36	28/28	
100. Fibers in alar plate of rhombomere 1			9/20	21/32	19/27	
101. Migrating cells in hippocampus				21/31	+	
102. Neurohypophysial evagination			2/23	16/37	30/31	
103. Mesenchyme between lens vesicle and surface ectoderm				14/35	32/32	
104. Hypothalamo-thalamic tract		3/23	4/12	2/8	8/12	
105. Posterior commissure			6/14	6/34	30/31	

Stage	15	16	17	18	19	Total
Total number	40	56	44	48	36	224
Good quality	26	39	32	35	23	155
Silver-treated	5	3	5	7	7	27
Greatest length (mm)	7.4±0.3	9.3±1.5	12.6±1.2	15±1.5	18.4±1.5	
Age (weeks)	5	$5\frac{1}{2}$	6		$6\frac{1}{2}$	
106. Cell islands in olfactory tubercle		13/31	28/31	35/35	23/23	
107. Mesenchymal skeleton in pharyngeal arch 2		7/37	29/31	35/35	23/23	
108. Blind nasal sac		4/39	31/32	35/35	23/23	
109. Primary lens fibers		5/35	27/31	35/35	23/23	
110. Crescentic lens cavity			29/31	35/35	23/23	
111. Fibers from olfactory field to amygdaloid body		5/10	9/23	35/35	23/23	
112. Habenulo-interpeduncular tract		4/16	14/24	35/35	23/23	
113. Intermediate layer in tectum mesencephali			22/31	35/35	23/23	
114. Cortical nucleus in amygdaloid body			22/31	35/35	23/23	
115. Definitive special visceral nucleus of 5			18/31	35/35	23/23	
116. Capillaries between adenohypophysis and hypothalamus			15/32	34/35	23/23	
117. Dorsal thalamus with intermediate layer			9/28	35/35	23/23	
118. Commissure of nerve 3			4/32	35/35	23/23	
119. Tractus solitarius separated			3/32	35/35	23/23	
120. Olfactory bulb and fibers from bulb to olfactory tubercle			3/25	25/26	23/23	
121. First signs of choroid plexus of lateral ventricle			2/32	34/35	23/23	
122. First signs of choroid plexus of fourth ventricle			2/32	31/35	23/23	
123. Follicles in epiphysis cerebri			3/32	25/31	20/21	
124. Adenohypophysis separated from pharynx		1/39	1/32	27/35	23/23	
125. Nerve fibers in retina			2/29	18/33	23/23	
126. Supraoptic commissure			2/32	15/32	22/23	
127. Vomeronasal ganglion				35/35	23/23	
128. Nucleus isthmi sends fibers to cerebellum				34/34	23/23	
129. Primordium of stapes surrounds stapedial a.				35/35	23/23	
130. Sensory nucleus of 5				32/32	23/23	
131. Internal cerebellar swelling				35/35	23/23	
132. Dentate nucleus				33/33	23/23	
133. Bucconasal membrane				34/35	23/23	
134. Medial ventricular elevation extends to preoptic sulcus				32/33	23/23	
135. Vomeronasal organ				33/35	23/23	
136. Mesenchymal nasal septum is condensed				33/35	23/23	
137. Nasolacrimal duct				33/35	23/23	
138. External cerebellar swelling and posterolateral fissure				28/32	23/23	

444

Stage	15	16	17	18	19	Total
Total number	40	56	44	48	36	224
Good quality	26	39	32	35	23	155
Silver-treated	5	3	5	7	7	27
Greatest length (mm)	7.4±0.3	9.3±1.5	12.6±1.2	15±1.5	18.4±1.5	
Age (weeks)	5	$5\frac{1}{2}$	6		$6\frac{1}{2}$	
139. Walls of neurohypophysis are folded				34/35	19/23	
140. At least two semicircular ducts have become individualized			2/31	29/35	23/23	
141. Medial ventricular elevation reaches septal area				25/30	22/23	
142. Olfactory bulb shows ventricular recess				22/34	20/23	
143. Cell migration in area dentata				24/30	12/23	
144. Plexus of fourth ventricle contains villi				14/35	23/23	
145. Cavity of lens vesicle slitlike or disappeared				18/35	17/23	
146. Mamillothalamic tract				11/32	19/22	
147. Choana				7/35	19/23	
148. Styloid process is cartilaginous				5/35	19/23	
149. Globus pallidus externus				2/25	22/23	
150. Area of nucleus accumbens projects into ventricle					16/16	
151. Nuclei of forebrain septum					22/23	
152. Subcommissural organ					16/17	
153. Cochlear nuclei					22/23	
154. Ganglion of nervus terminalis					20/23	
155. Orbital wing of sphenoid is cartilaginous					19/23	
156. Stria medullaris thalami				5/35	13/23	
157. Plexus of lateral ventricle possesses villi				1/35	16/23	
158. Cochlear duct turned "upward"				2/35	13/22	
159. Paraphysis is present as a button					16/22	
160. Mandible begins to ossify					15/23	
161. Thalamostriatal fibers				1/35	13/23	
162. Medial accessory olivary nucleus					13/23	
163. Fibers in optic chiasma					7/18	
164. Paraphysis with opening to ventricular cavity					8/22	
165. Maxilla is ossifying					5/23	
166. Stapedial artery is regressing					4/23	
167. Habenular commissure					2/17	

Appendix 1, Continued. Main Features from 7 to 8
Postfertilizational Weeks, Beyond the Study by Computer Ranking

Stage	Approximate age (days)	
20	47	Crossing fibers in optic chiasma
		Medial septal nucleus
		Nucleus of diagonal band
		Cuneate and gracile decussating fibers
		Olivo-arcuate migration
21	50	Lateral olfactory tract
		Cortical plate in cerebral hemispheres
		Pyramidal cells in hippocampus
		Globus pallidus internus (future entopeduncular nucleus)
		Cranial nerves with glial (olfactory and optic) and neurilemmal cells between nerve fibers
		Ventral part of lateral geniculate body
		Area of future dentate gyrus
		Dentate nucleus of cerebellum
22	52	Internal capsule present and three outlets forming
		Nerve fibers between neopallial subplate and internal capsule
		Claustrum
		Intereminential sulcus between medial and lateral ventricular eminences
		Roof of ventricle 3 becoming folded
		Intradural veins (dural sinuses) present
23	56	Hippocampus reaches temporal pole
		Insula
		Caudate nucleus and putamen
		Beginning of anterior commissure
		Optic tract reaches ventral part of lateral geniculate body
		Cerebellar commissures
		Principal nucleus of inferior olivary nuclei
		Olivocerebellar fibers
		Cells of area membranaceae cuboidal
		Pyramidal decussation
		Falx cerebri
		Most cisterns present
		Lateral parts of tentorium cerebelli
		No apertures in roof of ventricle 4

Appendix 2. Sequence and Stage of Appearance of Median Features of the Brain

	Preoptic recess (rostral end of neural plate) (stage 14)				
Neuromere	**Dorsocaudally** ↓	**Stage**	**Ventrocaudally** ↓		**Stage**
T	Lamina terminalis				
	Embryonic	11			
	Adult	15			
	Commissural plate				
	(situs neuroporicus)	12			
	Velum transversum	14			
D1			Chiasmatic plate		10
			Supraoptic commissure		17
			Postoptic recess		14
Par. r.			Infundibular region		13
Par. c.			Inframamillary recess		17
			Mamillary region		13
			Supramamillary recess		17
			(termination of sulcus limitans)		
Syn.	Epiphysis cerebri	16	Supramamillary commissure		15
	Posterior commissure	17			
M1	Commissure of superior				
	colliculi	15			
M2			Oculomotor decussation		17
Isth.	Trochlear decussation	15	Isthmic recess		16

Appendix 3. Sequence and Stage of Appearance of Tracts of the Brain

Tract	Stage	Tract	Stage
Lateral longitudinal	12	Crossed tectobulbar	16
Ventral longitudinal	13	Fibers from olfactory tubercle to amygdaloid body	16, 17
Common afferent[1]	13		
Medial longitudinal*	13	Habenulo-interpeduncular*	16, 17
Dorsal funiculus	14	Fibers from olfactory bulb to olfactory tubercle[4]	17
Preoptico-hypothalamic[2]	14		
Hypothalamotegmental	14, 15	Mamillothalamic	18
Mamillotegmental	15	Stria medullaris thalami*	18, 19
Medial forebrain bundle*	15, 16	Lateral lemniscus	18, 19
Tractus solitarius separates from common afferent tract	15, 16	Thalamostriatal[5]	19
		Tract of zona limitans intra-thalamica	19
Hypothalamo-thalamic	15, 16		
Tract of posterior commissure	15, 16	Central tegmental*[6]	19

[1] Containing fibers of the future tractus solitarius.
[2] Part of the basal forebrain bundle.
[3] Containing striatosubthalamic fibers.
[4] Part of the basal forebrain bundle.
[5] Synonyms: lateral forebrain bundle; *Stammbündel* (of His).
[6] Zecevic and Verney (1995).
* Pathways concerned with the transportation of monoamines.

Appendix 4. Sequence and Stage of Appearance of Features Associated with the Rhombencephalon

Stage	Age (weeks)	Neural Discs	Neural Crest	Ganglia	Nuclei	Nerve Fibers
9	3½	9 (otic)				
10	4	10 (arch 4)	5, 7, 9, 10(–11?)			
11			7–8	5, 7–8		
11–12					(5, 7, 9, 10–11, 12 eff.)*	
12				9 superior & 10 superior		5, 7, 9, 11 SVE; 12 GSE
12–13		7, 9, (arches 2 & 3)		9 inferior & 10 inferior	3, 4, eff.	5, 7 eff. 5, 7 GVA
13	4½	5 (arch 1)				3 GSE
13–14					6 eff.	
14						4 GSE; 5 mesenc. root; 8v eff. 9, 10–11 aff.
14–15	5					6 GSE
15–16					Sup. & inf. salivatory	
16	5½					8c
17	6				5 motor	
18					5 main sensory	
19	6½				8c ventral & dorsal	
20	7				10 dorsal eff.	
21					8v lateral	
22	7½				8v superior	

* Provisional location.
Abbreviations: aff., afferent; eff., efferent; GSE, general somatic efferent; GVA, general visceral afferent; SVE, special visceral efferent; 8c, 8v, cochlear and vestibular parts of cranial nerve 8, respectively.
Source: All the data are based on the authors' studies.

449

I N D E X

451

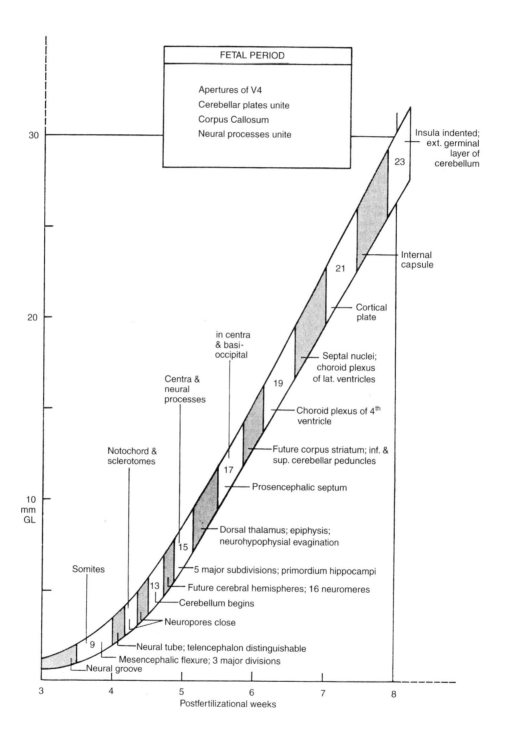

FETAL PERIOD

Apertures of V4
Cerebellar plates unite
Corpus Callosum
Neural processes unite

Insula indented;
ext. germinal
layer of
cerebellum

23

Internal
capsule

21

Cortical
plate

in centra
& basi-
occipital

Septal nuclei;
choroid plexus
of lat. ventricles

19

Centra &
neural
processes

Choroid plexus of 4th
ventricle

Future corpus striatum; inf. &
sup. cerebellar peduncles

17

Prosencephalic septum

Notochord &
sclerotomes

Dorsal thalamus; epiphysis;
neurohypophysial evagination

15

5 major subdivisions; primordium hippocampi

Somites

Future cerebral hemispheres; 16 neuromeres

13

Cerebellum begins

Neuropores close

9

Neural tube; telencephalon distinguishable

Mesencephalic flexure; 3 major divisions

Neural groove

30

20

10
mm
GL

3   4   5   6   7   8

Postfertilizational weeks